CARBOHYDRATE METABOLISM

Advances in Modern Nutrition

Editor
Myron A. Mehlman

1 Carolyn D. Berdanier

Carbohydrate Metabolism: Regulation and Physiological Role

IN PREPARATION

Howard M. Katzen
and Richard J. Mahler

Diabetes, Obesity, and Vascular Disease: Metabolic and Molecular Interrelationships

VOLUME 1

Advances in Modern Nutrition

CARBOHYDRATE METABOLISM
Regulation and Physiological Role

EDITED BY
CAROLYN D. BERDANIER
UNIVERSITY OF NEBRASKA COLLEGE OF MEDICINE

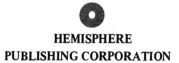

HEMISPHERE
PUBLISHING CORPORATION
Washington   London

A HALSTED PRESS BOOK

JOHN WILEY & SONS
New York   London   Sydney   Toronto

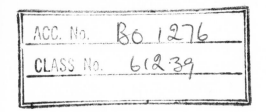
Hemisphere Publishing Corporation
1025 Vermont Ave., N.W., Washington, D.C. 20005

Distributed solely by Halsted Press, a Division of John Wiley & Sons, Inc.,
New York.

1 2 3 4 5 6 7 8 9 0   D O D O   7 8 4 3 2 1 0 9 8 7 6

ISBN 0-470-15047-5
LC No. 76-1564

Printed in the United States of America

CONTENTS

PREFACE

Until recently the carbohydrates as a nutrient class have been largely ignored. Nutritionists have been concerned with the provision of adequate amounts of protein, vitamins, and minerals and also with the type and amount of fat. Carbohydrates were added (almost indiscriminately) to provide the remaining needed energy. In the last ten years, however, nutritionists have begun to realize that the physiological responses depend on the nature or type of carbohydrates in the diet. Factors such as chemical conformation, taste, bioavailability, sex, age, stage of development, and genetic makeup have all been shown to affect carbohydrate metabolism. These factors together suggest that there is both a minimal and a maximal daily intake for each of the nutritionally significant carbohydrates and that much research is needed to delineate these limits. Recognition of the need for carbohydrate has come through the studies of the metabolic consequences of carbohydrate-free diets; however, the idea that there may be an upper limit to carbohydrate intake has not been so readily recognized or accepted.

This volume was designed to combine the major research areas in carbohydrates in order to present a diversity of thought with respect to carbohydrate nutrition. Leading authorities have contributed key chapters as have some newcomers to the field of carbohydrate nutrition and metabolism in an attempt to review the latest thinking in this important area. It is hoped that this work not only will be of value to research workers and advanced students of biochemistry, physiology, and nutrition but also will have a wider appeal to those engaged in the more practical aspects of patient management.

It is difficult for researchers to keep abreast of areas other than those of their own immediate concern. Thus while we are aware of the criticism that might be tendered against a multiauthored work, we feel sure that the reader will in the end benefit from the authoritative reviews herein presented. To the authors themselves and to the publishers a heartfelt thanks is extended.

Carolyn D. Berdanier

INTRODUCTION

Advances in Modern Nutrition is a series that reviews and assesses the state of the art and science in the field of nutrition. Chapters in these volumes are contributed by scientists who are experts in both broad and specific areas of nutrition such as cell biology, nutrition and genetics, biochemistry, toxicology of foods, pathology, physiology, medicine, economics, anthropology, epidemiology, behavioral sciences, food science, and endocrinology.

The objective of this series is to arrive at some understanding of

- The response of cells to changes in their environment when exposed to nutrients or biologically active materials
- The methods by which nutrients are transported into the cells
- The utilization of nutrients and the consequences of this utilization to normal and diseased organisms

The understanding of cell, tissue, and organ function at physiological and biochemical levels should result in the opening of new horizons in the prevention of disease through changes in dietary management.

We hope that these volumes will serve as a valuable resource for students, teachers, scientists, clinicians, and researchers by providing basic information and a review of up-to-date research findings and by outlining the future needs of nutritional efforts.

Myron A. Mehlman

ABBREVIATIONS

In today's fast-moving society, shortcuts in language have become commonplace, so common, in fact, that the same abbreviations can have several meanings. For this reason a list of abbreviations and their meanings as used in the volume is provided.

ATP	Adenosine triphosphate
ADP	Adenosine diphosphate
AMP	Adenosine monophosphate
cAMP	Cyclic 3',5'-adenosine monophosphate
CoA	Coenzyme A
EPI	Epinephrine
FFA	Free fatty acids
6-PGD	6-Phosphogluconate dehydrogenase
G6PD	Glucose-6-phosphate dehydrogenase
DNA	Deoxyribonucleic acid
RNA	Ribonucleic acid
NAD	Nicotinamide adenine dinucleotide
NADH	Nicotinamide adenine dinucleotide (reduced)
NADP	Nicotinamide adenine dinucleotide phosphate
NADPH	Nicotinamide adenine dinucleotide phosphate (reduced)
PEP	Phosphoenolpyruvate
PEPCK	Phosphoenolpyruvate carboxykinase
TCA cycle	Tricarboxylic acid cycle
UDP	Uridine diphospho- (usually linked to a sugar)

CARBOHYDRATE METABOLISM

Chapter 1

SOME PERSPECTIVES ON CARBOHYDRATE CONSUMPTION

Lilly Gardner
*Department of Foods, Nutrition
and Institution Administration
University of Maryland
College Park, Maryland*

INTRODUCTION

Prior to 1945, most advances made in nutrition concerned the discovery of vitamins, minerals, and amino acids and their respective roles in human health and disease. As a result of these discoveries food enrichment programs contributed greatly to decreasing the prevalence of deficiency diseases such as pellagra, scurvy, rickets, and kwashiorkor. In the following decade attention was focused on providing food and technical assistance to developing nations; little concern was given to the nutrition problems in the "western world." Adequate food supply did not guarantee adequate dietaries as was soon discovered.

The nutrition community was stirred from its complacency by several public health nutrition survey findings conducted in the 1960s (FAO, 1971; Kelsay, 1969; DHEW, 1972). These population studies exposed numerous deficiencies, excesses, and imbalances present in contemporary dietary patterns. Some of these situations resulted from rapid national economic development. In many instances, industrialization had forced rapid economic and social changes that, in turn, brought about changes in food habits and consumption patterns. Once again keen interest was generated in the relationship between nutrition and health, and noteworthy advances in normal and abnormal carbohydrate nutrition resulted from inquiries made into the consequences of an observed switch from starch to sucrose consumption (USDA, 1971; Wretlind, 1974). This dietary modification also appeared to be accompanied by a reduction in the fiber content of the diet (USDA, 1971). The physiologic effects of the switch from starch to sugar prompted nutritionists to take a closer look at the individual carbohydrates and to discard the notion that carbohydrates were essentially calorie providers with all types being nutritionally similar.

1

CARBOHYDRATES IN THE DIET

General Use

Eating practices reflect the physical, economic, social, technological, political, and ideological aspects of an existing culture. Present world dietary patterns, therefore, reflect considerable interregional variations, both in terms of overall sufficiency of the diet and in type of foods comprising the diet (Cesal et al., 1967). Carbohydrates have long been a mainstay in world dietaries, with starch, sucrose, and lactose being the major sources for human consumption (Herman, 1974). In regions where per capita incomes are low and the balance between food production and food demand close, consumption of cereals and starchy root vegetables largely meet the need for calories (FAO, 1971). Carbohydrates have been found to supply up to 90% of the calories consumed by persons in underdeveloped countries. When carbohydrate consumption is this high, it is cause for concern as these diets are apt to be deficient in essential vitamins, minerals, and protein (Cesal et al., 1967). In industrial nations carbohydrates may supply approximately half the energy requirements (FAO, 1971). These dietaries generally show a considerable margin of safety over minimum requirements for essential nutrients; problems that exist in these situations are most apt to be due to excesses rather than to deficiencies.

Food practices have been found to be more resistant to change than many other aspects of culture. They are often rooted in the past and are interwoven in custom, religious beliefs, and the educational achievements of a given society. To date, no one really knows precisely what motivates change in food habits or why some foods are accepted and others rejected. When speaking of food practices, nutritionists most often emphasize the habits themselves when, in fact, it may be the food that is changing society (Giff et al., 1972).

United States

Because of their fundamental place in all dietaries, carbohydrates have not, until quite recently, been considered etiological agents in clinical conditions. Cursory glances at consumption figures for carbohydrate usage show little change in total volume consumed over the past several decades. On close examination, however, alterations in carbohydrate consumption patterns in westernized countries show a drastic increase in the use of sugar at the expense of starch (USDA, 1971; Wretlind, 1974). Trends in consumption patterns also reflect a decline in dietary fiber intake since the midnineteenth century. It is estimated that in the United States fiber intake is only one-fifth what it was during the last century (National Dairy Council, 1975).

Trends shown in Table 1 indicate that the amount of carbohydrate used in the United States from 1909–1913 to 1968 has dropped about one-fourth (Page and Friend, 1974). Supplies of carbohydrates and use of grain products have decreased at a faster rate than total food use measured in calories (Friend and

Sports biomechanics

reducing injury + perfo

612.76/BAR

612/39/CAR

Carb metabolism.

TABLE 1 Calories, Fats, Carbohydrates, and
Total Sugars Available per Capita per Day
in the United States for Selected Periods

Year	Calories	Fats (g)	Carbohydrates (g)	Sugars (g)
1909–1913	3,484	125	492	157
1925–1929	3,466	135	476	198
1935–1939	3,270	133	436	190
1947–1949	3,230	141	403	193
1957–1959	3,133	143	374	190
1965	3,170	147	371	193
1974[a]	3,350	158	388	208

[a]Preliminary figures. Adapted from U.S. Department of
Agriculture (1970).

Marston, 1974). Over the past 65 years two food groups—flour/cereal products and sugar/syrup—have provided about three-fourths the total carbohydrate consumed. At the turn of the century flour and cereal provided about 56% and sugar and syrup about 22% of the total carbohydrate consumed. The examination of market disappearance data show that the proportionate contribution from each group has shifted over the years; the share now provided by flour and cereal products and by sugar and syrup is 35% and 38%, respectively. On a percentage basis the decrease in total starch since 1909–1913 is twice as great as the decrease in total carbohydrates. This shift is primarily the result of a sharp decline in the use of grain products (Pilgrim, 1961).

United States Department of Agriculture food disappearance data show a net gain in sucrose consumption since the early 1900s. This gain represents about half the overall increase for total sugars. Lactose, derived primarily from dairy products, accounts for about one-eighth the total sugars, compared with two-thirds contributed by sucrose. Glucose currently provides only one-twelfth the "total sugars," but it too is at its highest level since 1909–1913. In recent years corn syrup has contributed to this increase in glucose consumption. Maltose and fructose levels are also correlated with consumption of corn syrup. Fructose levels have remained fairly constant over the years as a decline in the use of fresh apples has offset any increases caused by a greater intake of corn syrup. A newly developed process for producing high fructose corn syrup from dextrose is currently finding favor with the food industry. Its appeal lies in the fact that it is much sweeter than any other syrups and, therefore, can be substituted by the industry for the more expensive sucrose (Mitchell, 1974). As industrial capacity for the production of fructose syrup increases, manufacturers will probably replace more sugar in formulations with ever-increasing amounts of high fructose syrup. In this event, the amount of fructose in the diet may well continue to rise.

Dietary fiber—a generic term referring to plant constituents resistant to digestion by nonruminant gastrointestinal secretions—includes a heterogenous group of carbohydrate compounds and the noncarbohydrate lignin. Consumption figures for fiber are difficult to tabulate as only a limited number of foods have been analyzed. The data that do exist are presented in United States Department of Agriculture (USDA) *Composition of Foods* (Watt and Merrill, 1963) as crude fiber. Crude fiber is defined as the insoluble material that remains after severe acid and base hydrolysis. Crude fiber data has been used as an index of dietary fiber in the analysis of nutrients for lack of better figures (National Dairy Council, 1975). It is thought that fiber content of the diet has decreased from 6 g per capita per day in 1909-1913 to 4 g per capita per day in 1971 (Friend and Marston, 1974).

Europe and Asia

Although carbohydrate consumption in European and Asian countries varies considerably, most countries have reported a continuous increase in the use of sugar over the past 35 yr. The most rapid increases are now being shown by countries that 25 yr ago had the lowest consumption (Yudkin and Morland, 1967). Between 1937 and 1957 average consumption increased by about 150% in the Near East and by 100% in Africa and Eastern Europe (Yudkin, 1968). In Europe the highest per capita consumption is found in Iceland, followed by Ireland, Holland, Denmark, and England (Cesal et al., 1967). In addition, the examination of disappearance data reflects trends that are quite similar to those mentioned for the United States (Wyden, 1965).

Many factors have contributed to this universal increase in sugar consumption, and any explanation for this increase must include cultural changes in food habits as well as disappearance data.

CULTURAL INFLUENCES ON CONSUMPTION PATTERNS

People are obviously eating differently than they did a number of years ago and for an assortment of reasons. It would be impossible to point to one single factor as a cause, for all aspects of a culture are interrelated and mutually reinforcing. The influences that tend to develop a greater variety in food choice are perhaps most apparent (Giff et al., 1972). As national economies develop, a larger portion of the population is able to pick and choose from a wider variety of foodstuffs, irrespective of season or geography. Higher per capita incomes permit a shift from choosing foods only to fill one's stomach to choosing foods to please one's palate. The rapid growth of science and technology has made it possible to add highly palatable "new" foods to the list of naturally preferred foods such as meat and fruit. A very large portion of the increase in sugar usage is due to the development of efficient methods for sugar refining and of methods of synthesizing materials that can be mixed and compounded with sugar. From about the early eighteenth century sugar ceased to be a luxury for the wealthy few and demand steadily increased through the world. Much sugar is now being consumed in the form of "convenience foods." The increased use of newly developed foods has contributed to the emergence of new food habits by changing much of the work in the home and freeing women for outside employment. This, in turn, has changed a woman's role in the family and altered many of the traditional practices observed in the family situation. When parental influence declines and a more casual eating pattern takes the place of the past structured three meals a day, knowledge and awareness of food is acquired through contact with mass media, peer group members, and a wider variety of social encounters. Although it has been shown (Giff et al., 1972) that the direct effect of audiovisual media on eating patterns is not substantial, the presence of television in the home causes certain changes in eating behavior in many families. Mealtimes are adjusted so that favorite programs can be watched, or meals are eaten hurriedly with a minimum of attention and conversation so that programs will not be missed or eaten on trays in front of the set. Snacks are frequently consumed while watching. One can only guess about the extent and the nutritional significance of the eating behavior that makes accommodation to the presence of TV. Many of the favorite snack foods contain large amounts of sucrose, thus facilitating piecemeal eating. The tendency to snacking, however, is only part of a larger pattern of changing food habits that include eating away from home and eating in a hurry.

Although providing food in the home is less costly and less burdensome than ever before, more people are eating more meals away from home (USDA, 1970). They eat in restaurants, cafeterias, lunchrooms, and fast-order food services or from vending machines. In a 1968 survey, approximately 20% of the total consumer expenditure for food and drink in the United States was spent away from home. Expenditures for meals eaten away from home in 1971 were up 9½%, more than three times the pace of the previous year. More eating away from home results in less control over food preparation; eating establishments have also increased their use of composite foods, ready-prepared foods, and soft drinks. For many individuals this will also result in more monotony in food choice.

Figure 1 shows the steadily increasing portion of sugar used by the food industry for confections, beverages, baked goods, etc. Beverages now comprise the largest single industry use of refined sugar, followed by cereal and baked goods (Page and Friend, 1974). These few food items account for over two-thirds the total refined sugar consumed in the United States (Page and Friend, 1974). Similar findings are being observed elsewhere. For example, in Germany the proportion of sugar used by industry was 35% in 1952–1953 and rose to 54% in 1968–1970 (USDA, 1971). In 1972 in Holland approximately 60% of the total sugar usage was by the food industry. Similar trends are noted in England (47%), Finland (34%), and Switzerland (34%). (These figures may not represent actual consumption by the specified nation, as a portion of this sugar finds its way into composite foods that are intended for export and data may not be recorded as such.)

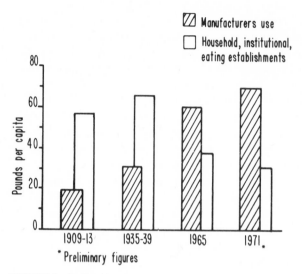

FIGURE 1 Refined sugar, estimated per capita use by manufacturers and household, institutional, and eating establishments for selected periods. Adapted from U.S. Department of Agriculture, Food Consumption Section (1968), and Page and Friend (1974). Figures for 1971 are preliminary.

The United Nations Food and Agriculture Organization in a series of commodity studies done in the 1970s confirmed this picture of world sugar consumption and reported a similar observation: There exists an ever-increasing human craving for sweetness (FAO, 1971). The food industry, it seems, is very willing to meet this demand and continually develops "new" products to entice the consumer. The use of sugar as a flavor enhancer in products not normally considered as "sweets" or the addition of thickening agents and stabilizers to inferior products in order to produce more "new" and less expensive items needs to be justified. These additions or deletions may often change the nutritive quality of the foods eaten, even when eating habits do not change. The consumer has the right to know if he is trading nutrition for convenience, superficial attractiveness, and possibly poor health.

NUTRITIONAL ASPECTS

From the viewpoint of nutrition, sugar functions as a readily available, concentrated source of energy for the body. It can easily be consumed beyond satiety in a way unlikely to occur with starch, fat, or protein. When the intake of sugar increases, the consumption of other foods containing essential nutrients probably decreases by an amount equal to the energy content of the ingested sugar (Wretlind, 1974). It has also been found that dietary increases of sugar in almost all cases are also accompanied by increases in fat consumption (McGandy et al., 1967). This combination, unfortunately, is not in tune with today's concepts of "good nutrition." The high incidence of obesity, especially in persons over 40, strongly suggests that the present dietary patterns are not suitable for the more sedentary consumer (Goldsmith, 1967b). In *The Overweight Society* Peter Wyden (1965) indicates from interviews conducted throughout the United States that an estimated 9.2 million persons were on some sort of reducing diets. Despite this large number of dieters, overweight is one of the great health problems in this prosperous country. Conditions of modern life, temptations of delicious foods, combined with sedentary living patterns, all predispose to this troublesome condition.

Poverty coexists with plenty and also exerts an influence on eating habits. Limitations on food choice that accompany inadequate income affect the kind and amount of pleasure in eating that is expected. Desire for preferred foods must be balanced against all other wants and in many instances results in a reshuffling of priorities that affect food choice (Giff et al., 1972).

Undoubtedly, most people are aware of a link between diet and health. The public has been made aware, to the point of being frightened, that certain foods increase one's susceptibility to heart attacks, obesity, etc. Motivated by advertisers and proponents of "natural foods" many individuals embrace one or another "food fad." Trends in consumer concerns indicate that the layman views certain foods as more of a danger than a blessing, (i.e., potatoes and pasta make one fat and eggs contain cholesterol). As a result, perceived information is frequently inaccurate or incomplete. This tendency to oversimplify cause and effect relationships is responsible, in part, for the decrease in starch consumption. Starch has been unjustifiably considered a villian among nutrients by laypeople. Many have altered their dietary patterns to eliminate these "fattening foods" only to consume the same amounts of alcohol and sugar (Leverton, 1964; Olson, 1958; Pilgrim, 1961).

DIETARY CARBOHYDRATES IN THE ETIOLOGY OF DISEASE

Man's total well-being depends on more than just food. It results from a complex interaction between his genetic endowments and the environmental climate in which he lives and develops (Giff et al., 1972). An individual's potential for well-being is determined by his hereditary makeup. The extent to which he reaches his potential depends on a variety of environmental factors, some within his control, others not. Environment in its total context includes physical, economic, and psychosocial elements. Food is only one component of the environment.

Environmental Factors

The role of refined carbohydrate foods in the etiology of dental caries has been known for some time. There is little doubt that the presence of carbohydrate in the mouth is essential for the development of dental caries; the quality of the carbohydrate as well as the quantity has been demonstrated to influence the rate of carie formation (Dalderup, 1967; Konig, 1968). In both animal-feeding experiments and human studies that dealt with comparative cariogenicity of different carbohydrates (sucrose, maltose, lactose, glucose, fructose, and starch), it has been clearly shown that sucrose is the most cariogenic and starch the least. Environmental factors, such as trace elements indigenous to the soil and food, temperature, and humidity, may influence regional food habits by influencing the amount of sugar-sweetened soft drinks consumed (Nizel, 1973). Undoubtedly, the increased consumption of sweets has increased the incidence of dental caries in the industrialized nations to the point of becoming an endemic disease. The introduction of snacking and piecemeal eating only serves to aggravate this situation. The more frequently carbohydrate and sugar are eaten, the more the caries activity is stimulated by prolonging oral sugar clearing time in hours per day (Dalderup, 1967; Jacobson, 1972).

Traditionally, carbohydrate intake has been linked to obesity. This group of foodstuffs is the one most frequently overindulged and the group considered safest to eliminate by physicians prescribing weight reduction diets. This does not imply that carbohydrates cause obesity. Carbohydrates provide calories, but no more than protein, and less than half that supplied by like amounts of fat. It is widely recognized that complex interactions of physiologic, psychological, and sociocultural factors in the etiology of the obesities make treatment extremely difficult (Goldblatt et al., 1965; Goldsmith, 1967a; Goth, 1973; Lopez-S. et al., 1966; Prugh, 1961; Stunkard, 1968; Young, 1973). Much remains to be learned before effective methods of prevention or treatment are available.

Intakes of dietary carbohydrate were implicated in impairment of glucose tolerance by Cohen et al. (1961) after observing Yemenite immigrants to Israel. Changes in dietary patterns resulting from the move to Israel were most dramatic in the increase in sugar consumption by old settlers. Animal experiments involving high-sucrose diets support the suggestion that a high proportion of sugar in the diet does indeed lead to early impairment of glucose tolerance (Blazquez and Quijada, 1969; Cohen and Teitelbaum, 1964).

States of overnutrition and obesity are generally accepted as potent factors in precipitating genetically predetermined diabetes. The incidence of obesity is known to be high in maturity-onset diabetes. The interrelationship between obesity and diabetes may, in fact, be causal as restriction of caloric intake alone often has a beneficial effect in the course of the diabetes, providing it is mild or moderate (Baird, 1973).

Much of our knowledge of atherosclerosis comes from epidemiologic observations. The data do not provide cause–effect relationships but can point the way to areas of investigation. Diet affects several risk factors associated with heart disease (Fig. 2) and as a result is the most attentive in terms of blame. Diet, because it can be modified and because it is a possible avenue of control of coronary heart disease, has become an attractive target for physicians and nutritionists (Mayer, 1960).

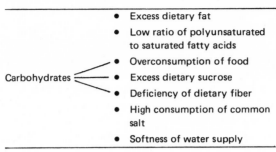

FIGURE 2   Dietary risk factors in coronary heart disease.
Adapted from British Advisory Panel (1975).

Through the study of the interrelationships between dietary carbohydrate and lipid metabolism, evidence has been found that indicates not only the amount but also the type of carbohydrate that influences metabolism. It has been demonstrated by researchers (Anderson, 1967; Herman, 1974; Kuo et al., 1967; Hodges and Krehl, 1965; Nestel et al., 1970) that the change from starch to sucrose causes an increase in plasma triglycerides, which can be even further elevated in hyperlipemic patients (Maruhama and Macdonald, 1973). In addition, these elevated serum lipids have been found to be highly correlated to atherosclerosis and clinical signs of heart disease. Average serum lipid levels and the rate of death from coronary heart disease have been shown to be highest in countries where a large proportion of the dietary carbohydrate is derived from sucrose, where intakes of total fat and cholesterol in the diet are high, and where the normal patterns of physical activity are sedentary (British Advisory Panel, 1975). Several theories have been proposed implicating sugar directly in the atherogenic process (Cohen et al., 1961; Leverton, 1964; Yudkin, 1968; Yudkin and Morland, 1967), but opinion concerning the validity of these theories is divided (British Advisory Panel, 1975). Any attempts to uniformly correlate heart disease with high sucrose intakes have been unsuccessful to date. No doubt this is due to the difficulty of separating the effects of dietary from nondietary risk factors.

The role fiber plays in the human diet is still rather nebulous. The immediate consequence of a low-fiber diet appears to be constipation, which may or may not lead to the development of diverticular disease (National Dairy Council, 1975). It has also been postulated that a diet high in refined carbohydrates may lead to high bacterial count and slow bowel movements, which in turn may enhance the likelihood of cancer of the colon (Darby, 1974; National Dairy Council, 1975). Serum cholesterol levels have been lowered with diets high in fiber. It has been hypothesized that fiber may sequester bile acids and prevent cholesterol and fat absorption (National Dairy Council, 1975). Most evidence on the reported association between dietary fiber and disease is epidemiologic. Until physiologic mechanisms are identified, recommendations for changes in diet relating to fiber are not being made.

Genetic Factors

Scientists have demonstrated time and again that genetic imperfections have a profound effect on well-being. The ability to synthesize adequate amounts of hormones and enzymes, utilize specific nutrients, and react to specific substances in the foods eaten are determined, at least in part, by genetics. Imperfections in the genetic constitution could result in allergies, diabetes, congenital disturbances in carbohydrate digestion and absorption, and a host of other disorders including the predisposition to such diseases as obesity, hypertension, and atherosclerosis. A recent coronary heart disease demography study suggests that major risk factors involved in the disease are under "polygenic control." Nutritional status and other environmental factors modulate, but do not override, the expression of genotype (Hatch, 1974). The important implications of this study rest in the fact that the disease, while not amenable to any specific preventive measure, may be minimized by multiple interventions against risk factors. Through the use of "individualized preventive medicine," a credible degree of success in reducing the incidence of the disease could be achieved; the fundamental genetic influence on risk, however, would remain in evidence (Hatch, 1974). The existence of persons who are metabolically prone to one or another diet-induced or related malady emphasizes the need to distinguish between the normal and the abnormal individual. Failure to appreciate the role of predisposition could lead to the imposition of unnecessary dietary restrictions on most people because metabolic abnormalities are present in a few (Darby, 1974).

CONCLUSION

The biological relationships between food and humans are a complex web of causes and effects. Relating present nutrition knowledge to present eating practices is a formidable task, for man's food patterns influence well-being in diverse ways and at times may seem to serve no useful purpose. Over the past 100 years, the consumption of sucrose in nearly all areas of the world has risen. The incidence of obesity, diabetes, and heart disease has risen along with it. As the results of investigations into the relationships between dietary carbohydrates and disease begin to accumulate, the rational scientific explanation of what to eat to maintain health may be ignored. Scientific facts accumulate rapidly in a laboratory environment, but man changes his habits slowly and for various reasons. Progress is many times almost imperceptible when dealing with the daily patterns of living. There is a real need to increase research on human behavior toward food and on how to interpret and disseminate information effectively about nutrition and food. Perhaps, in the final analysis, nutrition efforts will best be served by involving many disciplines ranging from biochemistry and medicine to statistics, anthropology, sociology, psychology, and public health.

REFERENCES

Advisory Panel of the British Committee on Medical Aspects of Food Policy (Nutrition) on Diet in Relation to Cardiovascular and Cerebrovascular Disease. 1975. *Nutr. Today* pp. 16–27.

Anderson, J. T. 1967. *Am. J. Clin. Nutr.* 20:168–175.

Baird, J. D. 1973. *Proc. Nutr. Soc.* 32:199–203.

Blazquez, E. and Quijada, C. L. 1969. *J. Endocrinol.* 44:107–113.

Cesal, L., Blakeslie, L., and Heady, E. O. 1967. *World review of nutrition and dietetics,* vol. 7, pp. 1–23. New York: Hafner.

Cohen, A. M., Bavly, S., and Poznanski, R. 1961. *Lancet* 2:1399.

Cohen, A. M., and Teitelbaum, A. 1964. *Am. J. Physiol.* 206:105–107.

Dalderup, L. M. 1967. *World review of nutrition and dietetics,* vol. 7, pp. 72–137. New York: Hafner.

Darby, W. J. 1974. *Sugars in nutrition,* pp. 11–16. New York: Academic Press.

Food and Agriculture Organization of the United Nations. 1971. *The state of food and agriculture.* Rome: FAO.

Friend, B. and Marston, R. 1974. *National food situation,* pp. 26–32. Washington, D.C.: U.S. Department of Agriculture.

Giff, H. H., Washbon, M. B., Harrison, G. G. 1972. *Nutrition, behavior, and change,* pp. 55–109, 187–211. Englewood Cliffs, N.J.: Prentice-Hall.

Goldblatt, P. B. and More, M. D. 1965. *J. Am. Med. Assoc.* 192:1039–1042.

Goldsmith, G. A. 1967a. *Metabolism* 6:407–409.

Goldsmith, G. A. 1967b. *Metabolism* 6:409–411.

Goth, E. 1973. *Proc. Nutr. Soc.* 32:175–179.

Hatch, F. T. 1974. *Am. J. Clin. Nutr.* 27:80–90.

Herman, R. 1974. *Sugars in nutrition,* p. 946. New York: Academic Press.

Hodges, R. E. and Krehl, W. A. 1965. *Am. J. Clin. Nutr.* 17:334–346.

Jacobson, M. F. 1972. *Eater's digest,* p. 181. Garden City, N.Y.: Doubleday.

Kelsay, J. 1969. *J. Nutr.* 99:123–141.

Konig, K. G. 1968. *Ala. J. Med. Sci.* 5:269–275.

Kuo, P. T., Feng, L., Cohen, N. N., Fitts, W. and Miller, L. D. 1967. *Am. J. Clin. Nutr.* 20:116–125.

Leverton, R. 1964. *J. Home Econ.* 56:317–321.

Lopez-S., A., Hodges, R. E. and Krehl, W. A. 1966. *Am. J. Clin. Nutr.* 18:149–154.

Maruhama, Y. and Macdonald, I. 1973. *Metabolism* 22:1205–1215.

Mayer, J. 1960. *Bull. N.Y. Acad. Med.* 36:323–325.

McGandy, R. B., Hegsted, D. M. and Stare, F. J. 1967. *N. Engl. J. Med.* 277:186.

Mitchell, E. L. 1974. *Sugars in nutrition,* pp. 127–133. New York: Academic Press.

National Dairy Council. 1975. *Natl. Dairy Counc. Digest* 46:1.

Nestel, P., Carroll, K. F. and Havenstein, N. 1970. *Metab. Clin. Sci.* 19:1–18.

Nizel, A. E. 1973. *World Rev. Nutr. Diet.* 16:226–253.

Olson, R. 1958. *Nutr. Rev.* 16:97–99.

Page, L. and Friend, B. 1974. *Sugars in nutrition,* pp. 93–107. New York: Academic Press.

Pilgrim, F. J. 1961. *J. Am. Diet. Assoc.* 38:439–443.

Prugh, D. E. 1961. *Am. J. Clin. Nutr.* 9:538–540.

Stunkard, A. 1968. *Fed. Proc.* 27:1367–1369.

U.S. Department of Agriculture, Agricultural Research Service. 1968. *Food consumption of households in the United States, spring 1965. Household food consumption survey, 1965–66.* Rep. No. 1. Washington, D.C.: U.S. Government Printing Office.

U.S. Department of Agriculture, Agricultural Research Service. 1971. *Food consumption, prices, and expenditures.* Agric. Econ. Rep. No. 138. Suppl. Washington, D.C.: USDA.

U.S. Department of Agriculture, Economic Research Service. 1970. *National food situation, NFS – 131, Feb. 1970,* p. 7. Washington, D.C.: U.S. Government Printing Office.

U.S. Department of Health, Education, and Welfare. 1972. *Ten state nutrition survey in the United States, 1968–1970,* vol. 72, pp. 8129–8134. Washington, D.C.: U.S. Government Printing Office.

Watt, B. K. and Merrill, A. L. 1963. *Composition of foods,* Handbook No. 8. Washington, D.C.: USDA.

Wretlind, A. 1974. *Sugars in nutrition,* pp. 26–32. New York: Academic Press.

Wyden, P. 1965. *The overweight society,* pp. 1–3. New York: Morrow.

Young, C. M. 1963. *J. Am. Med. Assoc.* 186:903–907.

Yudkin, J. 1968. *Carbohydrate metabolism and its disorders,* pp. 169–183. New York: Academic Press.

Yudkin, J. and Morland, J. 1967. *Am. J. Clin. Nutr.* 20:503–508.

Chapter 2

TASTE AND BIOAVAILABILITY OF SUGARS AS RELATED TO STRUCTURE

R. S. Shallenberger
New York State Agricultural Experiment Station
Cornell University
Geneva, New York

STRUCTURE

The stereochemical structure of the sugars is related not only to their organic chemical and physical properties but to their biochemical, biophysical, and physiological roles as well. Living cells utilize sugars as an energy source, and in the human body an integrated sequence of biochemical events—beginning with sweet taste upon ingestion, intestinal hydrolysis and absorption, and interconversion and transformation—takes place either to metabolize D-glucose or to generate D-glucose from other sources for subsequent utilization.

Recent developments in the knowledge of sugar structure are the subject of several texts (Pigman and Horton, 1972; Shallenberger and Birch, 1975; Stoddard, 1971). A "simple" sugar such as D-glucose is now recognized to be an aldohexose that exists in a hemiacetal six-membered (pyranose) ring in crystalline form. In solution it forms a dynamic equilibrium among configurational, ring, acyclic, and conformational isomers; to gain insight into the mechanism of biochemical events, the structures of the sugars must be considered. A survey of the salient features of sugar structure related to biological activity will be presented here with emphasis placed on the stereostructures of D-glucose.

As mentioned above D-glucose exists in the crystalline lattice as a six-membered ring form. Since this form has an asymmetric carbon atom at the point of ring closure, two D-glucoses with different biological properties are possible, both of which are known as crystalline substances. They are α-D- and β-D-glucose, as shown in (1), when either a or β equals OH.

The structure shown for α- and β-D-glucose is a formalized *perspective* formula that emphasizes the favored shape of the six-membered heterocyclic ring with the ring numbered in a clockwise direction when viewed from "above." In one sense it can also be considered to be a modified Haworth–Hirst

13

$$(1)$$

perspective formula (2). The latter was originally drawn with a portion of the

$$(2)$$

ring shaded to indicate to the reader that the structure is shown in three dimensions with the "lower" portion of the ring actually perpendicular to the plane of the paper. In other words, the C-5 to the ring oxygen bond is the only part of the structure "drawn" on the paper. Since the meaning of the shading of this formula is so well established, it is rarely necessary to elaborate its perspective nature by shading. Nevertheless, the significance of the formula is occasionally neglected and otherwise elegant schemes for the biologic properties or roles of the sugars become so muddled in transposing from one drawing to another for a given sugar that impossible sugar transformations are executed. Permissible operations with stereoformulas for the sugars will be presented later in this chapter since their manipulation is a relatively new requirement for explaining biological phenomena.

Configurational Isomers

Whenever sugars are capable of exhibiting isomerism about a chiral center, such as an asymmetric carbon atom, the two possible isomers are said to be *configurational* isomers or diastereoisomers. This is due to the fact that an asymmetric carbon atom can have two absolute configurations with the arrangement of atoms or substituents about one of them related to the other as an object is related to its nonsuperimposable mirror-image structure. For the ring forms of the sugars, configurational isomerism at carbon atom number one leads to the possibility of *anomers.*

Anomers. For each of the two ring forms possible for an aldohexose, two anomers are possible, designated, as shown previously for the pyranose ring of D-glucose as α-D and β-D. When referring to a specific sugar anomer, carbohydrate chemists insist that it must be accompanied with a chiral specification (D or L) since enantiomeric anomers have the opposite configuration about the hemiacetal carbon atom while, for example, α-D- and β-L-anomers have the same absolute anomeric carbon atom configuration (3). Some investigators apparently consider this to be a trivial point, but it is rather important when attempts are made to deduce the chemistry of biological events based on the varying behavior of enantiomers.

$$(3)$$

The distinction between the structure of an α-anomer and a β-anomer is not always an easy matter. The initial distinction was made on the basis of optical rotatory power. In the D-series of sugars the most dextrorotatory anomer was designated α and usually was found to have the same absolute configuration as that of the "reference" or enantiomeric carbon atom. For the L-series, the opposite was true. Many exceptions to the rules of "isorotation" (Hudson, 1909) subsequently have been found. When β-D-fructopyranose mutarotates it establishes an equilibrium mainly with the β-D-furanose form that is also more dextrorotatory. The approximate composition of certain sugar anomers in solution is given in Table 1. The distribution of anomers shown in this table may be influenced significantly by concentration, temperature, and polarity of the solvent in addition to the method employed for making the estimation.

Isbell and Pigman (1937) related the distinction between anomers to the geometry of the ring. Conformationally, an α-anomer is distinguished from the β-anomer in either the D- or L-series of sugars by the OH group equatorially disposed in the C1 conformation.

Epimers. Configurational isomerism at C-2 of the aldohexose sugars creates *epimers.* The term was originally intended to describe those diastereoisomers with the opposite configuration at the second carbon atom of the aldohexoses. Thus, D-mannose and glucose, D-allose and altrose, and D-galactose and talose are "2-epimers"; galactose and glucose are occasionally considered to be "4-epimers." Configurational isomerism at the second carbon atom of ketohexoses leads to the two anomeric forms of each ring that are possible.

TABLE 1 Distribution (%) of Sugar Anomers in Water at 20°C

Sugar	α-Pyranose	β-Pyranose	α-Furanose	β-Furanose
Glucose	31.1–37.4	64.0–67.9	–	–
Galactose	29.6–35.0	63.9–70.4	1.0	3.1
Mannose	64.0–68.9	31.1–36.0	–	–
Fructose	4.0	68.4–76.0	–	28.0–31.6

Enantiomers. Configurational isomerism at the highest numbered asymmetric carbon atom generates the two chiral families of the sugars. In this sense, D-glucose and L-idose are "5-epimers," as shown in (4) using Fischer projection formulas. Enantiomers, however, are the total mirror-image structures possible

$$
\begin{array}{cc}
\text{HC=O} & \text{HC=O} \\
| & | \\
\text{HC OH} & \text{HC OH} \\
| & | \\
\text{HOC H} & \text{HOC H} \\
| & | \quad\quad (4)\\
\text{HC OH} & \text{HCOH} \\
| & | \\
\text{HCOH} & \text{HOC H} \\
| & | \\
\text{CH}_2\text{OH} & \text{CH}_2\text{OH} \\
\text{D-Glucose} & \text{L-Idose}
\end{array}
$$

whenever an element or elements of chirality are possible and, therefore, are nonsuperposable. L-Glucose is shown in (5) in both the Haworth-Hirst and the conformational structures. The conformational structure of L-glucose clearly

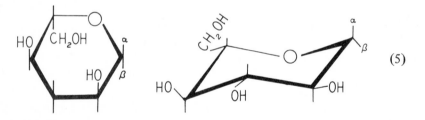

(5)

shows that in addition to being the configurational mirror-image structure of D-glucose, the chiral ring shape is a nonsuperposable mirror-image structure.

Ring Isomers

Ring or constitutional isomers of the sugars differ in size. The six-membered (pyranose) ring is usually encountered for the free hexoses and the free pentoses, but when a five-membered (furanose) ring form has a certain degree of conformational stability it too is sometimes encountered in the free state. Examples are β-D-galactofuranose (Shallenberger and Acree, 1966) and β-D-fructofuranose. Occasionally, a septanose (seven-membered) ring may be encountered if the aldose or ketose is suitably substituted (Stoddard, 1971).

Conformational Isomers

Ring conformational isomers. The sugars serve admirably as examples of the rapidly developing subject of "conformational isomerism." They serve not only as models for developing conformational concepts (and conceptual arguments) but also as examples of applications in chemical and biological phenomena that are conformationally directed. Literally, a conformational isomer is a *shape* isomer and is to be distinguished from configurational isomerism in that a single covalent bond must be severed and reformed in the latter, whereas conformational isomers are generated through simple rotation about single covalent bonds. This "sharp" distinction between configuration and conformation seems to work well for the sugars at present, but it is not generally applicable to other compounds.

The pyranose and the furanose rings for the sugars are themselves chiral. This is brought about conceptually by merely numbering the carbon atoms of the pyranose ring and actually by the fact that the substituent hydroxyl groups are not chemically equivalent. For example, sugar OH groups possess different acidities. The hydrogen atom of the anomeric hydroxyl group is the most acidic, the β-anomer of D-glucose being more acid than the α-anomer. For methyl-D-glucopyranoside, the acidity of the OH groups decreases in the order 2-OH $\gg$ 6-OH $>$ 3-OH $>$ 4-OH (Rendleman, 1973). Consequently, two pyranose ring structures are possible, which are related as nonsuperposable mirror images (6). The structures (6) B and C are mirror images of A, formed by placing

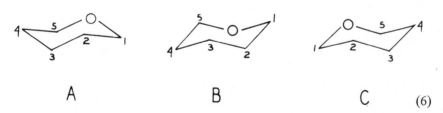

$$A \qquad\qquad B \qquad\qquad C \qquad (6)$$

the mirror either before or beneath **A**. That pyranose ring conformation is designated as C1 when the carbon atom sequence is numbered clockwise, beginning with the carbon following the ring oxygen atom that protrudes from the average plane of the ring (Shallenberger and Acree, 1971). When the carbon atom sequence is counterclockwise when viewed in the same manner, the conformation is 1C.

In (6), A is the C1 conformation and B and C are 1C, utilizing the principle of mirror-image symbols for mirror-image conformational structures. Stoddard (1971) uses the symbols $^4C_1$ and $^1C_4$ to describe these mirror-image conformations. In arriving at this latter set of conformational descriptors, the pyranoid ring is numbered. A reference plane is then chosen so that it contains four of the ring atoms, or it is chosen so that the lowest numbered carbon atom in the ring is displaced from that plane. Ring atoms that lie above the reference plane, numbering clockwise from above, are written as superscripts and precede the letter; ring atoms that lie below the reference plane are written as subscripts and immediately follow the letter. This method retains an element of the Reeves' (1950) system, which the present writer favors. Use of superscripts and subscripts, however, becomes quite necessary for describing the envelope and twist conformations for the furanoid sugars (Hall, 1963).

The pyranose ring structure for any *given* sugar can adopt either the C1 or the 1C conformation; as such, D-glucose can exist in two chair conformations. In the C1 conformer all bulky hydroxyl substituents are "equatorial" for the β-D-anomer (in the same plane as the average plane for the ring). In the 1C (7) conformation they are perpendicular ("axial").

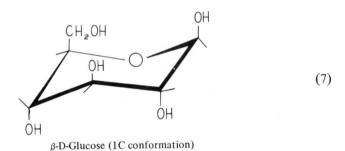

(7)

β-D-Glucose (1C conformation)

Because a sugar belonging to a given chiral family can exist in mirror-image ring conformations, the use of a conformational symbol such as Reeves' C1 or Stoddard's $^4C_1$ must be accompanied by a chiral designation (D or L) if the chiral family to which the sugar belongs has not been established. Otherwise, the use of mirror-image conformational symbols is ambiguous (Durette and Horton, 1971).

In terms of conformational analysis, β-D-glucopyranose in the C1 conformation serves as the model for the most highly favored (preferred) structure of any aldohexopyranose; the 1C conformation serves as the model for the least favored structure. Evidence for this statement is the ease with which the aldohexopyranoses form 1,6-anhydrohexopyranoses. Angyal and Dawes (1968) found that at equilibrium at 100°C only those sugars that, because of instability factors, contain appreciable amounts of the 1C conformation in solution, readily form 1,6-anhydrohexopyranoses. Thus, D-glucose forms levo-glucosan (8) least readily (0.2%), while altrose and idose generate them with ease (65 and 86%, respectively).

The disposition (axial or equatorial) of the hydroxyl groups on the C1 (D) ring structure for aldohexopyranoses and aldopentopyranoses is given in Table 2. The stereodispositions also apply to the favored 1C conformation of the L-series of sugars.

The conformational structures for the sugars have several significant features. For example, a significant consequence of enantiomerism is not

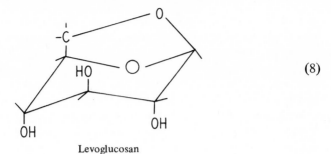

(8)

Levoglucosan

apparent from the Haworth–Hirst perspective formulas: Because the entire shape of the rings possesses a mirror-image relationship, enantiomerism involves more than mere transposition of configuration at individual chiral centers. Biochemical predictions based on the rationale that sugar enantiomers have the same ring conformation are, therefore, erroneous. It is unfortunate that this principle was perpetuated in the international carbohydrate chemical literature for several years resulting in misleading biochemical interpretations and ambiguous predictions.

TABLE 2 Disposition of OH Groups (Axial or Equatorial) on the Cl Conformation Ring Carbon Atoms of β-D-aldohexopyranoses (CH_2OH on C-5) and Aldopentopyranoses

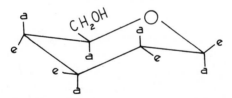

Sugar	Carbon atom number				
	1	2	3	4	5
Glucose	e	e	e	e	e
Mannose	e	a	e	e	e
Allose	e	e	a	e	e
Galactose	e	e	e	a	e
Altrose	e	a	a	e	e
Gulose	e	e	a	a	e
Talose	e	a	e	a	e
Idose	e	a	a	a	e
Xylose	e	e	e	e	—
Lyxose	e	a	e	e	—
Ribose	e	e	a	e	—
Arabinose	e	a	a	e	—

In addition to the two chair forms possible for the pyranose ring, a "flexible cycle" of boatlike structures and skew conformations is possible. These are intermediate forms encountered in the transposition from one chair structure to the alternate chair form. Boat conformations are described by the carbon atoms that occupy the "stem" positions of the boat. In the Reeves' system, the lowest numbered carbon atom at a stem position serves to describe the conformation and, as shown in (9), this system uses mirror-image conformational symbols to indicate mirror-image ring structures. With reference to the

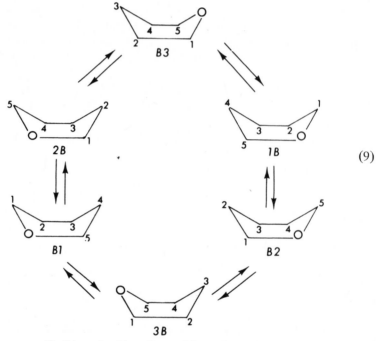

(9)

Flexible cycle of boat forms of the pyranose ring

overall boat conformation of the pyranose ring, carbon atoms that form the cockpit of the boat have substituents that are designated either *equatorial* or *axial*, while the carbon atom(s) that form the stems of the boat have substituents that are called *bowsprits* (b) or *flagpoles* (f), as shown in (10) for the B3 conformation.

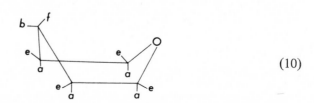

(10)

Although the boat and skew conformations of the pyranose ring are not as energetically favored as the chair forms, the possibility exists that one of them may indeed be the participating form in certain organic chemical and biological reactions. At present objective methods for determining the sugar conformation that participates in a particular chemical event are not available. Empirically, however, certain reactions of the sugars seem to have more complete descriptions through reference to one or more appropriate conformational forms. This is brought about by considering a second important attribute of ring conformational structures, the varying stereogeometry of hydroxyl groups either with relation to each other, or to the ring conformation.

α-Glycol conformations. Alterations in the ring conformation result in changes in the stereoposition that the carbon atom substituents have with respect to each other, and descriptive terms have evolved to describe these "partial" conformational features, particularly vicinal hydroxyl groups. Some of the vicinal glycol relations are shown in (11), using Newman projection formulas

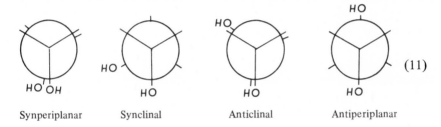

| Synperiplanar | Synclinal | Anticlinal | Antiperiplanar | (11) |

for the different torsion angles described. Other terms in common use are simply *anti* for antiperiplanar, *staggered* or *gauche* for the synclinal arrangement, and *eclipsed* for synperiplanar. Inverting the C1 ring conformation of β-D-glucose changes the individual OH groups from the equatorial to the axial disposition and the α-glycol conformation from synclinal to antiperiplanar.

The steric disposition of a single hydroxyl group, in relation to the overall shape of the ring, can have bearing on its individual chemical properties. An axial hydroxyl group at the anomeric center is oxidized by bromine water much more slowly than an equatorial hydroxyl group (Isbell, 1962).

For a reaction to proceed that requires two hydroxyl groups to reside within a certain minimum distance of each other may not only require an appropriate vicinal glycol configuration (e.g., *cis*) but an appropriate ring conformation as well. The reaction of the sugars with borate requires *cis* hydroxyl groups in the staggered (synclinal) conformation. For α-D-glucose this is possibly only on the furanose ring, or on the pyranose ring in the B3 conformation since the reaction is apparently a concerted reaction (12).

For a pair of adjacent hydroxyl groups to react with cuprammonium (Reeves, 1950, 1951), the hydroxyl groups must have a projected dihedral angle of 0° (eclipsed or synperiplanar) to 60° (the staggered conformation with either

(12)

Hypothetical interaction between borate and α-D-glucopyranose

the *cis* or the *trans* configuration). Vicinal hydroxyl groups in the antiperiplanar or the anticlinal conformations are inert toward cuprammonium reagent.

Several examples can be given where an appropriate spatial arrangement of three hydroxyl substituents is required to explain chemical events, such as the migration of the tridentate borate anion of epiinositol during electrophoresis (13). In this case, a conformational interconversion is required to permit the complex and to explain the migration rate (Angyal, 1973).

(13)

Epiinisitol   Borate anion

It is possible that an appropriate steric arrangement of three electronegative centers is required for bitter taste in the sugars and that many biologic substrate-receptor or substrate-carrier interactions involve a coordinated reaction between three or more sites. This leads to the development of the concept of "multiple group stereogeometry" (Birch and Shallenberger, 1973) and to the investigation of the behavior of enantiomers. A difference in the behavior of enantiomers indicates a tripartite or even higher order substrate-receptor interaction.

Permissible operations with perspective formulas. Because the Haworth-Hirst and the conformational structures for the sugars are perspective structures, they can be manipulated and illustrated at will. The manipulator, however, should not lose sight of the fact that only one single covalent bond can be drawn on the plane of the paper and that neither the conformation nor the configuration about the asymmetric centers is altered. In Fig. 1, α-D-gluco-pyranose in the C1 conformation, with only hydroxyl ring substituents indicated, is rotated in the plane of the ring, perpendicular to the plane of the paper, so that all possible forms where only one single covalent ring bond is written on the plane of the paper are presented.

In Fig. 2 the model has been turned over from left to right (A to B or toward the viewer, A to C). In neither case has the identity of the compound as α-D-glucose in the C1 or $^4C_1$ conformation been altered, although the formal convention for depicting the structure of the compound has been breached. These exercises can be applied to all of the sugars in any conformation. With practice, identifying the sugars or writing their structures in a variety of forms becomes intuitive.

TASTE RELATED TO STRUCTURE

Sweetness

According to dictionary definitions, sugars are sweet and usually crystal-line substances. However, some are bitter, and different sugars possess widely different degrees of sweetness. This latter observation was one of the first indications that the molecular formula for the hexoses ($C_6H_{12}O_6$) was not entirely adequate for describing their constitution (Wells, 1858). It was not until conformational principles were applied to the behavior of the sugars that some inkling as to reasons for their sweetness and its variability began to evolve (Shallenberger, 1963). Elaborating on the observation that saporous groups occur in pairs and that ethyl alcohol is not sweet while ethylene glycol (14) is quite sweet, it was reasoned that the ethylene glycol moiety or grouping in the

(14)

Ethylene glycol   Ethyl alcohol

sugars was the primary saporous unit for sweet taste, particularly when the conformation of that grouping was *staggered*. Based on individual sugar and model compound observations, it became apparent that the two extreme glycol conformations, eclipsed and antiperiplanar, were incapable of eliciting sweet taste. This relationship is shown in Fig. 3. The conformation of a glycol moiety of a sugar or sugar derivative is dictated by the conformation of the sugar ring and also by the ring size.

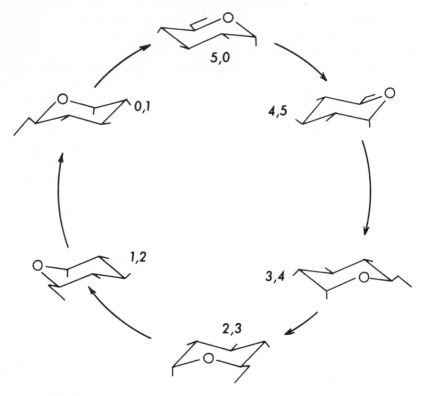

FIGURE 1   Rotational itinerary for the Cl conformation of α-D-glucopyranose.

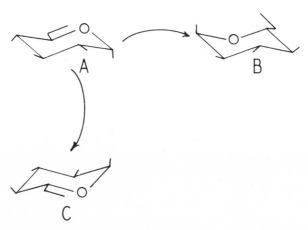

FIGURE 2   Inversion of the formal drawing of the α-D-gluco-
pyranose structure.

Deviation from the staggered α-glycol conformation results in lowered sugar sweetness for either of two reasons: Whenever hydroxyl groups approach the eclipsed conformation, they are sterically disposed to hydrogen bond to each other; the strength of the intramolecular hydrogen bond is inversely proportionate to the O-O distance (15). The formation of an intramolecular hydrogen

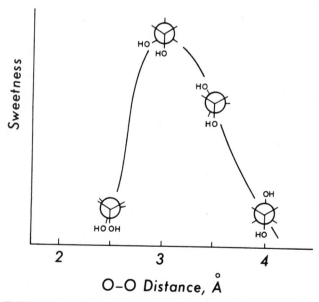

$$(15)$$

bond (or the potential for an intramolecular hydrogen bond) is associated with decreased sugar sweetness. Optimum sugar sweetness seems to occur at an O-O distance of 3 Å, where the potential for intramolecular hydrogen bonding is minimal. On the other hand, whenever vicinal OH groups are too far apart for intramolecular H-bond formation, sugar sweetness is again at a minimum. These seemingly opposed requirements for lack of sweet taste were rationalized by constructing a sweet taste receptor site that had stereochemical properties commensurate with those indicated by vicinal sugar hydroxyl groups in the staggered conformation and by viewing the initial chemistry of the sweet taste sensation as a concerted intermolecular hydrogen bond (Shallenberger and

FIGURE 3 Ability of various sugar α-glycol groups to elicit sweet taste.

Acree, 1967). With vicinal OH groups acting as AH and B of a hydrogen bonding system,[1] it was proposed that these OH groups react with a stereochemically appropriate AH,B system at the receptor site (Fig. 4).

The best evidence for assigning tastelessness to the antiperiplanar and the eclipsed α-glycol conformation is found in the intriguing behavior of the sweetness of D-fructose. In freshly prepared solutions, or when tasted as the crystalline material, β-D-fructopyranose is the sweetest naturally occurring sugar, and it is reported to be nearly twice as sweet as sucrose. Upon dissolution, however, the sweetness diminishes rapidly until it is only slightly sweeter than sucrose (Pangborn and Gee, 1961). In addition to an unusually rapid mutarotation for a reducing sugar, fructose exhibits a striking thermal mutarotation (Tsuzuki and Yamazaki, 1953), which is accompanied by rapid decrease in sweetness. These data, after Shallenberger (1973), are shown in Fig. 5.

At equilibrium at room temperature, the composition of a fructose solution is about 76% β-D-fructopyranose, 20% β-D-fructofuranose, and 4% of an additional tautomer believed to be α-D-fructopyranose (Shallenberger, 1973; Streefkerk et al., 1974). In any event, one of the fructose tautomers formed must be nearly tasteless, and β-D-fructofuranose (16) with *cis* and eclipsed or

(16)

[1] In a hydrogen-bonding system, A and B are electronegative atoms, usually oxygen or nitrogen. H is a proton attached to A through a single covalent bond. When AH is conveniently near a second electronegative atom B, H is delocalized and is said to "bond" to B also. While the energy of the H-bond is low, it is biologically significant.

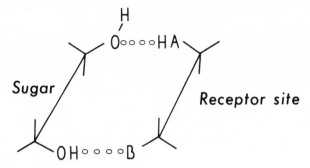

FIGURE 4 Concerted interaction of vicinal sugar OH groups, acting as AH and B of a hydrogen-bonding system, with a stereochemically appropriate AH,B unit of a taste bud receptor site.

trans and antiperiplanar OH groups is the logical candidate. Unfortunately, β-D-fructopyranose is the only crystalline form of D-fructose known; as such the tastelessness of β-D-fructofuranose has not as yet been directly proved.

A second case for decreased sugar sweetness occurs when one hydroxyl group of a glycol moiety is sterically disposed to a hydrogen bond elsewhere in the sugar molecule. The axial hydroxyl group of galactose and mannose can bond the ring oxygen atom (17), and the α-D-anomers of these hexoses are only about half as sweet as glucose.

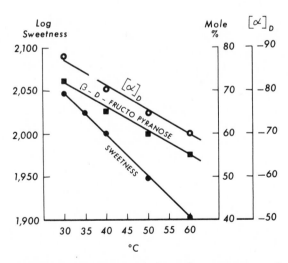

FIGURE 5 Change in optical rotation, sweetness, and concentration of β-D-fructopyranose during thermal mutarotation. After Shallenberger (1973). Published with permission of the American Chemical Society.

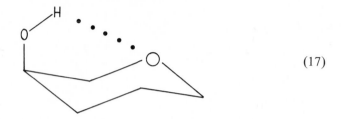

(17)

In the case of β-D-fructopyranose, the potential for an intramolecular hydrogen bond seems to be associated with enhanced sugar sweetness (18). In this case, the sugar AH,B system of prime importance is external to the ring (Birch and Lindley, 1973; Shallenberger and Acree, 1967). Lindley and Birch (1975) have suggested that since α-L-sorbose is not so sweet as fructose, the intramolecular H-bond in fructose serves to increase the acidity of OH_2 and, therefore, accentuates its function as AH.

β-D-Fructofuranose   α-L-Sorbopyranose

(18)

An AH,B system seems to be the primary unit for a compound to taste sweet, and the grouping has been demonstrated in a variety of substances, both organic and inorganic, that have this attribute. Examples are the D-series of amino acids, chloroform, unsaturated alcohols, lead acetate, salts of beryllium, saccharine, and the cyclamates (Shallenberger and Acree, 1967, 1971).

Further insight into the stereochemistry of sweet taste became available through an attempt to rationalize the fact that the D-forms of the alpha-amino acids generally taste sweet, while the L-forms (19) are usually tasteless or described as bitter (Solms et al., 1965).

$$
\begin{array}{cc}
\overset{\displaystyle O}{\underset{\displaystyle \|}{C}}-OH & \overset{\displaystyle O}{\underset{\displaystyle \|}{C}}-OH \\
| & | \\
H-C-NH_2 & H_2N-C-H \\
| & | \\
R & R
\end{array}
$$

(19)

D-Amino acid   L-Amino acid

Since the amino acids have a fixed AH,B unit consisting of $-NH_2$ as AH and the carbonyl oxygen atom of the carboxyl group as B, it was proposed

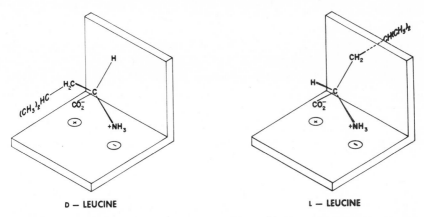

D — LEUCINE   L — LEUCINE

FIGURE 6 Positioning of the sweet unit of D-leucine over a hypothetical AH (+) and B (−) unit of a taste bud receptor site, and the inability to position that unit of L-leucine over the same site due to steric hindrance of a spatial barrier. After Shallenberger et al. (1969). Reproduced by permission of *Nature.*

(Shallenberger et al., 1969) that the AH,B unit of a D-amino acid could approach the sweet taste receptor site, while the L-amino acids, with an amino acid radical (R) larger than the ethyl group, could not do so. This could be explained by merely placing a spatial barrier at about 3–4 Å from the AH,B receptor. Thus, a sweet-tasting D-amino acid could be positioned over the receptor site, but an L-amino acid could not (Fig. 6).

That D- and L-amino acids have different tastes led Pasteur (1886) to suggest that the gustatory nerve endings must be dissymmetric because of their ability to differentiate enantiomers. Consequently, it has generally been accepted that since the D-series of sugars taste sweet, the L-series must be tasteless. The literature contains at least one report (Boyd and Matsubara, 1962) that supports this contention.

Because the sugar α-glycol group is bifunctional when viewed as an AH,B system, with an OH group able to function as either AH or B, there should be little difference in the sweetness of the enantiomeric sugars; in the presence of a spatial barrier at the taste bud receptor site, the same glycol pair of OH groups can still be positioned over the receptor site, although their identity as AH and B is transposed. When the sweetness of a series of enantiomeric pairs of sugars was evaluated (Shallenberger et al., 1969), it was found that a taste panel could not significantly distinguish the difference in sweetness intensity of 10% solutions of an enantiomeric pair of sugars.

Although it is known that there is a relation between the hydrophobic nature of a molecule and its ability to elicit sweet taste (Deutsch and Hansch, 1966), it is only recently that the role of hydrophobicity and the hydrophobic bond (Kauzmann, 1959) in the mechanism of sweet taste has been elucidated. One obvious role of the hydrophobic nature of a molecule is to impart a degree of lipophilicity to the compound for interaction, partition with, or passage through the lipoprotein structure of the tastebud cell membrane. This role for hydrophobicity is related to the "impact" time for the sweet taste response (Shallenberger and Acree, 1967, 1971).

In a study of the sweetness of the amino acids and other compounds, Kier (1972) deduced that in addition to the AH,B component prerequisite for sweetness, a sweet molecule has a third site that is electron-rich and thus capable of participating in some type of bonding involving the electron component, such as a dispersion interaction. The pattern of the atoms that impart sweet taste as described by Kier is as shown in (20).

$$
\begin{array}{c}
\text{X} \\
\\
\text{A} \qquad \text{B} \\
\text{H}
\end{array}
\qquad (20)
$$

Kier calculated from the preferred conformations of the amino acids that the distances of the tripartite saporous unit are A to X, 3.5 Å; X to B, 5.5 Å; and A to B, 2.6 Å. The angles described by this oblique relation are AXB, 30°, XAB, 104°, and ABX, 45°. The dispersion site in several other sweet molecules is

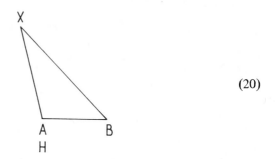

CYCLAMIC ACID   SACCHARINE

NEOHESPERIDIN DIHYDROCHALCONE

FIGURE 7   AH,B and the dispersion unit (X) of some sweet substances according to Kier (1972).

shown in Fig. 7. Using interaction energy calculations, Höltje and Kier (1974) found a good correlation between an isomorphic compound simulating the receptor features and the sweetness of a series of 2-amino-4-nitrobenzenes; the major contribution to those energies was due to dispersion forces.

The present writer prefers to consider that a third site for sweet taste is primarily hydrophobic in nature, and capable of participating in the hydrophobic bond. There is, of course, a dispersion element to the hydrophobic bond also. Since the spatial structure for the sugars is known as well as, and perhaps better than, any other class of compounds, the sugars were examined to see if they possessed a third site in order to develop further explanations for their sweet taste. The hydrophobic site in the sugars can be unambiguously identified. For the aldohexoses in pyranose ring form, it is the methylene carbon atom (CH_2) external to the ring. For aldoketoses, it is the ring methylene carbon atom. The relationship of AH to B to γ (indicating hydrophobicity) bears a very close relationship in terms of multiple group stereogeometry (Birch and Shallenberger, 1973) to the saporous unit (glucophore) of sweet-tasting compounds proposed by Kier (1972). In terms of dissymmetry, it is somewhat more slightly skewed, and the group distances (21) are AH to B, 3 Å; AH to γ, 3.13 Å; and γ to B, 5.25 Å. This multiple group

(21)

stereorelation is shown in (22) superimposed on β-D-glucopyranose, where AH is the OH group at carbon atom number four, B is the oxygen atom of the OH group at carbon atom number three, and γ is the methylene group of the sixth carbon atom. In line with this assignment is the finding that the hydroxyl group

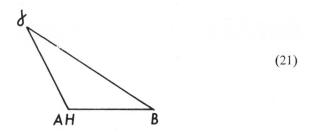

(22)

at C-4 is of special importance in the sweet taste of aldohexoses (Birch et al., 1970); similarly, the OH group at C-3 is important (Birch and Lee, 1974).

Galactose, then, would not be as sweet as glucose since the OH group at C-4 is bonded to the ring oxygen atom. It is another glycol moiety—one that does not bear the appropriate relation to γ—that must act as AH and B. Only the less intense quality characteristics of sweetness is elicited by this bipartite grouping. That is, AH,B is prerequisite for sweetness, but the tripartite structure or fit to the receptor site enhances the intensity of the sensation. Such reasoning has been used to explain the varying activity of drug substances (Nagwekar and Kostenbauder, 1970), as well as the odorous characteristics of volatile enantiomers (Shallenberger, 1972).

The multiple group stereogram for the sweet taste of the sweetest sugar, β-D-fructopyranose, is shown in (23). AH for this sugar is the anomeric OH group at C-2 (the most acidic of the sugar anomeric OH protons), B is the oxygen atom at C-1, and γ is the ring methylene carbon atom.

$$
\text{(structures)} \qquad (23)
$$

A receptor site for sweet taste using the tripartite multiple group structure needs to have the same skewness as suggested by the saporous unit, but differs from it in that AH and B are transposed (24). The initiation of the sweet taste sensation (strong sweet taste sensation) then is due to concerted intermolecular hydrogen bonding between AH and B of the saporous substance with B and AH of the receptor site and also a hydrophobic bond between γ of the sweet compound and γ of the receptor site (Fig. 8).

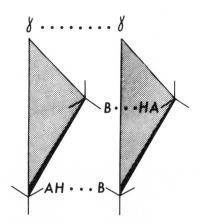

FIGURE 8 Tripartite interaction between AH,B and γ of a sweet-tasting compound and a chemically and geometrically appropriate receptor site.

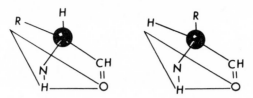

FIGURE 9   Superposition of a D- and an L-amino acid over a tripartite sweet taste receptor site.

(24)

Tripartite receptor site for sweet taste

Using the multiple group receptor site, the varying sweetness of amino acid enantiomers and the sugar enantiomers is explained in much the same way as before, but instead of a spatial barrier for the receptor site (Shallenberger et al., 1969), the varying sweetness of these compounds becomes a matter of the appropriateness of the tripartite fit to the receptor site. As shown in Fig. 9, a D-amino acid, with a hydrophobic side chain (R) may be superposed over the receptor site to yield a tripartite fit, but its enantiomer cannot. Since some sweetness would be expected using the scheme shown for the L-amino acids, the spatial barrier must still be invoked.

The enantiomeric sugars possess the same tripartite saporous unit. The stereogeometry of this fact is shown below using β-L-glucopyranose for comparison with β-D-glucopyranose (22). Only the direction of the functional groups AH, B, and γ, in respect to those of the receptor site (25) is transposed (away vs. toward).

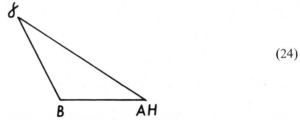

(25)

Bitterness

An interesting stereostructure–function problem is the distinctly bitter taste of β-D-mannose and gentiobiose (26). The taste of β-D-mannose is of

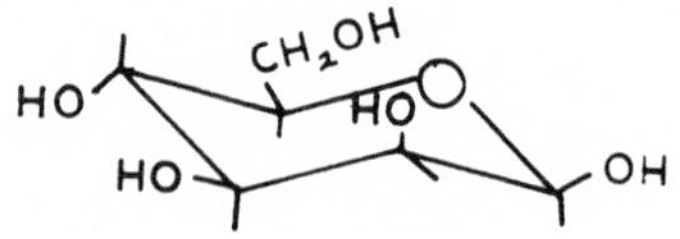

β-D-Mannose

(26)

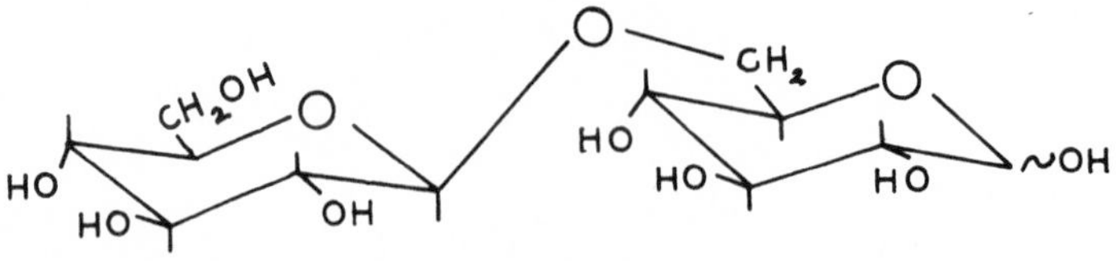

Gentiobiose

particular interest since it serves as a model (Stewart et al., 1971) to illustrate the high degree of stereospecificity exhibited by taste receptors.

In an attempt to specifically identify the AH,B sweet unit in the sugars, Birch et al. (1970) considered jointly the sweetness and the bitterness attributes of sugars and sugar derivatives. These results provide information on structural relations and requirements for bitterness. It was found that the depression of sweetness by bitterness, or bitterness by sweetness obeys a simple mathematical relationship that may be used to calculate the "true" sweetness of a bitter–sweet sugar. Bitterness and sweetness were found to interact according to the equation

$$\Delta T = K \log C/C_m$$

where ΔT = taste depression, either sweetness or bitterness

     C = concentration of additive producing the depression

   C_m = the maximum concentration of additive having no effect on the taste

    K = a constant

Application of this finding established that the anomeric center of methyl α- and β-D-glucopyranoside has no significance in determining their degree of sweetness although methyl β-D-glucopyranoside is distinctly more bitter.

In a study of deoxy sugars, methyl α-D-2,6-dideoxyribohexopyranoside and arabinohexopyranoside (27) were found to be very bitter. Birch and Lee

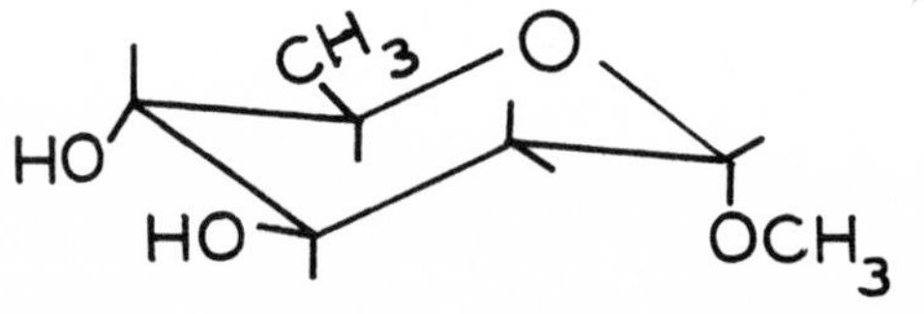

(27)

Methyl α-D-2,6-dideoxyarabinohexopyranoside

(1974) concluded that if the AH, B system for the sugars is made up of the third and fourth carbon atom OH substituents, then the first, second, fifth, and sixth carbon atom substituents provide lipophilic centers that may give rise to the bitter taste response. When two oxygen atoms are removed from a sugar ring, the molecule is never sweet and always bitter. The 1-deoxy derivatives of free sugars are always sweet and never bitter indicating, as previously found, that the anomeric oxygen atom, while not necessary for sweetness, is involved in the bitter response (Birch et al., 1975). In a study of critical molecular size for the bitterness of the aglycone portion of the glycosides, the sensory properties of a series of glycosides were recorded as shown in (28). The increasing size of the

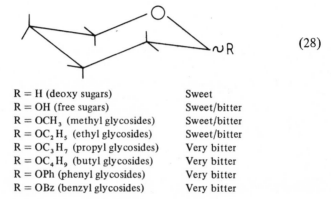

(28)

R = H (deoxy sugars)   Sweet
R = OH (free sugars)   Sweet/bitter
R = OCH$_3$ (methyl glycosides)   Sweet/bitter
R = OC$_2$H$_5$ (ethyl glycosides)   Sweet/bitter
R = OC$_3$H$_7$ (propyl glycosides)   Very bitter
R = OC$_4$H$_9$ (butyl glycosides)   Very bitter
R = OPh (phenyl glycosides)   Very bitter
R = OBz (benzyl glycosides)   Very bitter

aglycone, accompanied by increasing bitterness, indicates that there is no obvious limit to the size of the bitter receptor site and that bitterness increases with increasing lipophilicity.

One explanation for the bitterness of β-D-mannose has been offered (Shallenberger and Acree, 1971). The structure of this sugar contains three electronegative oxygen atoms that lie in the same plane, in the C1 or 1C conformation, with an O . . . O distance of 2.5 Å. This arrangement of electronegative centers seems to be associated with the bitter taste since the compound may be viewed as a "soft" base.

Kubota and Kubo (1969) have advanced the idea that while an intramolecular hydrogen bond is associated with decreased sweet taste of compounds, it can also be associated with increased bitterness, which presumably lowers sweet taste, as in the case of galactose. Along these lines it is interesting that gentiobiose can be structured so that nearly all of its hydroxyl groups are intramolecularly hydrogen bonded (29).

Given that bitterness in peptides (Matoba and Hata, 1972) and sugar derivatives can be related to hydrophobicity as well as to intramolecular hydrogen bonding, it is clear that bitterness can be elicited by compounds with chemical properties having more than one set of "common" features (Shallenberger and Acree, 1971).

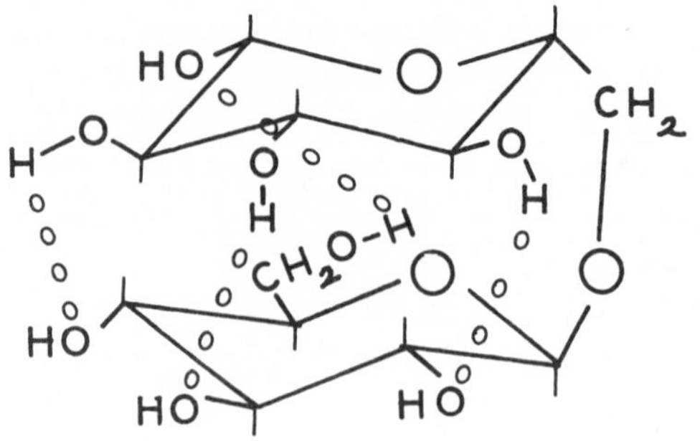

(29)

H-bonded gentiobiose

BIOAVAILABILITY

Occurrence in Foods

The most widely distributed sugar in nature is β-D-glucopyranose. It is the repeating unit of the plant cell wall substance cellulose, and in solutions of glucose it is the most abundant anomeric form. One teleological reason for its abundance rests in its pyranose form. The C1 conformation of this form with all bulky carbon atom substituents equatorially disposed is the most energetically favorable of the aldohexoses.

Foods of plant origin accumulate glucose, fructose, and sucrose as their major sugar components, probably because sucrose is the sugar most commonly translocated by plants following photosynthesis. It is also the first nonphosphorylated sugar produced by photosynthesis. In special cases, such as squash (Beitler and Hendrix, 1974), tetrasaccharide stachyose is translocated.

The amount of glucose, fructose, and sucrose accumulated in foods of plant origin varies considerably. Vegetables usually contain glucose and fructose in about equal amounts as well as sucrose; certain fruits, such as apples and pears, accumulate mainly fructose; leguminous foods, such as the lima and kidney beans, accumulate the raffinose family of oligosaccharides, raffinose, stachyose, and verbascose, in addition to sucrose. Tables that list the approximate sugar distribution in foods of plant origin are available (Lee et al., 1970; Hardinge et al., 1965; Shallenberger, 1974). The feature of the sugar distribution in foods of plant origin—one that is not always recognized—is that the sugars constitute a very significant portion of the total solids content of these foods. Some selected examples of fruits and vegetables are given in Table 3.

Lactose (30), the sugar of mammalian milk, accounts for 7.5% and 4.5% of the composition of human and cow's milk, respectively. Since lactose is a disaccharide made up of galactose and glucose (4-O-β-D-galactopyranosyl-D-glucose) and is hydrolyzed in the human intestine, it is the principal source of galactose in the diet.

TABLE 3 Distribution of Sugars in Fruits
and Vegetables as Percent of the Total Solids

	Solids (%)	Sugars, dry basis (%)		
		Glucose	Fructose	Sucrose
Apple	15.96	7.3	37.8	23.6
Peach	12.79	7.1	9.2	54.1
Pear	13.58	6.9	49.8	11.8
Sour cherry	15.05	28.5	21.7	2.6
Table beet	11.19	1.6	1.4	54.6
Carrot	12.00	7.0	7.0	35.3
Lettuce	4.97	5.0	9.2	2.0
Watermelon	9.57	12.3	36.9	24.5

Lactose (30)

With the relatively recent advent of processed foods and fabricated foods, the distribution of sugars in foods is changing. A spectrum of "rare food sugars" can now be found in the diet due either to the processing of the food or the addition of sugar syrup preparations, honey, or maple syrup. The quantities of these rare sugars are low and hardly detectable by the usual analytical techniques. Some, such as psicose (31), are formed by the rearrangement of

Psicose (31)

either glucose or fructose. Others, such as levoglucosan, are formed by intramolecular dehydration, especially under acid conditions. Recombination of the anhydro sugars, particularly those of glucose and fructose leads to a series of "reversion" products. Some of the resulting disaccharides due to the reversion of glucose are given, along with their common names, in Table 4.

TABLE 4   Reversion Disaccharides of
Glucose

Common name	Glucosidic linkage
α, α-Trehalose	$\alpha 1 \rightarrow \alpha 1$
Kojibiose	$\alpha 1 \rightarrow 2$
Nigerose	$\alpha 1 \rightarrow 3$
Maltose	$\alpha 1 \rightarrow 4$
Isomaltose	$\alpha 1 \rightarrow 6$
α, β-Trehalose	$\alpha 1 \rightarrow \beta 1$
β, β-Trehalose	$\beta 1 \rightarrow \beta 1$
Sophorose	$\beta 1 \rightarrow 2$
Laminaribose	$\beta 1 \rightarrow 3$
Cellobiose	$\beta 1 \rightarrow 4$
Gentiobiose	$\beta 1 \rightarrow 6$

The population spectrum of these disaccharides is related to the acid stability of the glucosidic linkage. This has been established by Bishop (1956) to be $(1 \rightarrow 6) > (1 \rightarrow 4) > (1 \rightarrow 3) > (1 \rightarrow 2)$; for glucose in 0.082 N hydrochloric acid, the predominant disaccharide reversion products were found to be isomaltose and gentiobiose in the β-D-anomeric configuration (Thompson et al., 1954). Higher molecular weight oligosaccharides which may also be encountered are isomaltotriose, tetraose and pentaose, panose, and isopanose. Ultimately, polymeric glucans made up of $\alpha 1 \rightarrow 6$ and $\alpha 1 \rightarrow 4$ linkages are formed.

Free fructose under acid conditions yields a series of eight possible "di-D-fructosedianhydrides" made up of α-D- and β-D-fructopyranose and fructofuranose 1,2'-anhydrides condensed by virtue of the elimination of water at these two positions to form a substituted dioxane ring (32) that is acid stable.

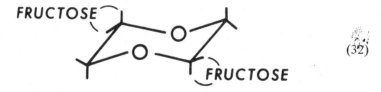

(32)

These compounds have been characterized by Binkley et al. (1973) not only with respect to the fructose structure (pyranose or furanose) but also in terms of the pyranose and furanose conformation.

Other rare food sugars made up by glucose and fructose combination, probably through enzymic transglycosylation are kestose, erlose, maltulose, theandose, and turanose.

Intestinal Absorption

Biologically available glycosidic linkages. The logical approach to determining the nutritional bioavailability of the various sugars that may be present in the diet would seem to be to establish the requirements for the hydrolysis of the various glycosidic linkages possible. A glycoside is a derivative of a sugar in which the hydrogen atom of the hemiacetal hydroxyl group has been replaced with another substituent that may or may not be another sugar or chain of sugars. The common disaccharide sucrose (33) is therefore either an α-D-gluco-pyranoside or a β-D-fructofuranoside.

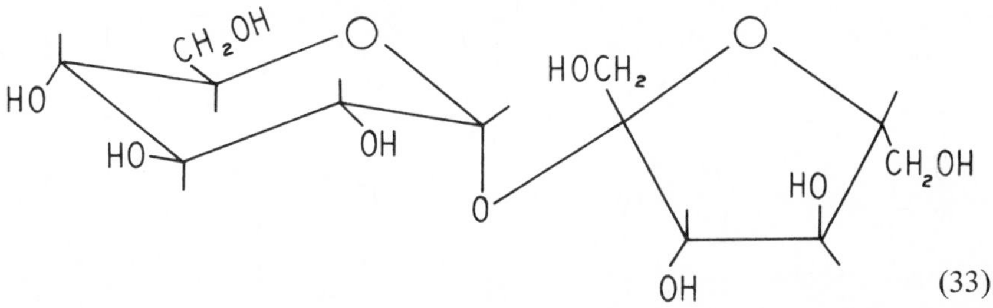

Sucrose

(33)

Teleological reasons given for the natural occurrence of glycosides are the lowering of osmotic activity, detoxification of the aglycone, and solubilization of an otherwise sparingly soluble metabolite. Enzymes that act on naturally occurring alkyl, aralkyl, and aryl glycosides are called glycosidases; those that hydrolyze carbohydrate polymers such as starch and cellulose are called polysaccharidases. In view of the wide range of carbohydrases present in nature, particularly microbial carbohydrases, this discussion will be restricted to the presence of the intrinsic carbohydrases of the human digestive tract.

According to Dahlqvist (1974) the intestinal brush borders contain at least five different "α-glucosidases" with overlapping activity. The enzymes, named according to their main substrate are isomaltase, with about half the activity toward maltose as for isomaltose; sucrase, with about one-quarter the ability to hydrolyze maltose as sucrose; two heat-stable maltases with about one-fifth the ability to hydrolyze isomaltose as maltose; a specific α,α-trehalase; lactase, with about an equal ability to hydrolyze lactose and cellobiose.

Asp et al. (1969) have determined that there are two β-D-galactosidases: disaccharidase as mentioned above (lactase) and "hetero" β-D-galactosidase, which acts on artificial substrates but not lactose.

It would appear then that the α-glucosidases of the intestinal brush borders have one or more of the following substrate requirements:

1. $R - O - R'$
2. $R - O -$
3. $- O - R'$

Number one is typical of the amylases and trehalase, number two is typical of the sucrase and maltase, and number three typifies isomaltase. The cellobiase can hardly be considered to be a β-D-glucosidase (cellulose is not attacked); it may be a 4-O-glucopyranosylase instead. In view of the diverse and overlapping nature of the α-glucosidases in the brush border, Dahlqvist (1974) suggests that they be named according to their main apparent substrate. It is not known at present whether or not the various glucosidic linkages possible, as shown in Table 4, are capable of being hydrolyzed, and the demonstration of an α-glucosidase in the digestive system for one particular type of linkage does not necessarily indicate that all such linkages are capable of being hydrolyzed.

The fate of other sugars in the diet is an important problem in treating certain types of sugar intolerance. The fate of melibiose, for example, cannot be easily predicted simply because an α-D-galactosidase is not a member of the intestinal disaccharidases. A 6-O-glucopyranosylase such as isomaltase may be able to hydrolyze it to the component monosaccharides galactose and glucose.

Structural requirements for intestinal transport. Under the appropriate conditions, which vary for individual sugars, monosaccharides may apparently be accumulated in the small intestinal tissues against a concentration gradient. This type of sugar transport is designated as "active," or energy dependent, and requires sodium for its operation. However, the designation of sugar transport as "active" is valid only from a relative point of view (Alvarado, 1966). In order of transport rate, glucose and galactose are considered to be about equal (Barnett et al., 1968); fructose is next, but apparently does not require sodium. Xylose is transported at about 1/100 the rate of glucose, and mannose is transported at an even slower rate.

As the result of the study of model compounds, it appears that the most favorable structure for rapid, sodium-dependent sugar intestinal transport is the D-glucose configuration in the C1 conformation with the equatorial OH group at C-2. This form is absolutely essential as is the considerable importance assigned to the presence of C-6 (34) (Barnett et al., 1968).

(34)

The original basic structure needed for active sugar transport was proposed by Crane (1960), but as stated previously, D-glucose itself is the ideal structure for active transport. If two or more hydroxyl groups, other than the one at C-2, are transposed or removed as in the deoxy sugars, then the compound is no longer "actively" transported. Later studies (Barnett et al., 1970) showed that the extent of accumulation correlated with the number of hydroxyl groups in the D-*gluco* configuration and that these probably formed hydrogen bonds with

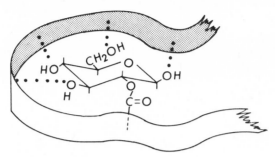

FIGURE 10 Binding of D-glucose to the intestinal sugar carrier according to Barnett et al. (1970).

the sugar carrier as shown in Fig. 10. The importance of the second hydroxyl group is assigned to the formation of an intermolecular ester. As deduced by the substitution of the sugar hydroxyl group with a proton, or by a halogen atom, the proton donor of the hydrogen bond is contributed by the intestinal receptor, and the proton acceptor group for the hydrogen bond is the oxygen atom of the sugar hydroxyl groups (Barnett, 1973).

$$\text{sugar - O .... } \overset{\text{H}}{\text{H}} \text{- X - protein receptor}$$

L-Glucose can be transported by such a system, but since the number of binding sites is reduced (Fig. 11), its active transport rate is reduced. The number of binding sites for L-glucose is reduced by orienting the enantiomer in Fig. 11 so that C-1, C-2, C-3, and C-6 of D-glucose are coincident with C-3, C-2, C-1, and C-6 of L-glucose, respectively (Barnett et al., 1968). The ring oxygen atom is not apparently involved in active transport since thio-D-glucose is a substrate for this transport mechanism (Critchley et al., 1970). It is possible (cf.

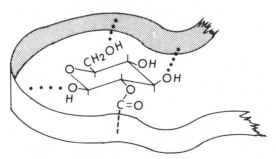

FIGURE 11 Binding of L-glucose to the intestinal sugar carrier according to Barnett et al. (1970).

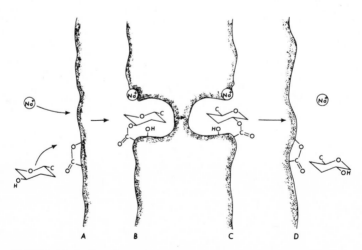

Thio-D-glucose

(35)

Barnett, 1973) that the H-bonding system between the OH group at C-4 of D-glucose and the receptor site is of the type

sugar – O – H . . . . X– protein receptor

In view of the importance of the equatorial OH group at C-2 of D-glucose in the C1 conformation (a consideration that indicates that it is the C1 conformation that is actively transported) Barnett et al. (1970) proposed that when a sugar is adsorbed on the carrier in the presence of sodium ion, the hydroxyl group at C-2 cleaves an intramolecular ester on the membrane to form an intermolecular ester bond between the sugar and the membrane. The intermolecular ester is regenerated with the release of the sugar to the inside of the cell in a low sodium environment. As shown in Fig. 12, the role of the sodium may be that of providing the proper conformation to the receptor site in order to provide for glucose binding (Caspary et al., 1969). In addition to the probable significance of intermolecular H-bonding, the ester bond, and conformational change of the membrane, it is also probable that a hydrophobic bond exists between the methylene at C-6 and the receptor site. The transfer of

FIGURE 12   Sodium-dependent mechanism for transporting D-glucose (A–D) across an intestinal cell wall membrane.

sodium from inside the cell to the intestinal lumen is believed to be a Na^+-K^+-dependent ATPase mechanism (Herman, 1974).

Fructose also appears to be transported *via* an active mechanism that is separate from that involved in the transfer of other actively transported sugars (Gracey et al., 1972); apparently, it is not Na^+ dependent. The special membrane mechanism for fructose transport is possibly dependent on hydrophobic factors.

REFERENCES

Alvarado, F. 1966. *Biochim. Biophys. Acta* 112:292.

Angyal, S. J. 1973. In *Carbohydrates in solution,* ed. R. F. Gould, pp. 106–120. Washington, D.C.: American Chemical Society.

Angyal, S. J. and Dawes, K. 1968. *Austr. J. Chem.* 21:2747.

Asp, N., Dahlqvist, A. and Koldovsky, O. 1969. *Biochem. J.* 114:351.

Barnett, J. E. G. 1973. In *Molecular structure and function of food carbohydrate,* ed. G. G. Birch and L. F. Green, pp. 216–234. London: Applied Science Publishers.

Barnett, J. E. G., Jarvis, W. T. S. and Munday, K. A. 1968. *Biochem. J.* 109:61.

Barnett, J. E. G., Ralph, A. and Munday, K. A. 1970. *Biochem. J.* 118:843.

Beitler, G. A. and Hendrix, J. E. 1974. *Plant Physiol.* 53:674.

Binkley, R. W., Binkley, W. W., Grey, A. A. and Wickberg, B. 1973. *Abstr. 164th Nat. Mtg. Am. Chem. Soc.* Carb. No. 15.

Birch, G. G. and Lee, C. K. 1974. *J. Food Sci.* 39:947.

Birch, G. G. and Lindley, M. G. 1973. *J. Food Sci.* 38:665.

Birch, G. G. and Shallenberger, R. S. 1973. In *Molecular structure and function of food carbohydrate,* ed. G. G. Birch and L. F. Green, pp. 9–20. London: Applied Science Publishers.

Birch, G. G., Lee, C. K. and Rolfe, E. J. 1970. *J. Sci. Food Agric.* 21:650.

Birch, G. G., Lee, C. K. and Lindley, M. G. 1975. *Stärke* 27:51.

Bishop, C. T. 1956. *Can. J. Chem.* 34:1255.

Boyd, W. C. and Matsubara, S. 1962. *Science* 137:669.

Caspary, W. F., Stevenson, N. R. and Crane, R. K. 1969. *Biochim. Biophys. Acta* 193:168.

Crane, R. K. 1960. *Physiol. Rev.* 40:789.

Critchley, D. R., Eichholz, A. and Crane, R. K. 1970. *Biochim. Biophys. Acta* 211:244.

Dahlqvist, A. 1974. In *Sugars in nutrition,* ed. H. L. Sipple and K. W. McNutt, pp. 189–214. New York: Academic Press.

Deutsch, E. W. and Hansch, C. 1966. *Nature* 211:75.

Durette, P. L. and Horton, D. 1971. *Adv. Carbohydr. Chem. Biochem.* 21:49.

Gracey, M., Burke, V. and Oshin, A. 1972. *Biochim. Biophys. Acta* 266:397.

Hall, L. D. 1963. *Chem. Inc.* 950.

Hardinge, M. G., Swarner, J. B. and Crooks, H. 1965. *J. Am. Diet. Assoc.* 46:197.

Herman, R. H. 1974. In *Sugars in nutrition,* ed. H. L. Sipple and K. W. McNutt, pp. 145–172. New York: Academic Press.

Höltje, H. -D. and Kier, L. B. 1974. *J. Pharmacol. Sci.* 63:1722.

Hudson, C. S. 1909. *J. Am. Chem. Soc.* 31:66.

Isbell, H. S. 1962. *J. Res. Natl. Bur. Stand.* 66A:233.

Isbell, H. S. and Pigman, W. W. 1973. *J. Res. Natl. Bur. Stand.* 18:141.

Kauzmann, W. 1959. *Adv. Protein Chem.* 14:1.
Kier, L. B. 1972. *J. Pharmacol. Sci.* 61:1394.
Kubota, T. and Kubo, I. 1969. *Nature* 223:97.
Lee, C. Y., Shallenberger, R. S. and Vittum, M. T. 1970. *N.Y. Food Life Sci. Bull. No. 1.* (Cornell University).
Lindley, M. G. and Birch, G. G. 1975. *J. Sci. Food Agric.* 26:117.
Matoba, T. and Hata, T. 1972. *Agric. Biol. Chem.* 36:1423.
Nagwekar, J. B. and Kostenbauder, H. B. 1970. *J. Pharmacol. Sci.* 59:751.
Pangborn, R. M. and Gee, S. C. 1961. *Nature* 191:810.
Pasteur, L. 1886. *Comp. Rend.* 103:138.
Pigman, W. W. and Horton, D., ed. 1972. *The carbohydrates,* vol. IA. New York: Academic Press.
Reeves, R. E. 1950. *Adv. Carbohydr. Chem.* 6:107.
Reeves, R. E. 1951. *J. Am. Chem. Soc.* 72:1499.
Rendleman, J. A., Jr. 1973. In *Carbohydrates in solution,* ed. R. F. Gould, pp. 51–69. Washington, D.C.: American Chemical Society.
Shallenberger, R. S. 1963. *J. Food Sci.* 28:584.
Shallenberger, R. S. 1972. *Proc. 5th Int. Congr. Pharmacol.* 5:22–30.
Shallenberger, R. S. 1973. In *Carbohydrates in solution,* ed. R. F. Gould, pp. 256–263. Washington, D.C.: American Chemical Society.
Shallenberger, R. S. 1974. In *Sugars in nutrition,* ed. H. L. Sipple and K. W. McNutt, pp. 67–80. New York: Academic Press.
Shallenberger, R. S. and Acree, T. E. 1966. *Carbohydr. Res.* 1:495.
Shallenberger, R. S. and Acree, T. E. 1967. *Nature* 216:480.
Shallenberger, R. S. and Acree, T. E. 1971. In *Handbook of sensory physiology,* ed. L. M. Beidler, vol. IV, part 2: *Taste,* pp. 221–277. Berlin: Springer-Verlag.
Shallenberger, R. S. and Birch, G. G. 1975. *Sugar chemistry.* Westport, Conn.: Avi Publishing Co.
Shallenberger, R. S., Acree, T. E. and Lee, C. Y. 1969. *Nature* 221:555.
Solms, J., Vuataz, L. and Egli, R. H. 1965. *Experientia* 21:692.
Stewart, R. A., Carrico, C. K. Webster, R. L. and Steinhardt, R. G., Jr. 1971. *Science* 234:220.
Stoddard, J. F. 1971. *Stereochemistry of carbohydrates.* New York: Wiley-Interscience.
Streefkerk, D. G., DeBie, M. J. A. and Vliegenthart, J. F. G. 1974. *Carbohydr. Res.* 33:250.
Thompson, A., Anno, K., Wolfrom, M. L. and Inatome, M. 1954. *J. Am. Chem. Soc.* 76:1309.
Tsuzuki, Y. and Yamazaki, J. 1953. *Biochem. Z.* 323:525.
Wells, D. A. 1858. *Principles and applications of chemistry.* New York: Ivison and Phinney.
Wolfrom, M. L. and Thompson, A. J. 1946. *J. Am. Chem. Soc.* 68:791.

Chapter 3

DIGESTION AND ABSORPTION
OF DIETARY CARBOHYDRATES

Sheldon Reiser

Nutrition Institute

U.S. Department of Agriculture

Beltsville, Maryland

INTRODUCTION

The fundamental roles of the small intestine in carbohydrate nutrition are the digestion and absorption of the various components of the carbohydrate diet. The current dietary intake of carbohydrate in the United States is estimated at about 380 g/day or approximately 46% of the total caloric intake (Page and Friend, 1974). Carbohydrates in foods such as cereals, grain products, and vegetables are classed as starches; carbohydrates in milk, fruits, and confections are classed as sugars. The sugar portion of the carbohydrate component is comprised primarily of sucrose (126 g/day), but also contains lactose (25 g/day), glucose (16 g/day), maltose (7 g/day), and fructose (6 g/day). The fundamental unit of carbohydrate absorption is generally believed to be the monosaccharide unit. Therefore, one of the primary functions of the small intestine is hydrolysis of the carbohydrate components of the meal that are not absorbable as such to their constituent monosaccharide units. The digestive function is carried out by a pancreatic enzyme secreted into the duodenum (α-amylase) and by the hydrolytic enzymes associated with the brush border membrane of the intestinal epithelial cell (glucoamylase, maltase, isomaltase, sucrase, and lactase). As a result of the action of these enzymes the monosaccharides (primarily glucose, galactose, and fructose) are liberated from the dietary poly- and disaccharides. The absorption of the monosaccharides occurs by at least two different transport pathways. Glucose and galactose are believed to be actively transported by the same pathway. Although a Na^+-gradient from the extracellular to the intracellular environment is believed to energize glucose transport, the exact molecular mechanism describing the entire process remains unknown. Fructose appears to be transported by a pathway exhibiting a different structural specificity than that mediating glucose and galactose transport. There is also some evidence to support a sugar transport system specific for disaccharides such as sucrose.

A portion of the carbohydrate diet is resistant to digestion by the enzymes found in the human gastrointestinal tract. This carbohydrate component has been defined as fiber and is present in the American diet in amounts ranging from 4 to 11 g/day as crude fiber (Friend and Marston, 1974; Hardinge et al., 1958). Fiber has been shown to be comprised of a group of compounds with distinct physical, chemical, and metabolic properties. It has been suggested that fiber plays an important role in the maintenance of the health of man through an action at the intestinal level.

In recent years it has become apparent that intestinal digestion and absorption may be influenced by many diverse factors. It has been shown that digestive enzymes and transport systems can adapt to the presence of specific dietary carbohydrates. The intestine has also been shown to respond to semistarvation, different patterns of food intake, and experimental diabetes with changes in digestive and absorptive parameters. The role of dietary glucose, compared with intravenously administered glucose, as a secretagogue of insulin has emphasized the important role of the intestine as an endocrine tissue. Intestinal digestion and absorption, therefore, appear to be of great importance in both initiating metabolic and physiological response to the ingestion of carbohydrate and in responding to the metabolic and physiological requirements for sugars originating in other tissues of the body.

DIGESTION OF DIETARY CARBOHYDRATE

Polysaccharides

The major dietary polysaccharide ingested by man is starch. Starch is a high molecular weight polymer composed of D-glucose units and is the principal reserve carbohydrate in plants. Most starches consist of a mixture of two types of polymers, amylose and amylopectin. Amylose is a linear polymer of glucose joined by α-1,4 linkages to yield chains that can attain molecular weights of several million (Geddes, 1969). Amylopectin has been shown to be a branched molecule with branching occurring every 24–30 glucose residues via α-1,6 glucose linkages. Some α-1,3 linkages have been reported in amylopectin (Wolfrom and Thompson, 1955). The ratio of amylose to amylopectin varies in different starches but is usually in the range of one amylose to three amylopectins (Pazur, 1965). Glycogen, an amylopectin-type storage carbohydrate found in the liver and muscle of animals, may also contribute somewhat to the total intake of digestible polysaccharide.

The process of starch digestion is facilitated by cooking food, a process that ruptures the starch granules and facilitates subsequent enzyme hydrolysis. The initial step in the digestion of dietary polysaccharides occurs in the mouth.

Saliva contains an α-amylase that splits α-1,4 glucosidic bonds in an apparently random fashion. Despite the presence of α-amylase in the saliva, it is doubtful that significant polysaccharide digestion occurs during chewing because of the short duration of contact between enzyme and substrate. The low pH of the stomach inactivates salivary amylase, thus terminating enzymic polysaccharide digestion. The low pH of the stomach does not appear to contribute significantly to acidic polysaccharide digestion (Gray, 1971). The major digestion of dietary polysaccharide occurs in the small intestine by the action of pancreatic α-amylase secreted into the duodenum. Pancreatic amylase initially splits the interior α-1,4 glucose linkages of starch and glycogen producing oligosaccharides. The final products of the action of α-amylase on amylose are maltose and maltotriose (Fisher and Stein, 1960; Roberts and Whelan, 1960). Since α-amylase is unable to hydrolyze the α-1,6 branching points and α-1,4 linkages adjacent to the branching points (Roberts and Whelan, 1960), the end products of amylopectin and glycogen hydrolysis by α-amylase also include low-molecular-weight branched oligosaccharides (Gardner et al., 1970; Gray, 1971). Pancreatic amylase can be adsorbed to the outer surface of the intestinal brush border membrane (Ugolev, 1965, 1972). The digestion of starch by membrane-bound α-amylase appears to be more efficient than the digestion of starch by intraluminal α-amylase (Jesuitova et al., 1964). The presence of small quantities of glucose among the products of starch digestion probably results from the action of a brush border-bound glucoamylase that liberates glucose directly from starch (Dahlqvist and Thomson, 1963a).

Oligosaccharides and Disaccharides

The final digestion of the oligosaccharides and disaccharides formed from the action of α-amylase on polysaccharides, as well as such dietary disaccharides as sucrose and lactose, is mediated by enzymes found in the brush border membrane of the intestinal epithelial cell. Specifically, the disaccharidases have been shown to be present in mushroom-shaped particles, 50–60 Å in diameter, located at the external surface of the brush border membrane (Johnson, 1969; Oda and Seki, 1965). Figure 1 shows an electron micrograph of these particles as they appear on negatively stained brush border preparations isolated from hamster intestine. The location of the hydrolytic enzyme in the brush border appears to be external to the site of monosaccharide transport, suggesting a functional organization of the digestive and absorptive processes in the epithelial cell membrane (Crane, 1967).

The disaccharidase activities of the intestinal brush border can be separated into at least five different α-glycosidases and one distinct β-glycosidase (Borgström and Dahlqvist, 1958; Dahlqvist, 1959, 1960). The α-glycosidases include at least three maltases with overlapping specificities for the products of the α-amylolytic digestion of starch and glycogen (Auricchio et al., 1972; Kolínská and Kraml, 1972). Two of the maltases are associated with sucrase and isomaltase activities (Cummins et al., 1968; Kolínská and Semenza, 1967); the

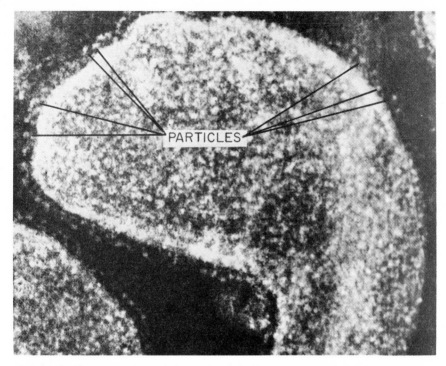

FIGURE 1 The intact, isolated brush border microvillus. The particles are visible as projections along the edge or as globules when visible head on. Negatively stained with 2% potassium phosphotungstate. Magnification is approximately × 96,000. Reprinted from *Fed. Proc.* 28:26–29, 1969 (Johnson, 1969).

third is associated with glucoamylase (Dahlqvist and Thomson, 1963a; Eggermont, 1969). The α-glycosidases catalyze the digestion of sugars such as low-molecular-weight oligosaccharides (limit dextrins), maltotriose, isomaltose, maltose, and sucrose into the component monosaccharides, which are the functional units of carbohydrate absorption. The β-glycosidase or lactase activity of the brush border catalyzes the digestion of lactose into glucose and galactose.

ABSORPTION OF DIETARY SUGARS

Glucose and Galactose

In spite of many studies the exact mechanism governing the intestinal transport of glucose and galactose remains relatively obscure. However, these studies have described many of the properties of the glucose transport pathway and have permitted several working hypotheses for this process to evolve.

Figure 2 describes the steps involved in the equilibrating translocation of glucose and galactose across the intestinal brush border. Transport of these sugars is believed to be mediated by a structurally specific binding site or carrier

(LeFevre, 1961; Wilbrandt and Rosenberg, 1961) located in the brush border of the intestinal epithelial cell. According to the concept of a mobile carrier (Crane, 1965; Alvarado, 1967), the first step is the binding of the monosaccharide to the carrier at the luminal side of the membrane. This step is not absolutely specific for glucose and galactose since many derivatives of these sugars, as well as other aldoses, appear to exhibit some affinity for the carrier. The formation of the sugar-carrier complex is analogous to the formation of a substrate-enzyme complex. A transformation or rearrangement of the sugar-carrier complex during or subsequent to binding has been suggested to explain the observation that certain sugars are bound to the carrier but not transported (Caspary et al.,

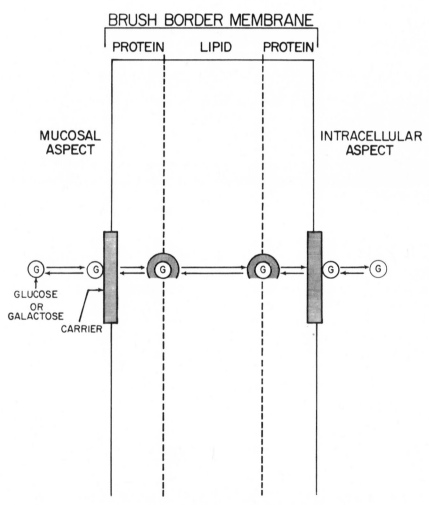

FIGURE 2 Representation of the steps mediating the equilibrating translocation of glucose across the intestinal brush border.

1969). The purpose of the transformation may be to mask the hydrophilic functions of the sugar and thus permit the water-soluble molecule to traverse the lipid-rich membrane in an energetically feasible manner (Csáky, 1963a). The sugar–carrier complex then translocates across the lipid portion of the membrane. Finally, the sugar–carrier complex dissociates at the intracellular aspect of the membrane to regenerate free carrier and liberate sugar into the intracellular fluid. This process is assumed to be freely reversible and is of itself capable only of equilibrating sugar across the membrane (i.e., facilitated diffusion). The mechanisms by which the energy necessary for the active transport of these sugars may be coupled to carrier-mediated transport will be described below.

Although no molecular entity with the properties ascribed to the carrier has as yet been isolated from the intestinal mucosa, the presence of such a mediating site is necessary to explain many of the properties of glucose and galactose transport. Glucose and galactose are too large to pass through the 4.0 Å pores that have been postulated to be present in membranes (Lindeman and Solomon, 1962), yet these sugars can penetrate across the cell membrane faster than can be attributed to simple diffusion. Moreover, at lower concentrations the rate of penetration is more rapid than at higher concentrations. The transport of glucose (Malathi et al., 1973) and galactose (Kimmich, 1970a) exhibits saturation kinetics described by apparent affinity constants and maximal capacities (Bihler, 1969; Crane et al., 1965; Goldner et al., 1969b; Schultz and Curran, 1970). Competitive inhibition is exhibited among glucose, galactose and other sugars sharing this transport pathway. These properties are consistent with the presence of structurally specific, saturable, rate-limiting steps in the intestinal transport of sugars as is postulated by a carrier-mediated process. In addition, sugars sharing the glucose transport pathway exhibit countertransport (substrate-induced counterflow) (Alvarado, 1965), a phenomenon predictable on the basis of transport mediated by a mobile carrier (Wilbrandt and Rosenberg, 1961).

A list of sugars that have been reported to be actively transported by the small intestine is given in Table 1. Most of these sugars are not of nutritional importance and represent derivatives of glucose and galactose. These sugars have, however, been useful in establishing the structural requirements necessary for active transport. Since these derivatives are not metabolized by the small intestine, their use in transport studies permits definitive distinctions between active transport and gradients established by metabolic utilization of the sugar. The concept of a minimal structural requirement for a sugar to be actively transported by the small intestine (Fig. 3) was proposed on the basis of earlier observations (Crane, 1960). Given that L-glucose (Caspary and Crane, 1968), D-fructose (Gracey et al., 1972; Macrae and Neudoerffer, 1972), D-mannose (Csáky and Ho, 1966; Bihler, 1969), D-xylose (Alvarado, 1966a; Csáky and Lassen, 1964), 5-thio-D-glucose (Critchley et al., 1970), and phenylglycosides (Alvarado and Crane, 1964) are actively transported, these structural requirements do not appear to be obligatory.

TABLE 1 Some Sugars and Sugar Derivatives Reported To Be Actively Transported by the Small Intestine

Sugar or derivative	Reference
D-Glucose	Fisher and Parsons, 1950
L-Glucose	Caspary and Crane, 1968
D-Galactose	Fisher and Parsons, 1953
D-Fructose	Gracey et al., 1972; Macrae and Neudoerffer, 1972
D-Mannose	Csáky and Ho, 1966; Bihler, 1969
D-Xylose	Csáky and Lassen, 1964; Alvarado, 1966a
D-Allose	Wilson and Crane, 1958
D-Glucoheptulose	Wilson and Crane, 1958
α-Methyl-D-glucoside	Wilson and Landau, 1960
1-Deoxy-D-glucose	Jorgensen et al., 1961
1,5-Anhydro-D-glucitol	Crane and Krane, 1956
2-C-Hydroxymethyl-D-glucose	Crane and Krane, 1959
3-O-Methyl-D-glucose	Campbell and Davson, 1948
3-Deoxy-D-glucose	Wilson and Landau, 1960
4-O-Methyl-D-galactose	Wilson and Landau, 1960
5-Thio-D-glucose	Critchley et al., 1970
6-Deoxy-D-glucose	Crane and Krane, 1956
6-Deoxy-D-galactose	Wilson and Crane, 1958
6-Deoxy-6-fluoro-D-glucose	Wilson and Landau, 1960
7-Deoxy-D-glucoheptulose	Wilson and Crane, 1958
Phenylglycosides	Alvarado and Crane, 1964

If it is assumed that a single carrier mediates the transport of all the actively transported sugars, it can be concluded that this carrier exhibits a very broad structural specificity. Recent findings, however, indicate that active sugar transport is mediated by more than one carrier. The major criteria used to determine whether a sugar is transported by the glucose pathway have been a

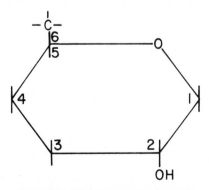

FIGURE 3 Minimal structural requirement for active intestinal transport (Crane, 1960).

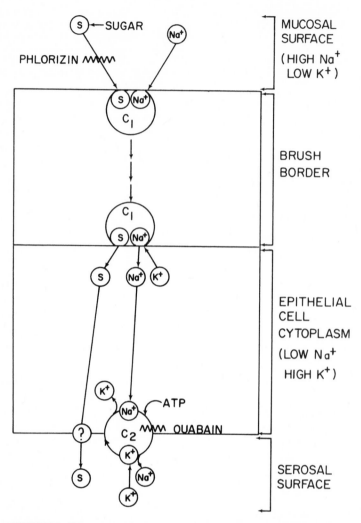

FIGURE 4 Schematic representation for active sugar transport across the intestinal epithelial cell as visualized by the Na⁺-gradient hypothesis.

mutual inhibition between glucose and the sugar in question and the ability of low concentrations of phlorizin added at the mucosal surface to competitively inhibit sugar transport (Alvarado and Crane, 1962; Newey et al., 1959), presumably by binding to the glucose carrier (Alvarado and Crane, 1964). On the basis of these criteria, fructose transport is mediated by a carrier system different from that utilized by glucose (see Fig. 4). Since 2-deoxy-D-glucose is not actively transported by the small intestine (Crane, 1960; Goldner et al., 1969a), the presence of a free hydroxy function at position C-2 may be a requirement for active transport by the carrier system mediating active glucose transport. A transport mechanism involving the formation of a covalent bond between the oxygen of this hydroxy group of glucose and the carrier has been ruled out (Swaminathan and Eichholz, 1973). It has been generally accepted that the other sugars and sugar derivatives listed in Table 1 are transported by a common glucose transport system. It now appears that there may be multiple carriers for the intestinal transport of such sugars as glucose, galactose, α-methyl-D-glucoside, 3-O-methyl-D-glucose, and 6-deoxy-D-glucose (Debnam and Levin, 1971; Honegger and Gershon, 1974; Honegger and Semenza, 1973; Levin and Syme, 1971; Newey et al., 1966).

The location of the carrier-mediated sugar transport in the brush border membrane of the epithelial cell has been substantiated by a number of observations. Following incubation of intact hamster small intestine, the concentration of sugar was found to be higher in the epithelial cell than in more underlying regions of the intestine (McDougal et al., 1960). Subsequently, the active accumulation of sugars by intestinal epithelial cells isolated from rabbit (Huang, 1965), rat (Stern, 1966), and chicken (Kimmich, 1970a) has been demonstrated. Autoradiographic studies have shown that the epithelial cell brush border is the site at which a concentration gradient of sugar is created during transport (Kinter and Wilson, 1965; Sterling and Kinter, 1967). More recently, it has been demonstrated that the properties binding glucose by isolated intestinal brush borders are very similar to those transporting glucose by intact intestine (Faust et al., 1968; Hopfer et al., 1973; Murer and Hopfer, 1974; Murer et al., 1974; Olsen and Rogers, 1971a).

Central to the mechanism by which energy transduction processes may be associated to carrier mediation to produce active sugar transport in the intestine is the role of Na^+. Na^+ has been shown to be required for the active transport of sugars by the small intestine (Clarkson and Rothstein, 1960; Csáky and Thale, 1960; Csáky and Zollicoffer, 1960; Riklis and Quastel, 1958). A relationship between the entry of sugar and Na^+ into the mucosal cell was shown in studies in which glucose produced an increase in the mucosal to serosal flux of Na^+ in rabbit (Curran, 1960) and rat (Clarkson et al., 1961) intestine. The increase in Na^+ transport could not be attributed to enhanced metabolism due to glucose since 3-O-methyl-D-glucose and galactose also increased Na^+ transport (Barry et al., 1962; Schacter and Britten, 1961). These results show that intestinal transport rather than metabolism is the major determinant in the acceleration of Na^+ transport by sugars. Cardiac glycosides such as ouabain have been shown to inhibit the active transport of sugars (Csáky, 1963b; Csáky and Hara, 1965; Csáky et al., 1961; Newey et al., 1968; Schultz et al., 1966). The ouabain inhibition is attributed to an inhibition of the $(Na^+ + K^+)$-dependent ATPase implicated in ion transport (Skou, 1965) and the subsequent decrease in the extrusion of Na^+ from the intracellular fluid (Glynn, 1964). The finding that ouabain inhibits specifically when present at the serosal rather than the mucosal aspect of the intestine (Csáky and Hara, 1965; Schultz and Zalusky, 1964a, b) places the Na^+ pump at a position in the epithelial cell apart from that of the sugar carrier located in the brush border. A role of Na^+ at the carrier level and in addition to its function in coupling metabolic energy to sugar transport is indicated by the finding that Na^+ facilitates sugar entry into the intestine under conditions where energy metabolism is inhibited (Bihler and Crane, 1962; Bihler et al., 1962). K^+ appears to exert a diphasic effect on Na^+-dependent sugar transport. In the absence of K^+ sugar transport is inhibited (Bihler and Crane, 1961; Riklis and Quastel, 1958). The K^+ requirement is probably related to the proper functioning of energy-yielding metabolic reactions such as the (Na^+ + K^+)-dependent ATPase. Optimal transport is usually observed at K^+ concentrations ranging from 4 to 15 mM (Schultz and Curran, 1970). Higher levels of K^+ have been shown to produce a greater inhibition of sugar transport than the same levels of other Na^+ replacements (Bihler and Adamic, 1967; Bosacková and Crane, 1965a, b). This inhibition is attributed to a competition by K^+ for the Na^+ binding site on the carrier (Bosacková and Crane, 1965a), resulting in a decreased affinity of the carrier for the sugar (Crane et al., 1965). These experimental observations provide the basis for the Na^+-gradient hypothesis for the active transport of sugars in the small intestine first proposed and subsequently elaborated by Crane (1962, 1965, 1968; Crane et al., 1961; see also Kimmich, 1973; Schultz and Curran, 1970). Figure 4 depicts a schematic representation of the active transport of sugars as visualized by the Na^+-gradient hypothesis. According to this hypothesis, a sugar–Na^+–carrier complex is formed at the brush border surface of the epithelial cell as a function of both the sugar and Na^+ concentrations. This carrier (C_1) confers structural specificity to sugar transport, and the formation of the sugar–carrier complex is competitively inhibited by phlorizin. Na^+ has been reported to increase the affinity of the sugar for the carrier (Bihler, 1969; Crane et al., 1965) or increase the maximum rate of sugar transport (Goldner et al., 1969b; Schultz and Zalusky, 1964b). The translocation of the ternary complex is favored by the lower Na^+ concentration present in the intracellular medium as compared with the mucosal medium (i.e., Na^+ gradient). At the intracellular aspect of the brush border membrane the low Na^+ concentration favors the dissociation of Na^+ from the complex. The resulting Na^+-free complex or sugar-K^+-carrier complex has a low affinity for the sugar, thus facilitating the dissociation of the sugar from the carrier and the accumulation of the sugar intracellularly. As the intracellular Na^+ concentration is increased, the energy-dependent, ouabain-sensitive Na^+ pump (C_2) located at or near the serosal aspect of the epithelial cell transports Na^+ out of the cell. The maintenance of the low intracellular Na^+ concentration by C_2 preserves the Na^+ gradient and prevents the equilibrating reverse transport of the accumulated sugar across the brush border membrane by C_1 from occurring. The mechanism by which the accumulated sugar leaves the cell at the serosal surface has not been studied in detail but is believed to be an energy-independent process (Crane, 1968), possibly Na^+-independent-facilitated diffusion (Bihler and Cybulsky, 1973; Naftalin and Curran, 1974). Consistent with this transport model is the finding that reversal of the Na^+ gradient (i.e., intracellular Na^+

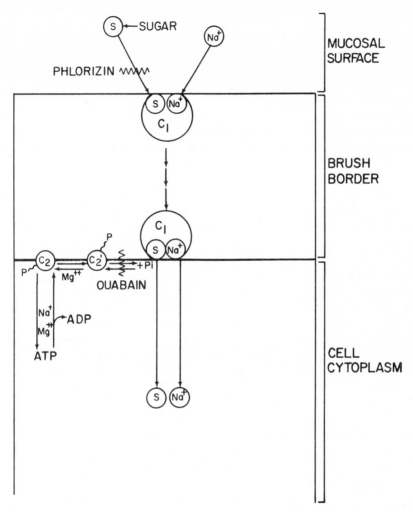

FIGURE 5 Schematic representation of active sugar transport based on direct input of metabolic energy.

greater than mucosal Na^+) results in the transport of sugars out of the cell against a concentration gradient (Crane, 1964; Goldner et al., 1972).

Although the Na^+-gradient hypothesis is generally accepted as explaining the coupling between Na^+ and sugar transport, other mechanisms have also been proposed to explain this interaction. Kimmich (1970b, 1973; Kimmich and Randles, 1973) has challenged the validity of the Na^+-gradient hypothesis after observing active galactose accumulation by isolated intestinal epithelial cells while the Na^+ gradient was reversed. An alternate mechansim has been suggested based on direct energy coupling between Na^+ and actively transported sugars (and amino acids) at the brush border membrane (Fig. 5). This mechanism proposes that a $(Na^+ + K^+)$-dependent ATPase reported to be present in intestinal brush border preparations (Quigley and Gotterer, 1969, 1972; Taylor, 1962) forms an energized intermediate $(C_2' \sim P)$ (Fahn et al., 1966; Sen et al., 1969). The energized intermediate is generated by reactions that require intracellular Na^+, Mg^{2+}, and ATP (Fujita et al., 1971; Sen et al., 1969) and is inhibited by ouabain (Post et al., 1969; Skou, 1965). Since the site of Na^+ action on the ATPase has been shown to be at the inner surface of the membrane (Garrahan and Glynn, 1967; Glynn, 1962; Whittam, 1962), intracellular Na^+ rather than extracellular Na^+ is suggested as being required for the energization of sugar transport. The energy associated with $C_2' \sim P$ is then utilized by the sugar–Na^+–carrier complex (C_1) to support the active transport of sugars. This mechanism does not reject an additional action of Na^+ at the mucosal aspect of the brush border to facilitate the equilibrating transport of sugar by C_1. Other reports suggest that the processes mediating active sugar transport are located at the serosal membrane of the epithelial cell (Esposito et al., 1973) and that glucose absorption is more likely to depend on the efflux of Na^+ from the epithelial cell to the tissue fluid than on either a Na^+ gradient at the brush border or on the concentration of intracellular Na^+ (Fisher and Gardner, 1974).

Interactions between sugar and amino acid transport. In recent years it has become apparent that a complex interaction exists between the intestinal transport of sugars and amino acids. Numerous studies have shown that sugars actively transported by the pathway specific for glucose can inhibit amino acid transport (Alvarado, 1966b; Alvarado et al., 1970; Bingham et al., 1966; Chez et al., 1966; Newey and Smyth, 1964; Read, 1967; Reiser and Christiansen, 1969, 1971; Saunders and Isselbacher, 1965). In general, the inhibition by galactose and the nonmetabolizable derivatives of glucose are more inhibitory than glucose. Conversely, amino acids have been shown to inhibit the active transport of sugars such as glucose, galactose, and xylose (Duthie and Hindmarsh, 1966; Hindmarsh et al., 1966). These interactions are not only of great potential nutritional and physiological significance but are also of interest at the mechanistic level since it is generally accepted that the carriers mediating the structurally specific binding of sugars and amino acids are different. The mechanisms by which the inhibitory interaction between Na^+-dependent sugar and amino acid transport occurs are still a subject of controversy. Possible explanations include competition for a common energy source (Kimmich, 1970b; Newey and Smyth, 1964), competition for a common polyfunctional carrier with resultant allosteric interactions (Alvarado, 1966b), and an accelerated efflux of amino acid from the epithelial cell across the mucosal border in the presence of sugars (Chez et al., 1966). In contrast to the inhibitory effect of other sugars, fructose appears to stimulate the intestinal transport of certain amino acids (Alvarado, 1968; Reiser and Christiansen, 1969, 1971; Reiser et al., 1975a). Since fructose has been reported to be actively transported in rat intestine by a Na^+-dependent process (Gracey et al., 1972) and poorly metabolized during transport (Mavrias and Mayer, 1973a), the activation by fructose is difficult to attribute to an increase in a rate-limiting energy supply. The nutritional and physiological significance of the fructose stimulation is also a subject for conjecture. Most of the fructose in the diet originates from sucrose, and it has been shown that sucrose digestion produces higher luminal levels of fructose than glucose (Miller and Crane, 1961a). Therefore, ingestion of sucrose may produce a localized luminal environment favoring the fructose stimulation rather than the glucose inhibition of amino acid transport.

Fructose

Fructose has now become a major dietary ingredient due to the use of large amounts of sucrose as a sweetener. Free fructose is also consumed in varying amounts in fruits and vegetables and especially in honey. The fructose content of fruits varies from 1 to 7%. Vegetables rarely exceed 3%, averaging about 1% of the fresh weight. The fructose content of honey has been estimated as 37% (Siddiqui, 1970). Dietary fructose is therefore introduced into the digestive tract primarily as sucrose but also as the free sugar. The absorption of fructose therefore depends to a large extent on the hydrolysis of the sucrose by sucrase. It appears that fructose liberated from sucrose and free fructose may not form a common pool in the intestinal lumen (Miller and Crane, 1961a). Fructose has been long known to be absorbed at rates intermediate between those of the actively transported sugars such as galactose and glucose and those sugars transported by passive diffusion (Cori, 1925). The greater rate of fructose absorption, compared with passively transported sugars, was formerly ascribed to the ability of the intestine to metabolize fructose to glucose. However, subsequent findings have shown that the conversion of fructose to glucose occurs only to a very limited extent in the small intestine of the rat (Ginsburg and Hers, 1960; Kiyasu and Chaikoff, 1957; Mavrias and Mayer, 1973a), chicken (Leveille et al., 1970), and man (Cook, 1969, 1971; Holdsworth and Dawson, 1965). It now appears that fructose transport in mammalian intestine is mediated by a relatively specific carrier mechanism with properties distinct from that of the carrier utilized by other monosaccharides (Table 2). In general, fructose transport has been found to be a Na^+-independent process that is not inhibited by phlorizin or glucose and is only slightly inhibited by the structurally similar ketose L-sorbose. By the criteria of transport against a concentration gradient and a dependence of transport on energy metabolism, there is evidence that fructose transport is an active process (Gracey et al., 1972; Macrae and Neudoerffer, 1972). There appear to be marked differences in the metabolism of fructose in the small intestine of various species. In the rat and man, fructose is minimally metabolized; in the guinea pig, fructose is mainly converted to glucose (Ginsburg and Hers, 1960; Kiyasu and Chaikoff, 1957; Mavrias and Mayer, 1973b). The hypertriglyceridemia observed after feeding fructose to man (Macdonald, 1967) and the rat (Nikkila and Ojala, 1965) but not the guinea pig (Bar-On and Stein, 1968) may be the consequence of these differences in

TABLE 2 Properties of Fructose Absorption in Mammalian Intestine

Mammal	D-Glucose	L-Sorbose	Phlorizin	Na⁺-dependent	Dinitrophenol	Reference
Rabbit	No inhibition	14% inhibition	No inhibition	No	—	Schultz and Strecker, 1970
Rat	No inhibition	No inhibition	No inhibition	No	—	Guy and Deren, 1971
Rabbit	—	No inhibition	No inhibition	—	—	
Rat	24% inhibition	31% inhibition	13–51% inhibition	Yes	33–47% inhibition	Gracey et al., 1972
Rat	32% inhibition	10% inhibition	No inhibition	Possibly	60% inhibition	Macrae and Neudoerffer, 1972
Hamster	No inhibition	No inhibition	No inhibition	No	—	Honegger and Semenza, 1973
Rat	No inhibition	No inhibition	No inhibition	No	—	Sigrist-Nelson and Hopfer, 1974

intestinal fructose metabolism and the resultant differences in the amount of free fructose appearing in the portal blood.

Disaccharides

Under normal conditions, disaccharides appear to be hydrolyzed during their transport into the intestinal epithelial cell. Thus 3 hr after the ingestion of 20 g sucrose or lactose by normal subjects, not more than 10 mg sucrose or 20 mg lactose was excreted in the urine (Fischer et al., 1965). It is now well accepted that dietary disaccharides are hydrolyzed by the disaccharidases bound to the external surface of the brush border membrane (Crane, 1969; Johnson, 1967; Miller and Crane, 1961a, b) rather than by intraluminal hydrolysis.

Typical of disaccharide transport is the finding of very low levels of luminal or mucosal glucose in relation to the amount liberated by the action of the disaccharidase (Gray and Ingelfinger, 1966; Miller and Crane, 1961a; Wilson and Vincent, 1955). In these studies the mucosal concentrations of fructose arising from the action of sucrase were from two to four times higher than that of glucose. Neither dilution of the mucosal medium nor the presence of glucose oxidase in the mucosal medium appreciably reduced the concentration of intracellular glucose and fructose arising from sucrose (Miller and Crane, 1961a). These results indicate that fructose and especially glucose liberated by the action of sucrase and maltase do not equilibrate with the mucosal medium. The intracellular concentrations of glucose and fructose arising from sucrose are much higher than can be accounted for by their transport by the mono-saccharide pathways at the prevailing mucosal concentrations. Fructose has been shown to be translocated across rat intestine more rapidly from sucrose than from the monosaccharide (Chain et al., 1960). On the basis of these and other results (Newey et al., 1963; Parsons and Prichard, 1968) it appears that disaccharide digestion is very closely associated with the mechanisms mediating the transport of the liberated monosaccharides. The concept of "kinetic advantage" (Crane, 1967) has been used to describe the close structural association between disaccharides such as sucrose and the pathways mediating the transport of glucose and fructose. The basis of this "kinetic advantage" may be the presence of a disaccharidase-associated glucose transport pathway in addition to and different from the Na^+-dependent monosaccharide transport system (Malathi et al., 1973; Ramaswamy et al., 1974). The major evidence for the existence of this transport system is:

(1) In the presence of saturating concentrations of glucose, total glucose uptake was increased in hamster intestine beyond the theoretical V_{max} for free glucose uptake in the presence of sucrose, maltose, and isomaltose but not glucose 1-phosphate.

(2) The transport of glucose from sucrose is substantially Na^+-independent.

(3) In the absence of Na⁺, glucose released from sucrose, maltose, isomaltose, and trehalose does not mix with a pool of glucose but is directly transported.

The structural relationships suggested by these experimental findings are presented in Fig. 6. Glucose transport as the monosaccharide is mediated by the Na⁺-dependent carrier I, previously described in detail. The disaccharidase A contributes to glucose transport by this pathway only insofar as the glucose liberated from disaccharide hydrolysis returns to the mucosal medium. Carrier II mediates the Na⁺-independent transport of glucose derived from the hydrolysis of the disaccharide and is in very close structural association with the site of disaccharide hydrolysis. The exact relationship between the disaccharidase and carrier II is not known. However, several properties of sucrase have raised the possibility that the disaccharidase itself may act as a carrier (A = II?). A purified

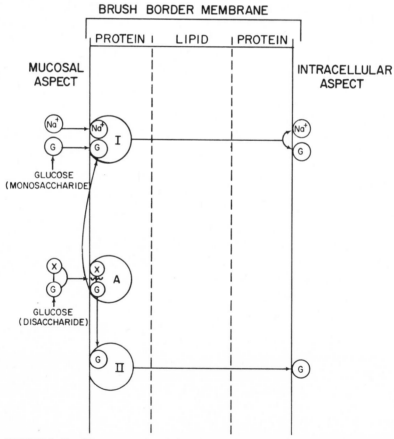

FIGURE 6 Possible structural and functional relationships between disaccharidases and glucose transport carriers.

sucrase–isomaltase complex incorporated into artificially reconstituted membranes that were essentially impermeable to sucrose, glucose, and fructose resulted in an increased permeability of sucrose (Storelli et al., 1972). The penetration by glucose and fructose derived from sucrose was greater than that for free glucose and fructose. The feeding of diets high in sucrose has been shown to produce an adaptive increase in the activity of intestinal sucrase (Blair et al., 1963; Deren et al., 1967; Reddy et al., 1968; Rosensweig and Herman, 1968). Sucrose feeding has also been shown to increase the intestinal transport of glucose, fructose, and sucrose (Reiser et al., 1975b), further suggesting a relationship between the activity of sucrase and sugar transport. From these findings it would be expected that the capacity for monosaccharide transport would be greater from a combination of dietary mono- and disaccharides than from an equivalent amount of these sugars as the monosaccharide alone. However, the physiologic significance of disaccharide transport in increasing the rate or capacity for monosaccharide transport is unresolved. An increase in the rate of glucose absorption from maltose as compared with an equivalent glucose solution has been reported in man (Cook, 1973). There also appear to be indications that monosaccharides reach higher levels in the blood after feeding the disaccharide than after feeding an equivalent amount of the component monosaccharides (Macdonald and Turner, 1968; Naismith and Rana, 1974). The concentration of fructose and, to a lesser extent, glucose in the portal blood of baboons was increased after adaptation to sucrose feeding (Crossley and Macdonald, 1970). The increased activity of hepatic lipogenic enzyme activity noted after feeding dietary disaccharides as compared with equivalent amounts of their component monosaccharides to rats (Michaelis and Szepesi, 1973, 1974; Naismith and Rana, 1974) is also consistent with a physiologically important disaccharide transport pathway. However, in the majority of studies on the rates of glucose or fructose transport from the disaccharides, compared with the component monosaccharides, no significant difference was observed in either man (Cook, 1970; Dencker et al., 1972; Gray and Ingelfinger, 1966; Gray and Santiago, 1966; Matthews et al., 1968; McMichael et al., 1967) or rats (Dahlqvist and Thomson, 1963b, c). The disaccharide transport system may not be present in all species since the process of disaccharide hydrolysis and transport of the component monosaccharides in amphibian intestine appear to be sequential and independent processes (Parsons and Prichard, 1971).

It has also been shown that not only is sucrase activated by Na^+ (Semenza et al., 1964) but that the kinetic properties of the Na^+ activation resemble the kinetic properties of the interaction of Na^+ with the glucose-transport carrier (Semenza, 1967, 1968a). Thus in hamster and rat, Na^+ increases the apparent affinity of sucrase for sucrose with no effect on the V_{max} of sucrose hydrolysis, while in rabbit and man Na^+ produces an increase in the V_{max} of sucrase with no change in K_m. The activation of monosaccharide transport by Na^+ in these species is the result of analogous changes in K_m and V_{max}. These findings cannot at present be explained on the basis that sucrase activity is a second property of the monosaccharide transport mechanism. Phlorizin, which inhibits monosaccharide transport, does not inhibit sucrase activity, and Tris, which inhibits sucrase activity, has no effect on monosaccharide transport. In addition, genetic defects that independently influence either sucrase activity or monosaccharide transport have been shown in man. These findings have raised the possibility that the sucrase and monosaccharide transport sites in the brush border are closely associated and share a common Na^+ site that can influence the kinetic behavior of hydrolysis and transport in a similar manner (Semenza, 1967, 1968a).

MALABSORPTION OF CARBOHYDRATES

Malabsorption syndromes caused by the inability to properly digest or absorb the components of the carbohydrate diet have now been recognized. These conditions are either due to a specific, congenital deficiency in a digestive enzyme or to an absorptive carrier or are the result of a generalized decrease in these components due to diseases that damage the small intestinal epithelium (e.g., celiac disease, tropical sprue, kwashiorkor). In all types of carbohydrate malabsorption, diarrhea is the main clinical symptom. The osmotic effect produced by the undigested disaccharide or unabsorbed monosaccharide attracts water into the intestinal lumen (Launiala, 1968). The bacterial metabolism of the nonabsorbed carbohydrate in the large intestine contributes to the diarrhea by further increasing the osmolarity of the intraluminal contents. In addition, the lactic acid formed lowers the intraluminal pH, thus impairing the absorption of water (Christopher and Bayless, 1969). The most prevalent form of carbohydrate malabsorption is the acquired primary lactase deficiency that develops after early childhood (Auricchio et al., 1963; Cook, 1967). It has been found that lactase deficiency is very high in many nonwhite ethnic groups including Asians, South and North American Indians, Africans, and Eskimos (Gray, 1971; Rosensweig, 1971). However, even in Caucasians the prevalence of lactase deficiency may reach 20% of the population (Gray, 1971). A similar incidence of lactase deficiency was observed in blacks whether living in Africa or the United States (Bayless and Rosensweig, 1968; Cook and Kajubi, 1966) and in Jews whether living in Israel or North America (Leichter, 1971). These results taken together with the inability to show adaptive increases in lactase activity after lactose feeding in humans (Keusch et al., 1969; Newcomer and McGill, 1967; Rosensweig and Herman, 1969a) suggest that lactase deficiency is due to genetic factors. In rats, however, it has been possible to produce an adaptive increase in lactase activity after lactose feeding (Bolin et al., 1969, 1971; Goldstein et al., 1971; Jones et al., 1972). Although lactose is not an essential component of the diet, lactase deficiency is a serious nutritional problem because it also prevents the proper utilization of the essential noncarbohydrate constituents found in dairy products (e.g., protein and calcium). The other forms of carbohydrate malabsorption due to congenital deficiencies in enzymes or carriers are very rare. A deficiency has been described in which both sucrase and isomaltase were shown to be absent (Anderson et al., 1963; Auricchio et al., 1962). Since these enzymes have been shown to exhibit distinctive catalytic activities but are closely associated in the brush border membrane (Semenza, 1968b), the genetic defect may involve the molecular organization of the enzymes in the membrane (Eggermont and Hers, 1969) or result from an alteration in a protein with more than one active site (Semenza, 1967). A congenital malabsorption of glucose and galactose has been described that appears to be due to the lack of the carrier mediating the transport of these sugars (Lindquist and Meeuwisse, 1963; Lindquist et al., 1962; Meeuwisse and Dahlqvist, 1968). The absorption of fructose and amino acids in these subjects is normal.

ADAPTIVE RESPONSES OF THE SMALL INTESTINE

It is now apparent that the small intestine of animals and humans can adapt to various nutritional and physiological stresses with changes in digestive, absorptive, and metabolic activities. Feeding diets containing the carbohydrate as sucrose or fructose, compared with glucose, increased the activities of sucrase and maltase but not lactase in human small intestine (Rosensweig and Herman, 1968). The increase in maltase activity due to sucrose or fructose feeding can be attributed to the maltolytic activity of intestinal sucrase (Auricchio et al., 1965; Dahlqvist et al., 1963; Kolínská and Kraml, 1972). The increase in sucrase activity occurred 2-5 days after subjects were changed from a glucose to a sucrose diet (Rosensweig and Herman, 1969b). Since this response time is similar to the estimated time for intestinal epithelial cell turnover (Bertalanffy and Nagy, 1961; MacDonald et al., 1964), it has been suggested that this dietary adaptation occurs at the crypt cell level (Rosensweig and Herman, 1969b). It is also possible that the synthesis or catabolism of disaccharidases may be modified in the mature villus cells (James et al., 1971). Increases in the activities of sucrase and maltase have also been observed in rat intestine as a function of the amount (Blair et al., 1963; Deren et al., 1967) and the nature (Reddy et al., 1968) of the dietary carbohydrate.

Intestinal transport processes also appear to respond to differences in the levels of specific nutrients in the diet. Increases in fructose transport that could not be attributed to fructose metabolism were observed in rats fed diets high in fructose (Crouzoulon-Bourcart et al., 1971; Mavrias and Mayer, 1973a). This adaptation occurred after only 3 days on diet (Mavrias and Mayer, 1973a). Rats accustomed to being fed diets high in sucrose showed increases in the intestinal transport of sucrose and its constituent monosaccharides as compared with rats fed a stock diet (Reiser et al., 1975b). Baboons adapted to diets high in sucrose also showed an increased transport capability for fructose and, to a lesser extent, glucose as measured by the increased appearance of these monosaccharides in the portal blood following a sucrose meal (Crossley and Macdonald, 1970). A significant increase in the absorption of 3-O-methyl glucose was observed in rats after a 48-hr intraduodenal perfusion of glucose or fructose, compared with an electrolyte solution (Roy and Dubois, 1972). This rapid increase in mono-saccharide transport appeared to occur independently of weight loss and caloric intake. Conversely, the transport of both glucose and galactose has been shown to be decreased by about 25% in rats fed carbohydrate-free diets (Ginsburg and Heggeness, 1968; Goldsmith et al., 1971). The processes governing amino acid transport also appear to respond to changes in the amount of protein or amino acids present in the diet. Thus, leucine (Scharrer, 1972) and histidine (Goldsmith et al., 1971) transport are both increased in rats fed diets high in protein as compared with diets low in protein. More specifically, methionine absorption was stimulated in rats fed high-methionine diets (Lis et al., 1972), and histidine absorption increased in rats fed a diet containing 5% histidine (Nakamura et al., 1972). The absorption of glucose and histidine in rat intestine was shown to follow circadian changes induced by the pattern of feeding, being highest at the time of feeding (Furuya and Yugari, 1974). These rhythmic changes were not induced by the presence of the dietary components in the gastrointestinal tract since the same rhythmic pattern of absorption continued for at least 24 hr after the animals had been starved. These results indicate that the enhanced absorption found in semistarved or starved rats (see below) should be carefully evaluated for the contribution of established dietary patterns.

Intestinal glycolytic enzymes have also been found to increase after feeding dietary sugars. Studies in rats (Shakespeare et al., 1969; Stifel et al., 1968a) and humans (Rosensweig et al., 1968a) have shown that fructose feeding produced the greatest increases in the activities of fructokinase and fructose phosphate aldolases; glucose feeding resulted in the greatest increase in hexokinase activity. Similarly, galactose feeding produced the greatest increase in the activities of galactose-metabolizing enzymes (Rosensweig et al., 1968b; Stifel et al., 1968b). These increases in enzymic activity occur very rapidly and are essentially complete after 1 day (Rosensweig et al., 1969a, b). It remains to be determined whether these increases in enzyme activity result from an adaptive increase in enzyme synthesis or, as in the case of hexokinase, are produced by intracellular shifts of enzyme type, secondary to increases in substrate concentration (Mayer et al., 1970; Weiser et al., 1971).

The capacity of the intestine to absorb nutrients appears to be influenced by the pattern of feeding and the caloric intake of the animal. Meal-fed rats (rats having access to food for a short, daily time period) showed an increased intestinal absorption of glucose and an increased weight of the small intestine as compared to rats fed *ad libitum* (Leveille and Chakrabarty, 1968; Tepperman and Tepperman, 1958). These intestinal changes may be important in permitting the meal-adapted animal to most efficiently cope with the dietary stress imposed by the introduction of large amounts of food in a short time period. Intermittent starvation, semistarvation, and caloric restriction have also been shown to increase the intestinal transport of glucose in rats and guinea pigs (Esposito et al., 1967; Hindmarsh et al., 1967; Kershaw et al., 1960; Kujalová and Fábry, 1960; Neame and Wiseman, 1959). The effect of a more prolonged food deprivation (e.g., a 3-day fast) on processes governing intestinal transport appears to be more complex. An increase in the affinity of the transport mechanism for glucose and galactose and a concurrent decrease in the maximum transfer capacity of these sugars has been reported in rats fasted for 72 hr (Debnam and Levin, 1971, 1973a,b). Hexose transport in the distal intestine, but not in the proximal intestine, has been shown to be stimulated in fasted rats (Newey et al., 1970; Sanford and Smyth, 1974). These results have been interpreted as indicating that fasting produces both an increase in hexose transport efficiency and a decrease in the energy supply required for hexose transport. In the jejunum where aerobic glycolysis predominates (Wilson and Wiseman, 1954) fasting decreases the energy supply (i.e., glucose) more than in the ileum where the oxidation of endogenous lipid predominates (Frizzell et al., 1974).

Animals with uncontrolled diabetes have been found to undergo adaptations in intestinal processes that may be necessary for their survival. Thus, to compensate for the loss of the equivalent of 60–80% of ingested carbohydrate as glucose in the urine (Younoszai and Schedl, 1972), the diabetic rat (Aulsebrook, 1965a; Axelrad et al., 1970; Crane, 1961; Flores and Schedl, 1968; Leese and Mansford, 1971; Olsen and Rosenberg, 1970; Schedl and Wilson, 1971) and rabbit (Fromm et al., 1969; Müller et al., 1967) have been found to show an increased absorption of hexoses. Comparable increases in glucose transport have been obtained in juvenile onset diabetes in humans (Vinnik et al., 1965). The increased rate of sugar transport by diabetic intestine does not depend on the metabolic fate of the sugar since nonmetabolized sugars (e.g., 6-deoxyglucose and 3-*O*-methyl glucose) are also transported more rapidly. The increase in hexose transport precedes the hyperphagia and intestinal hypertrophy (Jervis and Levin, 1966) found in diabetic animals. It appears that diabetes enhances transport by first rapidly increasing the activity per unit weight of intestine and then by increasing the total amount of intestine. The treatment of diabetic rats with insulin was found to reverse the increase in sugar transport (Olsen and Rosenberg, 1970). Thus, while insulin increases the rate of glucose transport in a variety of tissues, the intestine appears to be unique in that glucose transport is enhanced by a deficiency of insulin. Diabetes has also been found to increase the activities of intestinal disaccharidases in rats (Olsen and Rogers, 1971b; Younoszai and Schedl, 1972). It appears that the energy requirements of the diabetic intestine may be increased due to the increased active transport of sugars and amino acids (Lal and Schedl, 1974; Olsen and Rosenberg, 1970). It has been shown that the activities of various glycolytic enzymes and the rates of glucose utilization and lactate production are increased in the intestine of the diabetic rat (Anderson, 1974; Anderson and Zakim, 1970; Tyrrell and Anderson, 1971). These results are consistent with an increase in intestinal glycolysis that provides the energy required for the increased transport in the diabetic intestine.

While both fasting and diabetes have been shown to increase the intestinal transport of sugars, the metabolic responses of the intestine to these stresses appear to be different. The jejunum of the diabetic rat shows an increase in the rate of glycolysis, an increase in glycogen content (Anderson and Jones, 1974) but no increase in gluconeogenesis. In contrast, fasting decreases glycolytic rates and glycogen content and tends to increase gluconeogenesis in the intestine.

EFFECT OF HORMONES

The findings that the nature of the dietary components, circadian rhythms, semistarvation, starvation, and experimental diabetes modulate intestinal absorption suggest that hormonal interactions may affect this process. Hormones may act directly on the intestinal mucosal cells by affecting crypt mitosis, cell differentiation, and metabolic pathways. Changes in gastric emptying, intestinal motility, digestive secretions, appetite, and manner of eating represent some of the ways that hormones may indirectly influence absorption. It is, therefore, of interest to summarize the effects on carbohydrate absorption reported for some of the individual hormones (Table 3). Some of these conflicting results are probably due to differences in species, levels of hormone used, *in vivo* and *in vitro* effects, and transport parameters measured. For example, insulin reverses the increase in monosaccharide transport found in the diabetic intestine when injected into the whole animal (i.e., *in vivo*) but not

TABLE 3 Effect of Hormones on the Transport of Monosaccharides in Mammalian Intestine

Hormone	Type of study	Effect	Reference
Insulin	*In vivo*	None	Capps et al., 1966
		Increase	Manome and Kuriaki, 1961
		Increase	Mehnert et al., 1967
		Decrease	Beyreiss et al., 1964
		Decrease	Varró and Csernay, 1966
	In vitro	None	Dubois and Roy, 1969
		None (3-O-methyl glucose)	Love and Canavan, 1968
		Increase (glucose)	Love and Canavan, 1968
		Increase	Fromm et al., 1969
Glucagon	*In vivo*	Increase	Varró and Csernay, 1966
		Increase	Rudo and Rosenberg, 1973
	In vitro	None	Nagler et al., 1960
		None	Aulsebrook, 1965b
Growth hormone	*In vivo*	None	Fábry et al., 1959
		Decrease	Finkelstein and Schacter, 1962
Prostaglandins	*In vitro*	Decrease	Coupar and McColl, 1972
Adrenalin	*In vitro*	None	Halliday et al., 1962
		Increase	Aulsebrook, 1965b

when added to the fluid bathing the intestinal preparation (*in vitro*) (Flores and Schedl, 1968; Olsen and Rosenberg, 1970).

The mammalian small intestine has apparently evolved a receptor system that reacts to glucose ingested orally, but not given parenterally, by secreting an intestinal hormone or hormones that stimulate insulin secretion in the pancreas. The existence of an intestinal factor stimulating insulin secretion is supported by the findings that an oral glucose load elicits a significantly greater insulin secretory response than does the same amount of glucose given intravenously (Dupré, 1964; McIntyre et al., 1965) and that the insulin secretory response to oral glucose cannot be accounted for by the glycemic stimulus produced (Perley and Kipnis, 1967). The term *enteroinsular axis* has been used to describe the influence of intestinal hormones on the insulin-secreting activity of the pancreas (Unger and Eisentraut, 1969). It has been suggested that defects in the enteroinsular axis, such as an improper glucoreceptor mechanism, may contribute to the pathogenesis of diabetes (Kipnis, 1972; Unger and Eisentraut, 1969). Although gastrin, secretin, and several other well-characterized gastrointestinal hormones stimulate insulin secretion, these hormones cannot satisfactorily explain all of the features by which insulin release is stimulated by oral glucose. It appears more likely that the insulin-releasing enteric hormone(s) may be the recently isolated gastric inhibitory polypeptide (GIP) (Brown and Dryburgh, 1971; Cataland et al., 1974; Dupré et al., 1973) and/or insulin-releasing polypeptide (IRP) (Shabaan et al., 1974; Turner and Marks, 1972; Turner et al., 1973, 1974). Both GIP and IRP have been isolated from mammalian intestine free from contamination by secretin, cholecystokinin–pancreozymin, and enteroglucagon. These polypeptides enhance the release of insulin in response to intravenous glucose, improve glucose tolerance, and show increased secretion after oral administration of glucose. Since the purest preparation of IRP may be contaminated by GIP, the active component of these polypeptides may prove to be identical. It has been shown that dietary components can influence the ability of duodenal extracts to stimulate insulin secretion (Felber et al., 1974). These results suggest that an evaluation of the enteroinsular system under varying dietary conditions, particularly in carbohydrate sensitive models, may provide a basis for the abnormalities in carbohydrate metabolism provoked by nutritional stresses.

DIETARY FIBER

Dietary fiber has been defined as the structural components of plants present in the cell walls of the leaf, stem, root, and seed that, ingested as part of the diet, are resistant to digestion by the secretions of the human gastrointestinal tract (Trowell, 1972a). Most of the values for the fiber content of food are given as crude fiber or the portion resisting extraction with sulfuric acid, sodium hydroxide, water, alcohol, and ether (Kent-Jones and Amos, 1967). It is estimated that crude fiber values obtained by these extraction methods reflect only 16-20% of the nutritionally more relevant dietary fiber (Southgate, 1969). Chemically, fiber is classified as a carbohydrate since it is primarily comprised of cellulose, hemicelluloses (i.e., xylans, arabinans, galactans, mannans, glucans, glycuronans), and pectic substances. In addition, lignin, a polymer based on phenylpropane units, is also classified as a component of dietary fiber. Although present in the foods we consume, dietary fiber has long been neglected as an important factor in human nutrition since it is a negligible source of energy and no specific deficiency symptoms develop in its absence. Very recently, epidemiologic observations coupled to an increasing knowledge of the physiologic role of dietary fiber at the intestinal level has produced an hypothesis linking a variety of diseases prevalent in western civilization to a relative deficiency in dietary fiber (Burkitt et al., 1974; Trowell, 1972a). A discussion of the role of dietary fiber in human health appears pertinent in this section since fiber is a carbohydrate and, although not digested or absorbed, carries out its physiologic function at the intestinal level.

Many noninfective, degenerative diseases have become prevalent in western or affluent societies but are rare in less-developed countries. Table 4 lists a number of these diseases that are common in the United States but are rare in African populations living in a traditional manner. These diseases have a

TABLE 4   Noninfectious, Degenerative Diseases Prevalent
in the United States and Rare in African Populations
Living in a Traditional Manner

Disease	Reference
Ischemic heart disease	Cleave et al., 1969
	Seftel et al., 1970
	Schrire, 1971
	Trowell, 1972b
Diabetes	Wapnick et al., 1972
	Wicks and Jones, 1973
Obesity	Scotch, 1960
	Walker, 1964
	Cleave et al., 1969
Appendicitis	Burkitt, 1971a
	Walker et al., 1973
Diverticular disease	Trowell, 1960
	Painter and Burkitt, 1971
Hemorrhoids	Burkitt, 1972a
Cancer of colon and rectum	Burkitt, 1971b
	Walker, 1971
Hiatus hernia	Burkitt, 1972b
Varicose veins	Cleave et al., 1969
	Burkitt, 1972a
Gallstones	Heaton, 1972

comparable prevalence in white and black Americans, indicating that they are more dependent on environmental than on genetic factors. An environmental factor proposed to explain the prevalence of these diseases in western societies is the reduced level of dietary fiber consumed in comparison to that consumed in the underdeveloped areas of Africa (Burkitt et al., 1974; Cleave et al., 1969; Lubbe, 1971; Scala, 1974; Trowell, 1972b). It has been suggested that dietary fiber can influence the incidence of diverticular disease, appendicitis, and constipation by increasing the bulk of the food and decreasing the transit time required for the food to pass through the gut. These functions are accomplished by the water-absorbing properties of fiber, especially cellulose, and by formation of volatile fatty acids from unabsorbed cellulose and hemicellulose by bacteria in the colon (Cummings, 1973). Dietary fiber is believed to prevent the formation of venous disorders such as varicose veins, hemorrhoids, and venous thrombosis by decreasing the effort required to pass the food residue (Burkitt et al., 1974; Cleave, 1960). Fiber may protect against colonic cancer by altering the fecal bacterial flora resulting in a decreased degradation of bile salts to potential carcinogenic substances (Hill et al., 1971). In addition, any noxious substances formed would remain in contact with the bowel mucosa for shorter time periods in the presence of fiber. However, data for 37 countries indicate that cancer of the large intestine is correlated with dietary protein and fat and not with fiber (Drasar and Irving, 1973). There is evidence that dietary fiber increases the fecal excretion of bile salts in rats (Gustafsson and Norman, 1969; Portman and Murphy, 1958), monkeys (Portman, 1960), and humans (Antonis and Bersohn, 1962; Stanley et al., 1972), presumably by its ability to bind bile salts (Eastwood and Hamilton, 1968; Kritchevsky and Story, 1974; Morgan et al., 1974). Since the conversion to bile salts is a major metabolic pathway for body cholesterol, the protective role of dietary fiber in heart disease is attributed to the hypocholesteremia (deGroot et al., 1963; Mathur et al., 1968) that results from the inhibition of bile salt reabsorption. As the intake of dietary fiber is increased, the apparent availability of the other utilizable components of the diet is decreased (Southgate and Durnin, 1970). The decreased availability of components of the carbohydrate diet could prevent the steep increases in postprandial blood glucose and the associated strong stimulation of the insulin response associated with the ingestion of diets high in refined carbohydrates (Blazquez and Quijada, 1969; Cleave et al., 1969; Cohen et al., 1974; Reiser et al., 1975b; Szanto and Yudkin, 1969), thereby deterring the onset of diabetes. The removal of fiber from carbohydrate foods is also believed to lead to overconsumption and obesity (Cleave et al., 1969). Obesity is generally considered to be an important contributory factor in the causation of diabetes and heart disease. The interpretation of the epidemiologic studies linking dietary fiber to the various disease states is complicated by a variety of environmental factors including other dietary changes characteristic of western societies. However, the present evidence of a relationship between the intake of dietary fiber and the prevention of many serious diseases afflicting western societies represents an intriguing aspect of carbohydrate nutrition that warrants extensive study.

RESEARCH NEEDS

Continued studies are required to determine the exact mechanism by which sugars are actively transported by the intestinal epithelial cell. Isolation of membrane components or carriers that are responsible for the structurally specific binding of the sugars to the membrane is necessary to prove the validity of many of the hypotheses proposed to explain sugar transport. Analogous work on the isolation of the membrane components responsible for the digestion of sugars has been successful. Intestinal brush borders represent a good starting point for these studies since mediated sugar transport has been demonstrated in these membrane preparations. The elucidation of the organization of the digestive and absorptive components of the intestinal brush border and the functional interrelationships between these units is needed to explain differences in transport characteristics of sugars as disaccharide as compared with monosaccharide. An understanding of the fundamental processes of digestion and absorption would permit more definitive studies as to the mechanisms by which these intestinal functions adapt to various dietary and physiological stresses.

One of the most intriguing aspects of the changing pattern of carbohydrate consumption in urbanized cultures is the relationship between the increased intake of refined carbohydrates and the etiology of heart disease and diabetes. There appear to be two areas of carbohydrate nutrition that pertain primarily to intestinal events and that may provide a relationship between dietary carbohydrate and disease states. One involves the action of dietary fiber in lowering cholesterol levels and in apparently modulating the absorption of various dietary components. An understanding of the mechanism by which the individual components of dietary fiber affect the intestinal digestion and absorption of the diet, as well as the reabsorption of products secreted into the intestine, is required. The second area involves the action of dietary products, especially glucose, as secretagogues of an enteric hormone that stimulates the secretion of pancreatic insulin. A study of the effect of dietary carbohydrates on the secretion of the enteric hormone, particularly in carbohydrate-sensitive models, may provide an explanation for the abnormalities in insulin response and status found in a comparatively large segment of the population in urbanized cultures.

REFERENCES

Alvarado, F. 1965. *Biochim. Biophys. Acta* 109:478.
Alvarado, F. 1966a. *Biochim. Biophys. Acta* 112:292.
Alvarado, F. 1966b. *Science* 151:1010.
Alvarado, F. 1967. *Biochim. Biophys. Acta* 135:483.
Alvarado, F. 1968. *Nature* 219:276.

Alvarado, F., and Crane, R. K. 1962. *Biochim. Biophys. Acta* 56:170.
Alvarado, F., and Crane, R. K. 1964. *Biochim. Biophys. Acta* 93:116.
Alvarado, F., Torres-Pinedo, R., Mateu, L. and Robinson, J. W. L. 1970. *FEBS Lett.* 8:153.
Anderson, C. M., Messer, M., Townley, R. R. W. and Freeman, M. 1963. *Pediatrics* 31:1003.
Anderson, J. W. 1974. *Am. J. Physiol.* 226:226.
Anderson, J. W. and Jones, A. L. 1974. *Proc. Soc. Exp. Biol. Med.* 145:268.
Anderson, J. W. and Zakim, D. 1970. *Biochim. Biophys. Acta* 201:236.
Antonis, A., and Bersohn, I. 1962. *Am. J. Clin. Nutr.* 11:142.
Aulsebrook, K. A. 1965a. *Experientia* 21:346.
Aulsebrook, K. A. 1965b. *Biochem. Biophys. Res. Commun.* 18:165.
Auricchio, S., Dahlqvist, A., Murset, G. and Prader, A. 1962. *Lancet* 1:1303.
Auricchio, S., Rubino, A., Landolt, M., Semenza, G. and Prader, A. 1963. *Lancet* 2:324.
Auricchio, S., Semenza, G. and Rubino, A. 1965. *Biochim. Biophys. Acta* 96:498.
Auricchio, S., Ciccimarra, F., Moauro, L., Rey, F., Jos, J. and Rey, J. 1972. *Pediatr. Res.* 6:832.
Axelrad, A. D., Lawrence, A. L. and Hazelwood, R. L. 1970. *Am. J. Physiol.* 219:860.
Bar-On, H. and Stein, Y. 1968. *J. Nutr.* 94:95.
Barry, R. J. C., Matthews, J., Smyth, D. H. and Wright, E. M. 1962. *J. Physiol.* 161:17P.
Bayless, T. M. and Rosensweig, N. S. 1966. *J. Am. Med. Assoc.* 197:968.
Bertalanffy, F. D. and Nagy, K. P. 1961. *Acta Anat.* 45:362.
Beyreiss, K., Müller, F. and Strack, E. 1964. *Z. Ges. Exp. Med.* 138:277.
Bihler, I. 1969. *Biochim. Biophys. Acta* 183:169.
Bihler, I. and Adamic, S. 1967. *Biochim. Biophys. Acta* 135:466.
Bihler, I. and Crane, R. K. 1962. *Biochim. Biophys. Acta* 59:78.
Bihler, I. and Cybulsky, R. 1973. *Biochim. Biophys. Acta* 298:429.
Bihler, I., Hawkins, K. A. and Crane, R. K. 1962. *Biochim. Biophys. Acta* 59:94.
Bingham, J. K., Newey, H. and Smyth, D. H. 1966. *Biochim. Biophys. Acta* 120:314.
Blair, D. G., Yakimets, W. and Tuba, J. 1963. *Can. J. Biochem. Physiol.* 41:917.
Blazquez, E. and Quijada, C. L. 1969. *J. Endocrinol.* 44:107.
Bolin, T. D., Pirola, R. C. and Davis, A. E. 1969. *Gastroenterology* 57:406.
Bolin, T. D., McKern, A. and Davis, A. E. 1971. *Gastroenterology* 60:432.
Borgström, B. and Dahlqvist, A. 1958. *Acta Chem. Scand.* 12:1997.
Bosacková, J. and Crane, R. K. 1965a. *Biochim. Biophys. Acta* 102:423.
Bosacková, J. and Crane, R. K. 1965b. *Biochim. Biophys. Acta* 102:436.
Brown, J. C. and Dryburgh, J. R. 1971. *Can. J. Biochem.* 49:867.
Burkitt, D. P. 1971a. *Br. J. Surg.* 58:695.
Burkitt, D. P. 1971b. *Cancer* 28:3.
Burkitt, D. P. 1972a. *Br. Med. J.* 2:556.
Burkitt, D. P. 1972b. *The medical annual.* Bristol: Wright.
Burkitt, D. P., Walker, A. R. P. and Painter, N. S. 1974. *J. Am. Med. Assoc.* 229:1068.
Campbell, P. N. and Davson, H. 1948. *Biochem. J.* 43:426.
Capps, J. C., Shetlar, M. R. and Bradford, R. H. 1966. *Biochim. Biophys. Acta* 127:205.

Caspary, W. F. and Crane, R. K. 1968. *Biochim. Biophys. Acta* 163:395.
Caspary, W. F., Stevenson, N. R. and Crane, R. K. 1969. *Biochim. Biophys. Acta* 193:168.
Cataland, S., Crockett, S. E., Brown, J. C. and Mazzaferri, E. L. 1974. *J. Clin. Endocrinol. Metab.* 39:223.
Chain, E. B., Mansford, K. R. L. and Pocchiari, F. 1960. *J. Physiol.* 154:39.
Chez, R. A., Schultz, S. G. and Curran, P. F. 1966. *Science* 153:1012.
Christopher, N. L. and Bayless, J. M. 1969. *Gastroenterology* 56:1250.
Clarkson, T. W. and Rothstein, A. 1960. *Am. J. Physiol.* 199:898.
Clarkson, T. W., Cross, A. C. and Toole, S. R. 1961. *Am. J. Physiol.* 200:1233.
Cleave, T. L. 1960. *On the causation of varicose veins.* Bristol: Wright.
Cleave, T. L., Campbell, G. C. and Painter, N. S. 1969. *Diabetes, coronary thrombosis and the saccharine disease.* Bristol: Wright.
Cohen, A. M., Teitelbaum, A., Briller, S., Yanko, L., Rosenmann, E. and Shafrir, E. 1974. In *Sugars in nutrition,* ed. H. L. Sipple and K. W. McNutt, pp. 483–511. New York: Academic Press.
Cook, G. C. 1967. *Br. Med. J.* 1:527.
Cook, G. C. 1969. *Clin. Sci.* 37:675.
Cook, G. C. 1970. *Clin. Sci.* 38:687.
Cook, G. C. 1971. *Am. J. Clin Nutr.* 24:1302.
Cook, G. C. 1973. *Clin. Sci.* 44:425.
Cook, G. C. and Kajubi, S. K. 1966. *Lancet* 1:725.
Cori, C. F. 1925. *J. Biol. Chem.* 66:691.
Coupar, I. M. and McColl, I. 1972. *Pharm. Pharmacol.* 24:254.
Crane, R. K. 1960. *Physiol. Rev.* 40:789.
Crane, R. K. 1961. *Biochem. Biophys. Res. Commun.* 4:436.
Crane, R. K. 1962. *Fed. Proc.* 21:891.
Crane, R. K. 1964. *Biochem. Biophys. Res. Commun.* 17:481.
Crane, R. K. 1965. *Fed. Proc.* 24:1000.
Crane, R. K. 1967. In *Intracellular transport,* ed. K. B. Warren, vol. V, pp. 71–103. New York: Academic Press.
Crane, R. K. 1968. In *Alimentary canal,* vol. III, *Intestinal absorption,* ed. C. F. Code, pp. 1323–1351. Washington, D.C.: American Physiological Society.
Crane, R. K. 1969. *Am. J. Clin. Nutr.* 22:242.
Crane, R. K. and Krane, S. M. 1956. *Biochim. Biophys. Acta* 20:568.
Crane, R. K. and Krane, S. M. 1959. *Biochim. Biophys. Acta* 31:397.
Crane, R. K., Miller, D. and Bihler, I. 1961. In *Membrane transport and metabolism,* ed. A. Kleinzeller and A. Kotyk, pp. 439–449. New York: Academic Press.
Crane, R. K., Forstner, G. and Eichholz, A. 1965. *Biochim. Biophys. Acta* 109:467.
Critchley, D. R., Eichholz, A. and Crane, R. K. 1970. *Biochim. Biophys. Acta* 211:244.
Crossley, J. W. and Macdonald, I. 1970. *Nutr. Metab.* 12:171.
Crouzoulon-Bourcart, C., Crouzoulon, G. and Pèrés, G. 1971. *CR Soc. Bull.* 165:1071.
Csáky, T. Z. 1963a. *Fed. Proc.* 22:3.
Csáky, T. Z. 1963b. *Biochim. Biophys. Acta* 74:160.
Csáky, T. Z. and Hara, Y. 1965. *Am. J. Physiol.* 209:467.
Csáky, T. Z. and Ho, P. M. 1966. *Life Sci.* 5:1025.
Csáky, T. Z. and Lassen, U. V. 1964. *Biochim. Biophys. Acta* 82:215.
Csáky, T. Z. and Thale, M. 1960. *J. Physiol.* 151:59.

Csáky, T. Z. and Zollicoffer, L. 1960. *Am. J. Physiol.* 198:1056.
Csáky, T. Z., Hartog, H. G., III and Fernald, G. W. 1961. *Am. J. Physiol.* 200:459.
Cummings, J. H. 1973. *Gut* 14:69.
Cummins, D. L., Gitzelmann, R., Lindenmann, J. and Semenza, G. 1968. *Biochim. Biophys. Acta* 160:396.
Curran, P. F. 1960. *Am. J. Physiol.* 43:1137.
Dahlqvist, A. 1959. *Acta Chem. Scand.* 13:1817.
Dahlqvist, A. 1960. *Acta Chem. Scand.* 14:9.
Dahlqvist, A. and Thomson, D. L. 1963a. *Biochem. J.* 89:272.
Dahlqvist, A. and Thomson, D. L. 1963b. *Acta Physiol. Scand.* 59:111.
Dahlqvist, A. and Thomson, D. L. 1963c. *J. Physiol.* 167:193.
Dahlqvist, A., Auricchio, S., Semenza, G. and Prader, A. 1963. *J. Clin. Invest.* 42:556.
Debnam, E. S. and Levin, R. J. 1971. *J. Physiol.* 218:38P.
Debnam, E. S. and Levin, R. J. 1973a. *J. Physiol.* 235:81P.
Debnam, E. S. and Levin, R. J. 1973b. *J. Physiol.* 231:21P.
deGroot, A. P., Luyken, R. and Pikaar, N. A. 1963. *Lancet* 2:303.
Dencker, H., Johannesson, E., Meeuwisse, G., Norryd, C. and Tranberg, K-G. 1972. *Scand. J. Gastroenterol.* 7:707.
Deren, J. J., Broitman, S. A. and Zamcheck, N. 1967. *J. Clin. Invest.* 46:186.
Drasar, B. S. and Irving, D. 1973. *Br. J. Cancer* 27:167.
Dubois, R. S. and Roy, C. C. 1969. *Proc. Soc. Exp. Biol. Med.* 130:931.
Dupré, J. 1964. *Lancet* 2:672.
Dupré, J., Ross, S. A., Watson, D. and Brown, J. C. 1973. *J. Clin. Endocrinol. Metab.* 37:286.
Duthie, H. L. and Hindmarsh, J. T. 1966. *J. Physiol.* 187:195.
Eastwood, M. A. and Hamilton, D. 1968. *Biochim. Biophys. Acta* 152:165.
Eggermont, E. 1969. *Eur. J. Biochem.* 9:483.
Eggermont, E. and Hers, H. G. 1969. *Eur. J. Biochem.* 9:488.
Esposito, G., Faelli, A. and Caprano, V. 1967. *Arch. Int. Physiol. Biochem.* 75:601.
Esposito, G., Faelli, A. and Caprano, V. 1973. *Pflügers Arch.* 340:335.
Fábry, P., Kujalová, V. and Mosinger, B. 1959. *Endokrinologie* 38:152.
Fahn, S., Koval, G. J. and Albers, R. W. 1966. *J. Biol. Chem.* 241:1882.
Faust, R. G., Leadbetter, M. G. Plenge, R. K. and McCaslin, A. J. 1968. *J. Gen. Physiol.* 52:482.
Felber, J.-P., Zermatten, A. and Dick, J. 1974. *Lancet* 2:185.
Finkelstein, J. D. and Schacter, D. 1962. *Am. J. Physiol.* 203:873.
Fischer, R. A., Rosoff, B. M., Altshuler, J. H., Thayer, W. R. and Spiro, H. M. 1965. *Cancer* 18:278.
Fisher, E. H. and Stein, E. A. 1960. In *The enzymes*, ed. P. Boyer, H. Lardy, and K. M. Myrbäck, vol. 4, pp. 313–343. New York: Academic Press.
Fisher, R. B. and Gardner, M. L. G. 1974. *J. Physiol.* 241:235.
Fisher, R. B. and Parsons, D. S. 1950. *J. Physiol.* 110:281.
Fisher, R. B. and Parsons, D. S. 1953. *J. Physiol.* 119:224.
Flores, P. and Schedl, H. P. 1968. *Am. J. Physiol.* 214:725.
Friend, B. and Marston, R. 1974. *Natl. Food Situation* 150:26.
Frizzell, R. A., Markscheid-Kaspi, L. and Schultz, S. G. 1974. *Am. J. Physiol.* 226:1142.
Fromm, D., Field, M. and Silen, W. 1969. *Am. J. Physiol.* 217:53.
Fujita, M., Matsui, H., Nagaro, K. and Nagano, M. 1971. *Biochim. Biophys. Acta* 233:404.

Furuya, S. and Yugari, Y. 1974. *Biochim. Biophys. Acta* 343:558.

Gardner, J. D., Brown, M. S. and Laster, L. 1970. *New Engl. J. Med.* 283:1317.

Garrahan, P. J. and Glynn, I. M. 1967. *J. Physiol.* 192:217.

Geddes, R. 1969. *Q. Rev. Chem. Soc.* 23:57.

Ginsburg, J. M. and Heggeness, F. W. 1968. *J. Nutr.* 96:494.

Ginsburg, V. and Hers, H. G. 1960. *Biochim. Biophys. Acta* 38:427.

Glynn, I. M. 1962. *J. Physiol.* 160:18.

Glynn, I. M. 1964. *Pharmacol. Rev.* 16:381.

Goldner, A. M., Hajjar, J. J. and Curran, P. F. 1969a. *Biochim. Biophys. Acta* 173:572.

Goldner, A. M., Schultz, S. G. and Curran, P. F. 1969b. *J. Gen. Physiol.* 53:362.

Goldner, A. M., Hajjar, J. J. and Curran, P. F. 1972. *J. Membrane Biol.* 10:267.

Goldsmith, R. M., Munday, K. A. and Turner, M. R. 1971. *Proc. Nutr. Soc.* 30:80A.

Goldstein, R., Klein, T., Freier, S. F. and Menczel, J. 1971. *Am. J. Clin. Nutr.* 24:1224.

Gracey, M., Burke, V. and Oshin, A. 1972. *Biochim. Biophys. Acta* 266:397.

Gray, G. M. 1971. In *Annual review of medicine,* ed. A. C. Degraff, vol. 22, pp. 391–404. Palo Alto, Calif.: Annual Reviews, Inc.

Gray, G. M. and Ingelfinger, F. J. 1966. *J. Clin. Invest.* 45:388.

Gray, G. M. and Santiago, N. A. 1966. *Gastroenterology* 51:489.

Gustafsson, B. E. and Norman, A. 1969. *Br. J. Nutr.* 23:429.

Guy, M. J. and Deren, J. J. 1971. *Am. J. Physiol.* 221:1051.

Halliday, G. J., Howard, R. B. and Munro, A. F. 1962. *J. Physiol.* 164:28.

Hardinge, M. G., Chambers, A. C., Crooks, H. and Stare, F. J. 1958. *Am. J. Clin. Nutr.* 6:523.

Heaton, K. W. 1972. *Bile salts in health and disease,* p. 184. Edinburgh: Churchill Livingston.

Hill, M. J., Crowther, J. S., Drasar, B. S., Hawksworth, G., Aries, V. and Williams, R. E. O. 1971. *Lancet* 1:95.

Hindmarsh, J. T., Kilby, D. and Wiseman, G. 1966. *J. Physiol.* 186:166.

Hindmarsh, J. T., Kilby, D., Ross, B. and Wiseman, G. 1967. *J. Physiol.* 188:207.

Holdsworth, C. D. and Dawson, A. M. 1965. *Proc. Soc. Exp. Biol. Med.* 118:142.

Honegger, P. and Gershon, E. 1974. *Biochim. Biophys. Acta* 352:127.

Honegger, P. and Semenza, G. 1973. *Biochim. Biophys. Acta* 318:390.

Hopfer, U., Nelson, K., Perrotto, J. and Isselbacher, K. J. 1973. *J. Biol. Chem.* 248:25.

Huang, K. C. 1965. *Life Sci.* 4:1201.

James, W. P. T., Alpers, D. H., Gerber, J. E. and Isselbacher, K. J. 1971. *Biochim. Biophys. Acta* 230:194.

Jervis, E. L. and Levin, R. J. 1966. *Nature* 210:391.

Jesuitova, N. N., De Laey, P. and Ugolev, A. M. 1964. *Biochim. Biophys. Acta* 86:205.

Johnson, C. F. 1967. *Science* 155:1670.

Johnson, C. F. 1969. *Fed. Proc.* 28:26.

Jones, D. P., Sosa, F. R. and Skromak, E. 1972. *J. Lab. Clin. Med.* 79:19.

Jorgensen, C. R., Landau, B. R. and Wilson, T. H. 1961. *Am. J. Physiol.* 200:111.

Kent-Jones, D. W. and Amos, A. J. 1967. *Modern cereal chemistry.* London: Food Trade Press.
Kershaw, T. G., Neame, K. D. and Wiseman, G. 1960. *J. Physiol.* 152:182.
Keusch, G. T., Troncale, F. J., Thavaramara, B., Prinyanont, P., Anderson, R. P. and Bhamarapravathi, N. 1969. *Am. J. Clin. Nutr.* 22:638.
Kimmich, G. A. 1970a. *Biochemistry* 9:3659.
Kimmich, G. A. 1970b. *Biochemistry* 9:3669.
Kimmich, G. A. 1973. *Biochim. Biophys. Acta* 300:31.
Kimmich, G. A. and Randles, J. 1973. *J. Membrane Biol.* 12:47.
Kinter, W. B. and Wilson, T. H. 1965. *J. Cell Biol.* 25:19.
Kipnis, D. M. 1972. *Diabetes* 21(suppl. 2):606.
Kiyasu, J. T. and Chaikoff, I. L. 1957. *J. Biol. Chem.* 224:935.
Kolínská, J. and Kraml, J. 1972. *Biochim. Biophys. Acta* 284:235.
Kolínská, J. and Semenza, G. 1967. *Biochim. Biophys. Acta* 146:181.
Kritchevsky, D. and Story, J. A. 1974. *J. Nutr.* 104:458.
Kujalová, V. and Fábry, P. 1960. *Physiol. Bohemoslov.* 9:35.
Lal, D. and Schedl, H. 1974. *Am. J. Physiol.* 227:827.
Launiala, K. 1968. *Acta Paediatr. Scand.* 57:425.
Leese, H. J. and Mansford, K. R. L. 1971. *J. Physiol.* 212:819.
LeFevre, P. G. 1961. *Pharmacol. Rev.* 13:39.
Leichter, J. 1971. *Dig. Dis.* 16:1123.
Leveille, G. A. and Chakrabarty, K. 1968. *J. Nutr.* 96:69.
Leveille, G. A., Atkinbami, K. and Ikediobi, C. O. 1970. *Proc. Soc. Exp. Biol. Med.* 135:483.
Levin, R. J. and Syme, G. 1971. *J. Physiol.* 213:46P.
Lindeman, B. and Solomon, A. K. 1962. *J. Gen. Physiol.* 45:801.
Lindquist, B. and Meeuwisse, G. 1963. *Acta Paediatr. Scand.* 146(suppl. 1):110.
Lindquist, B., Meeuwisse, G. and Melin, K. 1962. *Lancet* 2:666.
Lis, M. T., Crampton, R. F. and Matthews, D. M. 1972. *Br. J. Nutr.* 27:159.
Love, A. H. G. and Canavan, D. A. 1968. *Lancet* 2:1325.
Lubbe, A. M. 1971. *S. Afr. Med. J.* 45:1289.
Macdonald, I. 1967. *Am. J. Clin. Nutr.* 20:185.
Macdonald, I. and Turner, J. L. 1968. *Lancet* 1:841.
MacDonald, W. C., Trier, J. S. and Everett, N. B. 1964. *Gastroenterology* 46:405.
Macrae, A. R. and Neudoerffer, T. S. 1972. *Biochim. Biophys. Acta* 288:137.
Malathi, P., Ramaswamy, K., Caspary, W. F. and Crane, R. K. 1973. *Biochim. Biophys. Acta* 307:613.
Manome, S. H. and Kuriaki, K. 1961. *Arch. Int. Pharmocodyn. Ther.* 130:187.
Mathur, K. S., Khan, M. A. and Sharma, R. D. 1968. *Br. Med. J.* 1:30.
Matthews, D. M., Craft, I. L. and Crampton, R. F. 1968. *Lancet* 2:49.
Mavrias, D. A. and Mayer, R. J. 1973a. *Biochim. Biophys. Acta* 291:531.
Mavrias, D. A. and Mayer, R. J. 1973b. *Biochim. Biophys. Acta* 291:538.
Mayer, R. J., Shakespeare, P. and Hübscher, G. 1970. *Biochem. J.* 116:43.
McDougal, D. B., Jr., Little, K. S. and Crane, R. K. 1960. *Biochim. Biophys. Acta* 45:483.
McIntyre, N., Holdsworth, C. D. and Turner, D. S. 1965. *J. Clin. Endocrinol.* 25:1317.
McMichael, H. B., Webb, J. and Dawson, A. M. 1967. *Clin. Sci.* 33:135.
Meeuwisse, G. and Dahlqvist, A. 1968. *Acta Paediatr. Scand.* 57:273.
Mehnert, H., Forster, H. and Haslbeck, G. 1967. *Diabetologia* 3:23.

Michaelis, O. E., IV and Szepesi, B. 1973. *J. Nutr.* 103:697.
Michaelis, O. E., IV and Szepesi, B. 1974. *J. Nutr.* 104:1597.
Miller, D. and Crane, R. K. 1961a. *Biochim. Biophys. Acta* 52:281.
Miller, D. and Crane, R. K. 1961b. *Biochim. Biophys. Acta* 52:293.
Morgan, B., Heald, M., Atkin, S. D., Green, J. and Chain, E. B. 1974. *Br. J. Nutr.* 32:447.
Müller, F., Beyreiss, K., Dettmer, D. and Hartenstein, H. 1967. *Acta Biol. Med. Ger.* 19:673.
Murer, H. and Hopfer, U. 1974. *Proc. Natl. Acad. Sci. U.S.A.* 71:484.
Murer, H., Hopfer, U., Kinne-Saffran, E. and Kinne, R. 1974. *Biochim. Biophys. Acta* 345:170.
Naftalin, R. and Curran, P. F. 1974. *J. Membrane Biol.* 16:257.
Nagler, R., Forrest, W. J. and Shapiro, H. N. 1960. *Am. J. Physiol.* 198:1323.
Naismith, P. J. and Rana, I. A. 1974. *Nutr. Metab.* 16:285.
Nakamura, Y., Yasumoto, K. and Mitsuda, H. 1972. *J. Nutr.* 102:359.
Neame, K. D. and Wiseman, G. 1959. *J. Physiol.* 146:10P.
Newcomer, A. D. and McGill, D. B. 1967. *Gastroenterology* 53:881.
Newey, H. and Smyth, D. H. 1964. *Nature* 202:400.
Newey, H., Parsons, B. J. and Smyth, D. H. 1959. *J. Physiol.* 148:83.
Newey, H., Sanford, P. A. and Smyth, D. H. 1963. *J. Physiol.* 168:423.
Newey, H., Sanford, P. A. and Smyth, D. H. 1966. *J. Physiol.* 186:493.
Newey, H., Sanford, P. A. and Smyth, D. H. 1968. *J. Physiol.* 194:237.
Newey, H., Sanford, P. A. and Smyth, D. H. 1970. *J. Physiol.* 208:705.
Nikkila, E. A. and Ojala, K. 1965. *Life Sci.* 4:937.
Oda, T. and Seki, S. 1965. *J. Electronmicrosc.* 14:210.
Olsen, W. A. and Rogers, L. 1971a. *Comp. Biochem. Physiol.* 39B:617.
Olsen, W. A. and Rogers, L. 1971b. *J. Lab. Clin. Med.* 77:838.
Olsen, W. A. and Rosenberg, T. H. 1970. *J. Clin. Invest.* 49:96.
Page, L. and Friend, B. 1974. In *Sugars in nutrition,* ed. H. Sipple and K. McNutt, chap. 7, pp. 93–107. New York: Academic Press.
Painter, N. S. and Burkitt, D. P. 1971. *Br. Med. J.* 2:450.
Parsons, D. S. and Prichard, J. S. 1968. *J. Physiol.* 199:137.
Parsons, D. S. and Prichard, J. S. 1971. *J. Physiol.* 212:299.
Pazur, J. H. 1965. In *Starch: Chemistry and technology, fundamental aspects,* ed. R. L. Wistler and E. F. Paschall, vol. 1, pp. 133–175. New York: Academic Press.
Perley, M. and Kipnis, D. M. 1967. *J. Clin. Invest.* 46:1054.
Portman, O. W. 1960. *Am. J. Clin. Nutr.* 8:462.
Portman, O. W. and Murphy, D. 1958. *Arch. Biochem.* 76:367.
Post, R. L., Kune, S., Tobin, T., Orcutt, B. and Sen, A. K. 1969. *J. Gen. Physiol.* 54:3065.
Quigley, J. P. and Gotterer, G. S. 1969. *Biochim. Biophys. Acta* 173:469.
Quigley, J. P. and Gotterer, G. S. 1972. *Biochim. Biophys. Acta* 255:107.
Ramaswamy, K., Malathi, P., Caspary, W. F. and Crane, R. K. 1974. *Biochim. Biophys. Acta* 345:39.
Read, C. P. 1967. *Biol. Bull.* 133:630.
Reddy, B. S., Pleasants, J. R. and Wostmann, B. S. 1968. *J. Nutr.* 95:413.
Reiser, S. and Christiansen, P. C. 1969. *Am. J. Physiol.* 216:915.
Reiser, S. and Christiansen, P. C. 1971. *Biochim. Biophys. Acta* 225:123.
Reiser, S., Michaelis O. E., IV, and Hallfrisch, J. 1975a. *Proc. Soc. Exp. Biol. Med.* 150:110.
Reiser, S., Michaelis, O. E., IV, Putney, J. and Hallfrisch, J. 1975b. *J. Nutr.* 105:894.

Riklis, E. and Quastel, J. H. 1958. *Can. J. Biochem. Physiol.* 36:347.

Roberts, P. J. P. and Whelan, W. J. 1960. *Biochem. J.* 76:246.

Rosensweig, N. S. 1971. *Gastroenterology* 60:464.

Rosensweig, N. S. and Herman, R. H. 1968. *J. Clin. Invest.* 47:2253.

Rosensweig, N. S. and Herman, R. H. 1969a. *Am. J. Clin. Nutr.* 22:99.

Rosensweig, N. S. and Herman, R. H. 1969b. *Gastroenterology* 56:500.

Rosensweig, N. S., Stifel, F. B., Herman, R. H. and Zakim, D. 1968a. *Biochim. Biophys. Acta* 170:228.

Rosensweig, N. S., Stifel, F. B. and Herman, R. H. 1968b. *J. Lab. Clin. Med.* 72:1009.

Rosensweig, N. S., Stifel, F. B., Herman, R. H. and Zakim, D. 1969a. *Fed. Proc.* 28:323.

Rosensweig, N. S., Stifel, F. B., Zakim, D. and Herman, R. H. 1969b. *Gastroenterology* 57:143.

Roy, C. C. and Dubois, R. S. 1972. *Proc. Soc. Exp. Biol. Med.* 139:883.

Rudo, N. D. and Rosenberg, I. H. 1973. *Proc. Soc. Exp. Biol. Med.* 142:521.

Sanford, P. A. and Smyth, D. H. 1974. *J. Physiol.* 239:285.

Saunders, S. J. and Isselbacher, K. J. 1965. *Biochim. Biophys. Acta* 102:397.

Scala, J. 1974. *Food Tech.* 28:34.

Schachter, D. and Britten, J. S. 1961. *Fed. Proc.* 20:137.

Scharrer, E. 1972. *Experientia* 28:267.

Schedl, H. P. and Wilson, H. D. 1971. *Am. J. Physiol.* 220:1739.

Schrire, V. 1971. *S. Afr. Med. J.* 45:634.

Schultz, S. G. and Curran, P. F. 1970. *Physiol. Rev.* 50:637.

Schultz, S. G. and Strecker, C. K. 1970. *Biochim. Biophys. Acta* 211:586.

Schultz, S. G. and Zalusky, R. 1964a. *J. Gen. Physiol.* 47:567.

Schultz, S. G. and Zalusky, R. 1964b. *J. Gen. Physiol.* 47:1043.

Schultz, S. G., Fuisz, R. E. and Curran, P. F. 1966. *J. Gen. Physiol.* 49:849.

Scotch, N. A. 1960. *Ann. N.Y. Acad. Sci.* 84:1000.

Seftel, H. C., Dew, M. C. and Bersohn, I. 1970. *S. Afr. Med. J.* 44:8.

Semenza, G. 1967. In *Protides of the biological fluids,* vol. 15, pp. 201–208. Amsterdam: Elsevier.

Semenza, G. 1968a. In *Modern problems in pediatrics,* ed. A. Hottinger and H. Berger, pp. 32–47. Basel: Karger.

Semenza, G. 1968b. In *Handbook of physiology,* ed. C. F. Code, vol. 5, pp. 2543–2566. Washington, D.C.: American Physiological Society.

Semenza, G., Tosi, R., Valloton-Delachaux, M. C. and Mühlhaupt, E. 1964. *Biochim. Biophys. Acta* 89:109.

Sen, A. K., Tobin, T. and Post, R. L. 1969. *J. Biol. Chem.* 244:6596.

Shabaan, A. A., Turner, D. S. and Marks, V. 1974. *Diabetes* 23:902.

Shakespeare, P., Srivastava, L. M. and Hübscher, G. 1969. *Biochem. J.* 111:63.

Siddiqui, I. R. 1970. *Adv. Carbohydr. Chem. Biochem.* 25:285.

Sigrist-Nelson, K. and Hopfer, U. 1974. *Biochim. Biophys. Acta* 367:247.

Skou, J. C. 1965. *Physiol. Rev.* 45:596.

Southgate, D. A. T. 1969. *J. Sci. Food Agric.* 20:331.

Southgate, D. A. T. and Durnin, J. V. G. A. 1970. *Br. J. Nutr.* 24:517.

Stanley, M., Paul, D., Gacke, D. and Murphy, J. 1972. *Gastroenterology* 62:816.

Sterling, C. E. and Kinter, W. B. 1967. *J. Cell Biol.* 35:585.

Stern, B. K. 1966. *Gastroenterology* 51:855.

Stifel, F. B., Rosensweig, N. S., Zakim, D. and Herman, R. 1968a. *Biochim. Biophys. Acta* 170:221.

Stifel, F. B., Herman, R. H. and Rosensweig, N. S. 1968b. *Science* 162:692.

78 S. Reiser

Storelli, C., Vögeli, H. and Semenza, G. 1972. *FEBS Lett.* 24:287.
Swaminathan, N. and Eichholz, A. 1973. *Biochim. Biophys. Acta* 298:724.
Szanto, S. and Yudkin, J. 1969. *Postgrad. Med. J.* 45:602.
Taylor, C. B. 1962. *Biochim. Biophys. Acta* 60:437.
Tepperman, J. and Tepperman, H. M. 1958. *Am. J. Physiol.* 193:55.
Trowell, H. C. 1960. *Non-infective diseases in Africa.* London: Arnold.
Trowell, H. C. 1972a. *Atherosclerosis* 16:138.
Trowell, H. C. 1972b. *Am. J. Clin. Nutr.* 25:926.
Turner, D. S. and Marks, V. 1972. *Lancet* 1:1095.
Turner, D. S., Shabaan, A., Etheridge, L. and Marks, V. 1973. *Endocrinology* 93:1323.
Turner, D. S., Etheridge, L., Jones, J., Marks, V., Meldrum, B., Bloom, S. R. and Brown, J. C. 1974. *Clin. Endocrinol.* 3:489.
Tyrrell, J. B. and Anderson, J. A. 1971. *Endocrinology* 89:1178.
Ugolev, A. M. 1965. *Physiol. Rev.* 45:555.
Ugolev, A. M. 1972. *Gut* 13:735.
Unger, R. H. and Eisentraut, A. M. 1969. *Arch Intern. Med.* 123:261.
Varró, V. and Csernay, L. 1966. *Scand. J. Gastroenterol.* 1:231.
Vinnik, I. E., Kern, F., Jr. and Sussman, K. E. 1965. *J. Lab. Clin. Med.* 66:131.
Walker, A. R. P. 1964. *Am. Heart J.* 68:581.
Walker, A. R. P. 1971. *S. Afr. Med. J.* 45:377.
Walker, A. R. P., Richardson, B. D., Walker, B. F. and Woolford, A. 1973. *Postgrad. Med. J.* 49:187.
Wapnick, S., Kanengoni, E., Wicks, A. C. B. and Jones, J. J. 1972. *Lancet* 2:300.
Weiser, M. M., Quill, H. and Isselbacher, K. J. 1971. *Am. J. Physiol.* 221:844.
Whittam, R. 1962. *Biochem. J.* 84:110.
Wicks, A. C. B. and Jones, J. J. 1973. *Br. Med. J.* 1:773.
Wilbrandt, W. and Rosenberg, T. 1961. *Pharmacol. Rev.* 13:109.
Wilson, T. H. and Crane, R. K. 1958. *Biochim. Biophys. Acta* 29:30.
Wilson, T. H. and Landau, B. R. 1960. *Am. J. Physiol.* 198:99.
Wilson, T. H. and Vincent, T. N. 1955. *J. Biol. Chem.* 216:851.
Wilson, T. H. and Wiseman, G. 1954. *J. Physiol.* 123:126.
Wolfrom, M. L. and Thompson, A. 1955. *J. Am. Chem. Soc.* 77:6403.
Younoszai, M. K., and Schedl, H. P. 1972. *J. Lab. Clin. Med.* 79:579.

Chapter 4

INSULIN/GLUCAGON RATIO—A DETERMINANT OF GLUCOSE HOMEOSTASIS

Elizabeth Bossong Spannhake
Department of Biological Sciences
University of New Orleans
New Orleans, Louisiana

INTRODUCTION

The evolution of higher vertebrates has been associated with the development of a complicated set of hormonal controls that monitor cell processes. The continuous activity of endocrine glands provides a chronic level of cellular regulation, whereas the capacity of the glands to secrete increasing amounts of hormones as needed permits acute regulation. The combination of chronic and acute regulation at multicellular levels contributes to the integrated behavior of organ systems, resulting in the delicate balance within the animal known as homeostasis. This manner in which homeostasis is attained and maintained is best explained in terms of "control" theory. At all levels of cellular organization, control factors influence the direction and route of metabolism. They affect the rate of transport and synthesis as well as the overall metabolism of carbohydrates, fats, and proteins.

INSULIN AND GLUCAGON: COFACTORS REGULATING PLASMA GLUCOSE LEVELS

A starting point for integrating and correlating the acute effects of hormones upon carbohydrate metabolism is illustrated by the rapid control of blood sugar concentration. The blood sugar levels in postabsorptive animals are indicators of the overall balance of glucose production and utilization. They reflect the balance between hepatic glucose release and the metabolic demands of other tissues under the influence of intracellular and hormonal controls (Litwack, 1970). The immediate hyperglycemic effects of glucagon on blood glucose are balanced by the hypoglycemia produced by the increased secretion

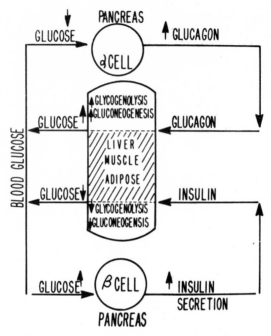

FIGURE 1   Schematic representation of the control
of blood glucose levels by insulin and glucagon.

of insulin (Karlson and Serkeris, 1966). In the normal animal with sufficient
carbohydrate precursor pools, insulin and glucagon share a major role in the
control of blood glucose concentration (Fig. 1).

Control of Metabolic Homeostasis

Exton and Park (1968c) and Mackrell and Sokal (1969) have clearly
demonstrated the opposing actions of glucagon and insulin on glucose balance.
Luyckx and Lefebvre (1970) have reported similar opposition on adipose tissue
fuel balance. It is, therefore, clear that by varying the relative concentrations of
glucagon and insulin, these hormones possess the biologic capability not only to
control the balance of glucose across the liver and of fuel across the adipose
tissue but also to direct the disposition of the gluconeogenic amino acids. Amino
acids of both endogenous and exogenous origin are distributed either into
glucose production or into protein synthesis in accordance with prevailing need
(Tata, 1968). A rise in the ratio of insulin to glucagon promotes storage of
ingested nutrients of all types. Under these conditions, gluconeogenesis and
lipolysis is inhibited and protein biosynthesis is favored (Unger, 1971). On the
other hand, a decline in the insulin to glucagon ratio favors the mobilization of
stored nutrients with an increase in hepatic glucose production from glycogen
and available amino acids (Unger, 1971). This gluconeogenesis occurs at the

expense of protein stores. Nitrogen balance is shifted toward negative with an increased production of urea. The release of free fatty acids and glycerol from adipose tissue is also increased (Unger, 1971).

The administration of glucagon lowers liver glycogen levels. The glycogen serves as a reservoir of glucose and glucagon, by stimulating the adenyl cyclase mechanism to increase tissue levels of cyclic $3',5'$-adenosine monophosphate (cAMP), promotes glycogenolysis (Frieden and Lipner, 1971). The opposing hypoglycemic effect of insulin is manifested at numerous key metabolic junctions. The effects include increased glycogenesis and glucose uptake by many tissues, as well as reduced gluconeogenesis. Some of these effects occur through a dampening of the adenylate cyclase system decreasing tissue cAMP levels (Exton and Park, 1969).

Insulin and glucagon also exert significant effects on lipid metabolism through the control of lipolysis and the release of free fatty acids from the lipid stores (Robison et al., 1971b). Glucagon through the stimulation of cAMP levels exerts a control over rates of lipolysis, i.e., the stimulation of lipid breakdown and utilization of the activating lipase that catalyzes the hydrolysis of triglycerides for the release of fatty acids (Robison et al., 1971). The augmentation of fat oxidation resulting from glucagon action represents a potential adaptor response since fat can then be used as an auxillary source of energy, conserving or supplementing glucose. The primary balance in conserving triglycerides is provided by insulin. In promoting glucose uptake by adipose tissue, insulin increases the supply and utilization of carbohydrate for energy and for the synthesis of triglycerides and cholesterol (Frieden and Lipner, 1971). The insulin effect in regulating this inverse relation between glucose and lipid metabolism depends highly on adequate dietary carbohydrate (Eaton and Kipnis, 1969a, b).

Recent studies have demonstrated that dietary uptake of carbohydrate can work to alter the insulin and glucagon concentrations within the organism (Eaton and Kipnis, 1969a, b). More importantly, dietary carbohydrate can shift the ratio of these hormones, inducing varied as well as abnormal metabolic responses. The shifting of insulin/glucagon ratios has a dramatic effect on tissue cAMP levels and, hence, affects numerous metabolic processes (Unger, 1971). The balance among gluconeogenesis, glycogenolysis, and glycolysis, as well as between lipogenesis and lipolysis, within hepatic tissues has been shown to be greatly dependent on the cAMP levels (Robison et al., 1971a). It is probable that under most conditions, the level of cAMP is also a function of the ratio of insulin to glucagon (Fig. 2). The intracellular cAMP concentration regulated by glucagon and insulin is therefore an important factor in the minute-to-minute control of carbohydrate and lipid homeostasis. Subtle shifts in the balance between these two hormones are probably more important than large changes in the absolute levels of either hormone in regard to their influence on metabolic balance. Increasing recognition of the importance of the role of the insulin/ glucagon ratio in the moment-to-moment regulation of nutrient homeostasis

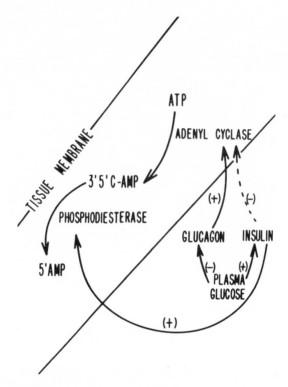

FIGURE 2   Schematic representation of the role of
insulin/glucagon ratios in the regulation of tissue cAMP
levels.

may help to reconcile a considerable body of diverse biochemical, physiologic,
and clinical data, thus providing rational explanations for previously irreconcil-
able observations.

INTRACELLULAR EVENTS OF GLYCOGENOLYSIS
AND GLUCONEOGENESIS

Glucagon Regulation of Glycogenolysis and Gluconeogenesis

Until recently, the effects of glucagon upon carbohydrate metabolism
appeared to be less important than those of insulin. However, it is now evident
that the function of glucagon is as significant as that of insulin. Glucagon
provides glucose for the organism when there is a need for this substance as an
energy source. The mechanism of action of glucagon as a powerful hepatic
glycogenolytic inducer has been studied in detail (Newsholme and Start,
1973; Robison et al., 1971a). Glucagon stimulates the synthesis of cAMP by
activating the enzyme adenyl cyclase (Robison et al., 1971a). cAMP

promotes the conversion of inactive phosphorylase to active phosphorylase, an enzyme that participates in the breakdown of glycogen to glucose. Sokal (1966) has demonstrated that glucagon is a more potent glycogenolytic agent than epinephrine and postulates that it is the only humoral factor that could function as a physiologic regulation of hepatic glycogenolysis. The hormone is effective in the liver at a concentration of 3×10^{-11} *M*, its onset of action is rapid and its duration of action is quite short (approximately 30 min). In addition to its stimulatory effect on glycogen degradation, glucagon reverses the activation of glycogen synthetase induced in dog liver by the administration of glucose and insulin (Sokal, 1966). This action prevents glucose from being stored in the liver, thus remaining available for use as a fuel.

The responsiveness of the hepatic phosphorylase and synthetase systems to glucagon administration has been recently studied by Curnow et al. (1975). The data indicate that glucagon when administered alone, induced a rapid increase in hepatic cAMP concentration with a concomitant rapid activation of phosphorylase and attendant glycogenolysis. In the fasted state, glycogen synthetase activity was low and could not be further decreased by glucagon. The results also indicate that relatively small increases in cAMP concentration are needed for maximal phosphorylase activation. As reported by Bishop et al. (1971), glucagon could increase cAMP concentration and reverse the enzymic effects of sustained glucose infusion. Despite the large increase in phosphophosphorylase activity and a decrease in synthetase I activity that resulted from the administration of glucagon (Curnow et al., 1975), there were no decreases in hepatic glycogen concentration when glucagon was given in the absence of glucose.

Glucagon also enhances gluconeogenesis, especially from alanine, lactate, and pyruvate (Eisenstein and Strack, 1968). The hormone induces this effect when present at physiologic concentrations of 10^{-9} *M*. The action of glucagon on gluconeogenesis can be totally reproduced by the administration of cAMP, and the data indicate that glucagon functions to promote gluconeogenesis by activating adenyl cyclase in the plasma membrane. The hormonal control of hepatic gluconeogenesis has been studied in detail. Precursors for hepatic glucose synthesis include lactate, pyruvate, several amino acids, as well as endogenous liver protein. Gluconeogenesis from these precursors can be stimulated by either glucagon or cAMP. However, the mechanisms through which cAMP acts are poorly understood. Exton and Park (1968b, c) have studied the control of gluconeogenesis in the isolated perfused liver. They have reported that saturating concentrations of fructose or dihydroxyacetone led to a rate of gluconeogenesis twice that observed with saturating concentrations of lactate or pyruvate. Glucagon and exogenous cAMP stimulated gluconeogenesis from lactate or pyruvate but not from fructose and dihydroxyacetone (Exton and Park, 1968c). These observations point to the conclucion that the rate-limiting steps that regulate gluconeogenesis from lactate and pyruvate likely occurred between the conversion of pyruvate to phosphoenolpyruvate and that the stimulatory effect of cAMP was probably exerted at this level.

Glucagon Regulation of Lipolysis

Glucagon stimulates lipolysis in adipose tissue and liver. As a result, there is an increased release of long- and short-chain fatty acid CoA esters. Intravenous injection of glucagon produced an immediate but transient rise followed by a fall in plasma levels of free fatty acids (FFA) (Sokal and Abdulla, 1966). The depression of plasma FFA that follows glucagon results from the stimulation of insulin secretion since the effect can be abolished by an infusion of antiinsulin serum along with glucagon (Sokal and Abdulla, 1966). Conversely, it has been shown in recent studies (Edwards et al., 1972; Eisenstein and Strack, 1968) that FFA may contribute significantly to the control of glucagon secretion. Elevation of plasma FFA levels has been demonstrated to decrease plasma glucagon levels (Edwards et al., 1969; Himsworth, 1935), whereas the depression of plasma FFA causes an increase in plasma glucagon concentrations (Luyckx and Lefebvre, 1970). Gerich et al. (1974c) have shown that rather small alterations in plasma FFA levels within the physiologic range have a significant effect on glucagon secretion in man.

In liver the lipolytic effect of glucagon is powerful and rapid. Several studies have shown that enhanced lipolysis may be responsible for the stimulation of gluconeogenesis and ketogenesis observed following a glucagon administration. Carboxylation of pyruvate to oxaloacetate is increased by the enhanced availability of acetyl CoA, thus accounting for the stimulation of gluconeogenesis (Renold et al., 1965). In isolated liver perfusions, additions of fatty acids increased the rate of gluconeogenesis from lactate and pyruvate. The effects of glucagon on fat metabolism have been produced with rather large doses of glucagon, and it appears that physiologic levels of the hormone may not significantly alter the lipid metabolism. Furthermore, since glucagon stimulates insulin secretion, the resulting anti-lipolytic action of insulin counteracts glucagon-induced fat mobilization.

It has long been suspected that the regulation of fatty acid oxidation in hepatic tissue is closely involved with some facet of carbohydrate metabolism (Lossow and Chaikoff, 1954; Lossow et al., 1956; Weinhouse et al., 1949). Alterations in the metabolism of carbohydrate could then be related to the management of ketogenic potentiation in the liver as well. Since hepatic carbohydrate metabolism, which plays a central role in glucose homeostasis, appears to be under the bihormonal regulation of insulin and glucagon (Cherrington and Vranic, 1974; Mackrell and Sokal, 1969; Parrilla et al., 1974; Unger, 1974), the possibility exists that shifts in the molar ratio of these two hormones could represent major determinants in hepatic ketogenic capacity.

In an attempt to investigate these interrelationships, McGarry and Foster (1974) treated nonketogenic rats with antiinsulin serum and with glucagon. Insulin antibody caused immediate hyperglycemia and increased plasma free fatty acid concentrations and ketosis; glucagon, even in very high doses, had little effect on these parameters. However, after only 1 hr of either treatment, hepatic metabolism in these animals changed from a nonketogenic to a ketogenic state. Thus, for the first time, a liver with a high ketogenic capacity was obtained from a nonketogenic animal. While the nature of the on-off signal for this reaction is completely unknown, the mechanism of the enhanced capacity for ketone body production appears to be an activation of the carnitine acyltransferase step. This reaction catalyzes the transfer of long-chain fatty acids across the mitochondrial membrane (McGarry and Foster, 1974).

Glucagon Stimulation of cAMP Release

The overall response to glucagon resembles that of epinephrine, which is understandable if cAMP functions as the second messenger for both hormones. The nature of this response and the evidence that cAMP mediates the response to glucagon can be summarized briefly.

Glucagon stimulates adenyl cyclase activity in washed particulate preparations from the livers of all species studied (Bitensky et al., 1967; Makman and Sutherland, 1964; Pohl et al., 1969). The stimulatory effect of glucagon on hepatic adenyl cyclase activity has been reported to occur at all levels of ATP and Mg^{2+} and to persist even through dialysis. According to Bitensky and co-workers (1967), there is a factor or factors in liver extracts capable of reversing the effect of glucagon on adenyl cyclase. Acidic phospholipids also play a critical part in the activation of adenyl cyclase by glucagon. It is postulated that phospholipids promote the necessary configurational shift in the catalytic site following the binding of glucagon to its receptor and, by this means, couples the receptor to the catalytic site (Rodbell et al., 1971).

To investigate the requirements for phospholipids in the activation mechanism and the relationship of binding to enzyme activation, Levey (1975) used a soluble preparation of myocardial adenyl cyclase. From these data, Levey proposed that glucagon binding occurred in the dissociation of the receptor site. Dissociation is succeeded by the activation of the enzyme adenyl cyclase, when the "critical" phospholipids are present to induce the configurational modification (Storm and Dolginowyd, 1973). Levey also reported glucagon binding and receptor dissociation in the solubilized preparation free of detergent, but in the absence of phospholipid. In this case, the activation of adenyl cyclase did not occur, presumably due to the lack of the key phospholipids and the resultant failure to obtain the necessary shift in the catalytic site.

Glucagon induces a prompt increase in the intracellular level of cAMP upon addition to isolated perfused rat livers (Fig. 3) (Exton and Park, 1968a). By measuring the amount of cAMP released into the perfusate, Lewis et al. (1970) were able to observe the effects of glucagon at concentrations (10^{-10} M) even lower (10^{-8} M) than those shown by Robison et al. (1971a) (Fig. 4). Stimulation of cAMP concentration is the earliest effect of glucagon on liver that has been measured and precedes changes in gluconeogenesis, glycogenolysis, amino acid uptake, potassium efflux, urea production and the increases in

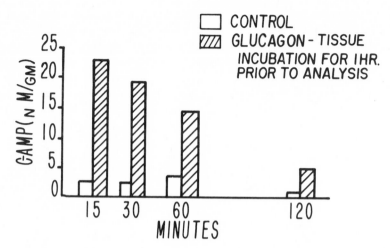

FIGURE 3 Effect of glucagon on the intracellular levels of cAMP in isolated perfused rat livers. Adapted from data reported by Siddle et al. (1973).

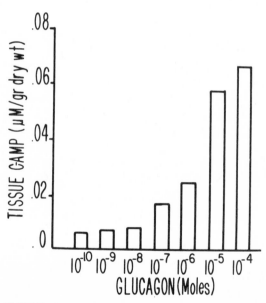

FIGURE 4 Changes in hepatic cAMP levels in response to different levels of glucagon. Tissues were incubated with the given dose of glucagon 1 hr prior to analysis. Adapted from data reported by Siddle et al. (1973) and Robison et al. (1971a).

tyrosine amino transferase activity. All of these changes can be induced by cAMP (Mallette et al., 1969; Wicks et al., 1969).

It is interesting to compare the dose response for glucagon upon cAMP and glucose release. It can be observed that the concentration of glucagon that results in a maximal stimulation of glucose production is quite small relative to the concentration required to produce a maximal effect on the level of cAMP. The concentration of glucagon that produces a maximal effect on glucose production is close to the highest blood glucagon level that has been reported to occur under physiologic conditions (Exton and Park, 1969). This means that under normal conditions *in vivo* the hepatic receptors for glucagon are presumably never saturated. The majority of these receptors comprise something of a reverse and can be referred to as spare receptors (Ariens, 1966). For any given effective concentration of glucagon the level of cAMP in the liver remains high as long as the glucagon is present in the perfusing medium and begins to fall toward the control level as soon as the hormone is removed.

Glucagon—A Hormone of Glucose Need

Since physiologic concentrations of glucagon have been demonstrated to be capable of stimulating the production and release of glucose by the liver, it seemed reasonable for many years to assume that glucagon might function as a hormone of glucose need (Samols et al., 1969). Although questioned for a time, this interpretation now seems to be well supported by experimental data. Thus, by increasing the concentration of glucose in the incubation medium, one finds an inhibition of release of glucagon from isolated pancreatic islets (Buchanan and McKiddie, 1967). An intravenous infusion of glucose produces a fall in the concentration of glucagon in the pancreatic duodenal vein of intact animals (Ohneda et al., 1968). Conversely, insulin-induced hypoglycemia is associated with an increase in the level of pancreatic vein glucagon (Ohneda et al., 1968). Decreased levels of circulating immunoreactive glucagon in response to intravenous glucose have also been detected in human volunteers (Aquilar-Parada et al., 1969). These and other observations imply that glucagon could function as a hormone of glucose need, possibly as part of a relatively simple feedback system. A fall in the level of blood glucose reaching the pancreas would stimulate hepatic glucose production. The resulting increase in blood glucose would then return to the pancreas to inhibit the release of glucagon.

The contradictory finding that glucagon could stimulate the release of insulin was dismissed by some investigators on the basis that most of the early experiments demonstrating this effect had made use of pharmacologic rather than physiologic doses of glucagon. It was later shown that intraportal injection of very small doses of glucagon did cause in increase in insulin levels (Buchanan and McKiddie, 1967). It seems plausible, therefore, that even circulating levels of glucagon, not to mention the higher levels likely to be in contact with pancreatic beta cells, could have an effect of the rate of release of insulin.

The ability of glucagon to stimulate the release of insulin from the pancreas, as well as glucose from the liver, seemed all the more puzzling in view of the evidence that insulin produced some of its effects in hepatic and adipose tissue by suppressing the accumulation of cAMP. The picture developed of one hormone, glucagon, stimulating adenyl cyclase in at least two types of cells. This action in the pancreas led to the release of a hormone that tended to oppose the action of glucagon in the liver.

Upon reflection, it is possible to view this arrangement as having a certain amount of survival value for the animal in which it occurs. It should be noted that the low blood glucose levels that presumably constitute the normal stimulus for pancreatic glucagon release in adult animals might be insufficient to permit the concomitant release of insulin. Because of the important requirement of a minimum glucose level for insulin release, glucagon and glucose could participate in the feedback system, despite the tendency of glucagon to stimulate insulin release at higher levels of blood glucose. Higher levels of glucose returning to the pancreas would, of course, tend to stimulate the release of insulin at the same time that glucagon release was being suppressed and that might have the beneficial effect of dampening the oscillations in blood glucose levels that might otherwise occur. It is also possible that enough insulin could at times be released with glucagon to affect adipose tissues without preventing the hepatic effects of glucagon because adipose tissue, at least in young rats, is more sensitive to insulin than is the liver (Robison et al., 1971a). The possibility that this might occur is not altered by the fact that the liver is also exposed to higher concentrations of insulin than other tissues. To the extent that this does occur, glucagon would function to shunt glucose from the liver to other tissues, thus differing from the catecholamines that tend to shunt glucose from the liver to the brain.

Insulin Regulation of Glycogenolysis and Gluconeogenesis

In studies in which insulin has been reported to diminish hepatic glucose production, inhibition of gluconeogenesis and/or glycogenolysis has been suggested. However, only indirect evidence could be cited to separate the pathway that was primarily responsible for the decreased glucose production. Insulin inhibition of urea production has been employed in the past to support decreases in gluconeogenesis (Exton et al., 1966; Glinsmann et al., 1969). The major effect of insulin on the gluconeogenic pathway is probably to induce decreased hepatic proteolysis (Mortimore and Mondon, 1970). While shifts in the concentration of urea may reflect availability of substrates for glucose production, they are inadequate measure of gluconeogenic activity. Possibly a more direct measure of gluconeogenic inhibition could come from studies of the cori cycle that showed decreases in radioactive lactate incorporation into glucose by the perfused liver (Haft, 1967). Work by Davidson and Berliner (1974) showed that insulin inhibits glucose production from glycerol. Experiments with

[^{14}C] glycerol demonstrated that only 26% of the inhibition of glucose production by insulin could be accounted for through the shunting of glycerol to glycogen via glucose. The additional glycerol converted to tissue lipids represented only 3% of the difference in [^{14}C] glucose production due to insulin. From this, Davidson and Berliner conclude that insulin must have a direct effect on gluconeogenesis.

The mechanism by which insulin influences glucose metabolism in the liver is not fully understood. It has been suggested, however, that hepatic glucose production is determined by the balance between insulin and glucagon. The effect of glucagon to stimulate glycogenolysis and gluconeogenesis by increasing hepatic cAMP is opposed by insulin that inhibits cAMP synthesis or increases cAMP degradation.

It has also been postulated that given appropriate conditions, insulin can modulate the glycogen pathways independent of glucagon. Basal glucose production in liver slices from fasted rats has been shown to be due to glycogenolysis. Insulin retards glucose release by inhibiting the breakdown of glycogen and/or by increasing the conversion of glucose to glycogen. Since glucagon does not affect basal glucose production (Rinard et al., 1969; Ross et al., 1967), this is an example in which insulin functions without the opposing actions of glucagon.

Studies by Bergman and Bucolo (1974) also confirm the insulin inhibition of glucose output from livers from fasted animals. The reaction proceeds slowly, and no data were found to support a rapid shift from net glucose production to net glucose intake through insulin action. The slow effect of insulin to decrease hepatic glucose release is due to insulin-mediated diminution of glycogenolysis and gluconeogenesis possibly because of lowered intracellular cAMP. The gradual onset of this reaction suggests that it may be at the point of *de novo* synthesis of RNA. Similarly, the effect of insulin in enhancing the stimulation of glucose uptake may involve the synthesis of new protein. Bergman and Bucolo's study (1974) suggests that glucose and insulin are important components in the regulation of glucose homeostasis. Insulin exerts an effect on the liver, causing the liver to be more or less sensitive to glucose. This regulation by insulin exists on a continuum from insulin-deficient diabetes, where the liver is insensitive to glucose; through fasting, where it is moderately sensitive; to the feeding of simple carbohydrates, where sensitivity is maximal.

Insulin also participates in the enzyme changes promoted by glucose administration. Curnow's (Curnow et al., 1974) study indicates that intravenous insulin, like glucose, is capable of inducing rapid and significant alterations in both glycogen synthetase and phosphorylase systems in the liver. Insulin causes very rapid decreases in phosphophosphorylase activities and a more gradual increase in synthetase I activities. The effect of insulin was, however, of short duration and probably was the result of the counterinsulin reaction consequent to induced hypoglycemia. Similar to Curnow's observations, Hers and co-workers (1969) have reported that intravenous insulin administration decreased phosphophosphorylase activity in the intact anesthetized rat. It has been suggested that the action of insulin upon these enzyme systems was modulated by decreases in cAMP concentration (Park et al., 1972). Insulin may also be acting to decrease the sensitivity of protein kinase to cAMP (Miller and Larner, 1973) and to stimulate synthetase phosphorylase (Bishop et al., 1971).

Insulin thus dramatically affects the control of glucose uptake and output by the liver. Insulin inhibits both glycogenolysis and gluconeogenesis, while promoting the uptake of glucose and its conversion to glycogen or tissue lipids.

Insulin and Inhibition of cAMP Levels

The capability of insulin to lower the intracellular concentrations of cAMP in the liver has been demonstrated under appropriate conditions. The normal level of cAMP in the unstimulated liver ranges from 400 to 700 picomoles per gram of tissue. This amount of cAMP, when evenly distributed throughout the intracellular water, leads to a concentration of the nucleotide sufficient to maximally stimulate glycogenolysis and gluconeogenesis and to virtually eliminate glycogen synthesis. That these conditions do not prevail infers that in the unstimulated liver, cAMP is present largely in a bound or sequestered form, or else that intracellular cAMP is effectively antagonized by other metabolites (Unger, 1971). In any event, insulin does not seem to be capable of reducing hepatic cAMP levels below this baseline level. When the control levels of cAMP are increased, as in normal livers in the presence of glucagon, however, the cAMP lowering effect of insulin can be readily demonstrated (Lewis et al., 1970).

Apparently, under normal physiologic conditions, insulin exerts a continuous damping effect on the hepatic level of cAMP. Exton and co-workers (Exton and Park, 1968a; Exton et al., 1966) have suggested that glucose output by the liver may depend on a balance between an agent such as glucagon that increases cAMP levels and insulin that lowers these levels. This interpretation is well supported by experimental evidence. Jefferson et al. (1968) reported that a rise in hepatic cAMP occurred in normal rats following the injection of insulin antibodies. cAMP levels were also increased in livers from fasted rats and from rats made diabetic thorugh the injection of alloxan. The data from this experiment also demonstrated that the administration of insulin to diabetic animals led to a prompt restoration of the normal cAMP levels. Although it now seems likely that insulin has other effects, most of its known effects in the liver can be accounted for in terms of its ability to lower the intracellular levels of cAMP.

Current research has suggested that insulin in some ways also affects lipolysis through decreased cAMP levels. Butcher et al. (1966) found that insulin lowered cAMP levels significantly and rapidly in fat pads. The effect of insulin in suppressing cAMP accumulation in fat appeared to be specific for native insulin. In addition, insulin lowered the increased levels of cAMP found in fat pads incubated with glucagon and ACTH as well as epinephrine in intact fat pads of isolated cells (Butcher and Baird, 1969). Corbin et al. (1970) later studied the effects of insulin on glycerol release and cAMP levels in isolated fat cells. In the presence of a mild lipolytic stimulus (5.5 μM epinephrine) insulin caused significant decreases in both cAMP levels and lipolysis, supporting the idea of a causal relationship between these effects of insulin.

From the many studies concerning the action of glucagon and insulin, it is recognized that these hormones are integral components of the cAMP system. The study of the "directing" role of insulin and glucagon on cAMP may aid in assisting our knowledge and understanding of both normal and abnormal carbohydrate metabolic patterns.

EFFECT OF DIETARY CARBOHYDRATE ON INSULIN AND GLUCAGON SECRETION

Dietary carbohydrate has been repeatedly demonstrated to influence carbohydrate and lipid intermediary metabolism in man and in animals (Brunzell et al., 1971; Eaton and Kipnis, 1969a, b). "Adequate" dietary carbohydrate will improve glucose tolerance when compared with carbohydrate "deficient" antecedent diets (Brunzell et al., 1971; Eaton and Kipnis, 1969b), while excessive carbohydrate ingestion will produce a transient endogenous lipemia (Eaton and Kipnis, 1969a). The mechanisms involved in these metabolic responses to the carbohydrate content of the diet have not been resolved, but a participation of hormones in these events has been postulated (Eaton and Kipnis, 1969a). One of the most important routes through which the dietary availability of carbohydrate regulates metabolism is through the pancreatic secretion and action of glucagon and insulin. Pancreatic glucagon secretion is suppressed by exposure to glucose, while pancreatic insulin secretion is augmented by the same stimuli both *in vivo* and *in vitro* (Müller et al., 1971; Unger et al., 1970).

Carbohydrate Stimulation of Insulin Secretion

Studies of a glucose-stimulated secretion by the perfused rat pancreas have demonstrated a biphasic pattern of insulin release (Curry et al., 1968) (Fig. 5). There appears to be an early response lasting approximately 5 min and a sustained later increase continuing for over 1 hr. Most studies concerned with the glucose effect have been involved with secretion over periods considerably longer than 5 min. These studies were related more to the mechanism of the sustained response. The relationship between glucose concentration and insulin release has been characterized so as to produce information dealing with the nature of the pancreatic glucoreceptor mechanism. Clearly, the latter should be capable of responding to changes in glucose concentration in the same range as those that stimulate insulin release. To this end, the glucose concentration resulting in a half maximum stimulation of release has been found to be in the region of 10-20 mmol/liter with a threshold at about 5 mmol/liter (Weir et al., 1974). While the argument relating to the range of receptor sensitivity is sound, that utilizing the maximum rate of release is not. Maximum rates of insulin

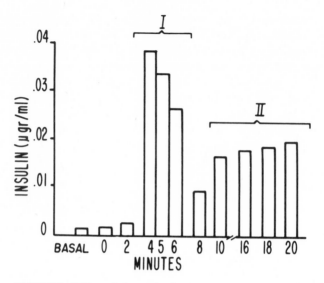

FIGURE 5 Effect of glucose load on the *in vitro* insulin release by isolated perfused rat pancreas. Adapted from the data reported by Curry et al. (1968), Litwack (1970), and Weir et al. (1974).

release may well be imposed by the release mechanism itself and not related to the saturation of the glucoreceptor in the pancreas.

In man and experimental animals the plasma insulin concentration rapidly increases when the blood glucose levels are elevated above the fasting range (60–100 mg/100 ml) by oral or intravenous glucose. Similarly, in the perfused rat pancreas the rate of insulin release increases when the glucose concentration is increased above 35–50 mg/100 ml (Litwack, 1970). The *in vitro* studies show that the glucose effect does not depend on extrapancreatic tissue and suggest, but do not entirely prove, that the sugar acts directly on beta cells.

The effects of other sugars on insulin release are summarized in Table 1. Mannose was the only other sugar with a marked stimulatory effect: glucosamine had a small effect, as did fructose at high concentrations (Coore and Randle, 1964; Grodsky et al., 1965). Much of the evidence that intracellular glucose metabolism is required in the production of a signal mediating the stimulation of insulin release has come from the inhibition of the process by mannoheptulose, a seven-carbon sugar. This sugar inhibits glucose phosphorylation by the liver hexokinase (EC 2.7.1.1) and is though to act similarly in the beta cell. Consistent with the theory that glucose metabolism is essential for the stimulation of insulin release are the observations that the mannose effect is similar to that of glucose but that the less metabolizable sugars, such as fructose, galactose, and 2-deoxyglucose, have little or no effect on insulin release (Coore and Randle, 1964; Grodsky et al., 1965).

After the discovery of insulin, much of the work in comparing sugars was devoted to demonstrating that fructose followed a different metabolic pathway from that of glucose. Cook and Jacobson (1971) have reported that there is an individual variation in fructose metabolism in man. If one examines the glucose tolerance curves presented in a paper by Cohen et al. in 1966, a great deal of variation among the different subjects will be noted. Differences in serum lipid responses to high-fructose and -sucrose diets have been observed in normal subjects as well as those with hypertriglyceridemia (Kaufmann et al., 1966). Carbohydrate effects have been shown to vary in different strains of rats (Chang et al., 1971; Durand et al., 1968). Berdanier et al. (1971a, b) reported that there are differences in insulin and glucose levels in different strains of rats.

Two important considerations of the mechanics of the glucoreceptor are its apparent ability to adapt to the relative intake of carbohydrate. Carbohydrate deprivation induces a decrease in the glucose stimulation of insulin secretion. This loss occurs at a time when the islet insulin concentration has not fallen significantly (Karam et al., 1963). Conversely, obese subjects (Karam et al., 1963) and rats with experimental obesity (Hales and Kennedy, 1964) show an increased insulin response to glucose. It was suggested that the latter change could be caused by the increased carbohydrate intake that led to adaptive changes in the metabolism of the beta cell.

Characteristics considered in obesity are the presence of hyper-glyceridemia, increased plasma insulin levels, and an antagonism to the action of insulin (Mueller et al., 1965). On the other hand, continuous ingestion of diets rich in sucrose are thought to result in obesity, hypertriglyceridemia, and an antagonsim to the action of insulin (Mackrell and Sokal, 1969). Apart from the peripheral factors that inhibit the action of insulin on the uptake of glucose in

TABLE 1 Effect of Sugars on
Insulin Release[a]

Sugar	Effect[b]
Glucose	+
Mannose	+
Fructose	+
Galactose	NE
2-Deoxyglucose	NE
Glucosamine	+
D-Ribose	NE
D-Xylose	NE
Mannoheptulose	—

[a]Based on data collected by Coore and Randle (1964).
[b]+ = stimulates; NE = no effect; — = inhibits.

animals fed a high-sucrose diet, there are other circumstances at the cellular level that antagonize the activity of this hormone.

In rats fed a high-carbohydrate diet, the plasma insulin levels were higher than those in control rats. After 17–20 hr of starvation, the glucose levels were reduced, and the plasma insulin concentrations remained high. This increased plasma insulin concentration present in the face of basal values of plasma glucose may be due to a peripheral antagonism to insulin (Blazquez and Quijada, 1968). However, Anderson and Marks (1973) reported a decrease in fasting plasma insulin concentration and in total insulin response to a glucose load as the percentage of calories from glucose was increased. When 80% of the calories came from sucrose, there was a reduction in fasting insulin levels, but not in the summed insulin reponses.

Because studies concerned with the effects of sucrose intake upon glucose and insulin response have given conflicting results, Kelsay et al. (1974) studied a group of young women consuming diets containing either glucose or sucrose in order to determine whether consumption of these diets would alter fasting glucose and insulin levels and/or glucose and insulin responses to a glucose load.

The increased insulin levels found after the consumption of high-sugar diets in Kelsay's study are similar to those reported by Szanto and Yudkin (1969), for men fed high-sucrose diets. Szanto and Yudkin found increased levels of insulin in response to a glucose load. They suggest that an increased insulin response occurs only in a fraction of the population. It may then be expected that subjects who have an increased insulin response following sucrose consumption would have an even greater response to glucose feeding, as a glucose load elicits a greater insulin response than does a sucrose load (Swan et al., 1966).

In Kelsay's study, the consumption of the high-glucose and -sucrose diets may have incurred a reduction in insulin sensitivity in these particular subjects. As the blood glucose was maintained at normal levels, more insulin may have been required for the removal of glucose to proceed at the same rate. The elevated fasting glucose and insulin levels observed at the conclusion of this study combined with increased insulin response to a glucose load are probably the first effects of a high-glucose or -sucrose diet. An increased insulin response to a glucose load may follow if the diet is continued.

Reports indicate that the utilization of sucrose is different from that of its component monosaccharides. Caspary (1972) has reviewed evidence for a sodium-independent transport system for glucose derived from disaccharides that offers substantiation for the postulation that glucose moieties from disaccharides are more efficiently absorbed than from the monosaccharide. Also, Curry et al. (1972) reported that in isolated perfused rat pancreas preparations, insulin release after the addition of fructose occurred when a stimulatory concentration of glucose was present, but not with fructose alone. Michaelis and Szepesi (1973) and Veech et al. (1973) have presented evidence that indicates that the sucrose molecule is more effective than either glucose or fructose in increasing certain enzyme activity levels in rat liver. Thus, sucrose might result in responses in the human subject that would be greater than with glucose.

In animal feeding studies, sucrose has been shown to have an effect on glucose and insulin blood levels. Bruckdorfer et al. (1972) reported that rats fed a sucrose or fructose diet had plasma insulin levels that were comparable to each other but were lower than those of rats fed glucose. Vrana et al. (1971) determined that feeding a high-sucrose diet to rats did not alter the serum concentration of insulin or the insulin-degrading activity of liver extracts, but did reduce the insulin sensitivity of adipose tissue, compared with that of rats fed wheat starch.

Carbohydrate Stimulation and Inhibition of Glucagon Secretion

While much research in the past has focused on the effect of glucose upon insulin secretion, a new emphasis is now being placed on the response of glucagon to glucose stimulation. Vance et al. (1968) have reported that as the glucose concentration in the media is raised from 30 to 300 mg/100 ml, there is a decreased secretion of glucagon and an increased secretion of insulin by the pancreas. The addition of 2-deoxyglucose and mannoheptulose to the media inhibited insulin release, but had no effect on glucagon release. Chesney and Schofield (1969) have also studied the effect of glucose on glucagon release. The effect of variation of glucose concentration in the incubation medium on the release of glucagon was studied. Glucagon release at 1.67 or 3.3 mmol glucose was significantly greater than at 16.7 mmol glucose. The residual glucagon of islets incubated in 1.67 mmol glucose was 68% greater than islets incubated in 16.7 mmol glucose. The percentage of total glucagon released in the presence of 1.67 or 3.3 mmol glucose was twice that released at 16.7 mmol glucose. The effect of glucose on the rate of release of glucagon from islets observed in this study agree with the *in vitro* findings of Vance et al. (1968) and the *in vivo* findings of Unger (1971).

It has been shown that glucose exerts an important control of alpha cell secretion in a manner almost the reverse of its control of insulin release from the beta cell. At low levels, glucagon secretion is enhanced and at high levels suppressed. This has been demonstrated both *in vivo* (Gerich et al., 1973; Mackrell and Sokal, 1969; Samols et al., 1969) and *in vitro* (Iverson, 1971; Luyckx, 1972; Malaisse et al., 1969). The details of the timing and magnitude of glucagon release in response to varying glucose concentrations remain incompletely defined. Weir et al. (1974) have observed that when perfused glucose was acutely dropped from 100 to 25 mg/100 ml, glucagon was released in a biphasic pattern with an early spike and a later plateau-like response (Fig. 6).

Although glucose is an important determinant of immunoreactive glucagon secretion (Unger et al., 1972), the mechanism by which it regulates pancreatic alpha cell function is poorly defined. It has been suggested that glucose may directly stimulate glucagon release via a glucoreceptor (Cerasi and Luft, 1970;

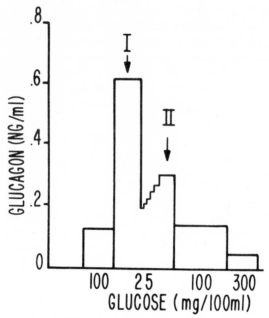

FIGURE 6 Effect of reductions in glucose level on glucagon release by isolated perfused rat pancreas. Adapted from data reported by Weir et al. (1974).

Edwards et al., 1972). In 1970, Edwards and Taylor observed that glucagon secretion could be diminished by energy yielding fuels, such as glucose, free fatty acids, and ketones *in vitro*. This suppression could also be prevented by blocking ATP formation. These results corresponded to *in vivo* data in which agents that inhibit intracellular glucose metabolism, such as 2-deoxyglucose or mannoheptulose, result in paradoxical hyperglucagonemia despite extracellular hyperglycemia (Müller et al., 1971). Insulin deficiency, whether induced by antiinsulin serum (Müller et al., 1971), alloxan (Müller et al., 1971), or streptozotocin (Meier et al., 1972), also resulted in hyperglucagonemia irrespective of the degree of hyperglycemia. It has also been demonstrated that glucagon release is greatly exaggerated during insulin insufficiency (Santeusanio et al., 1973). In experimental diabetes, loss of the glucagon response to extracellular hyperglycemia is instantly corrected with insulin. This suggests that the alpha cell may be an insulin-requiring cell. Severe insulin deficiency may therefore cause basal and stimulated hyperglucagonemia. In the total absence of insulin, the alpha cell could be incapable of responding appropriately to glucose need—behaving as if hypoglycemia were present (Unger, 1974). In 1974, Gerich attempted to further characterize the effects of glucose on the pancreatic alpha cell. His results demonstrate that the pancreatic alpha cell is also highly responsive to glucose. The K_i for glucose-induced inhibition of glucagon release was 5–6 mM or 90–110 mg/100 ml. This suggests that at or around physiologic levels glucose as well as insulin is an effective regulator of the alpha cell function.

To examine the concept that altered glucagon and insulin regulation may be involved in the metabolic alterations of chronic carbohydrate ingestion, Eaton et al. (1974) examined the secretion of these hormones in rats subjected to chronic glucose feeding. The results appear to indicate states of relative glucagon deficiency and insulin excess as glucagon secretion is significantly reduced. These results are consistent with a study conducted by Müller et al. (1971) who observed that an antecedent diet containing excessive carbohydrate results in reduced basal and stimulated serum glucagon concentrations in man. In the chronically glucose-fed animal, the reduction in the hyperglycemic action of glucagon may explain Eaton's demonstration of increased biologic activity of insulin in terms of glucose tolerance.

These observations emphasize the importance of the role of glucagon-insulin relationships in the maintenance of glucose homeostasis. Unger (1974) has recently reviewed this concept in detail in the clinical situation, while Exton et al. (1966) and Mackrell and Sokal (1969) have clearly shown in animal preparations the opposing actions of insulin and glucagon on hepatic glucose regulation.

Unger's research provides considerable evidence that the molar ratio of insulin to glucagon is inversely related to the need for endogenous glucose supply. In normal subjects, the insulin-to-glucagon ratio after an overnight fast ranges between 2.5 and 3.8. However, if the need for glucose is increased by a week of low-carbohydrate feeding, the overnight fasting insulin-to-glucagon ratio declines to 1.6, a bihormonal setting that favors an enhanced rate of hepatic glucose production. If the need for glucose is further increased by total starvation, the insulin-to-glucagon ratio is below 1.0. At the other extreme when the need for glucose is abolished by the infusion of glucose, the insulin-to-glucagon ratio soars to more than 15.

The effect of high-carbohydrate diets on glucose tolerance has fascinated medical research since the original clinical reports of this event by Himsworth in 1935. In 1940 Conn investigated this relationship in diabetic patients and established criteria for adequate carbohydrate intake prior to the testing for glucose intolerance. Brunzell et al. (1971) more recently illustrated that this response can be demonstrated in normal as well as mildly diabetic patients and is associated with a reduced basal and glucose-stimulated insulin secretion. This is in contrast to the results of Kelsay et al. (1974), Vrana et al. (1971), Szanto and Yudkin (1969), Blazquez and Quijada (1968) who suggested that in normal or nondiabetic humans or rats, carbohydrate-rich diets reduce the peripheral tissue sensitivity to insulin. Brunzell and co-workers suggested that a possible effect of carbohydrate-enriched diets in mild diabetics is to increase the sensitivity of tissue sites to insulin and its action. Eaton's research now proposes an hormonally directed explanation for an increased sensitivity to insulin—a reduction in the concentration of glucagon with a resulting decrease in glucagon-mediated opposition to the peripheral actions of insulin (Eaton et al., 1974).

EFFECT OF SOMATOSTATIN ON INSULIN AND GLUCAGON SECRETION AND METABOLIC CONSEQUENCES

Somatostatin, a hypothalamic peptide and inhibitory factor, has been reported to suppress the pancreatic secretion of insulin and glucagon (Yen et al., 1974). It has recently been discovered that these effects are the product of the direct action of somatostatin on alpha and beta cells (Okamoto et al., 1975). While it has been thought that natural somatostatin was confined to the hypothalamus and pituitary, Polak et al. (1975) have recently reported somatostatin to be a natural component of D-cells in both the gut and pancreas. If this can be further confirmed, somatostatin may function as a fundamental physiologic determinant in the control of pancreatic endocrine secretion.

Influence of Somatostatin on Glucagon Secretion

Thus far, the effect of somatostatin on glucagon release has received the greatest emphasis. The possibility of inducing experimental glucagon deficiency in man was suggested by the observation that infusion of somatostatin lowered plasma glucagon and glucose levels in baboons (Koerker et al., 1974). Gerich et al. (1974d) demonstrated that somatostatin directly inhibited glucagon secretion from the *in vitro* perfused rat pancreas. Gerich et al. (1975a) showed that infusion of somatostatin diminished glucagon secretion and plasma glucagon levels not only in normal volunteers but also in diabetic subjects. Infusion of 500 μg somatostatin over 1 hr in six normal subjects resulted in a rapid and reversible fall in plasma glucagon to approximately one-third the preinfusion levels. Concurrently, the plasma glucose concentration decreased to 30 mg/100 ml. Several observations indicate that this fall in plasma glucose is due to the concurrent inhibition of glucagon release. This suggests that glucagon may play a major role in glucose homeostasis.

Overall changes in plasma glucose closely parallels those of glucagon: A significant decrease in plasma glucose levels occurred with or was preceded by suppression of plasma glucagon levels. Discontinuation of somatostatin resulted in a rapid return to control levels. Koerker et al. (1974) have reported that during infusion of somatostatin in the baboon, hepatic glucose output diminished to zero. Since glucagon functions primarily by stimulating hepatic glycogenolysis (Sokal and Ezdenli, 1967) and gluconeogenesis (Exton and Park, 1968c), one would expect this to occur if the mechanism responsible for the fall in plasma glucose were inhibition of glucagon secretion.

Gerich et al. (1975) recently have suggested that glucagon may be a major contributor to the hyperglycemia observed in diabetes mellitus. In human diabetes, glucagon secretion is inappropriately high relative to the plasma glucose level (Unger and Orci, 1975) and is suppressed by neither hyperglycemia nor large amounts of exogenous insulin (Unger et al., 1972). In Gerich's study (Gerich et al., 1975a), the infusion of somatostatin resulted in a fall in both plasma glucagon and plasma glucose levels in a hypophysectomized diabetic. This observation implies that glucagon may contribute to the maintenance of diabetic hyperglycemia. This being the case, somatostatin could prove useful as an adjunct to insulin in the management of insulin-dependent diabetes.

The downswing of hopes for a therapeutic role for somatostatin has been accelerated by reports of acute thrombocytopenia in baboons (Koerker et al., 1974) and impaired platelet aggregation (Goodner, 1975) with increased concentration of a fibrin degradation product in man. Other drawbacks for the use of somatostatin as a therapeutic modulator are multiple: Somatostatin must be infused; its duration of activity is short; somatostatin is not selective among hormones it inhibits; and somatostatin may induce latent hemorrhage.

Influence of Somatostatin on Insulin Secretion

It has been demonstrated that somatostatin can suppress a glucose-induced increase of plasma insulin concentration (Alberti et al., 1973; Mortimore et al., 1974) and inhibits insulin release from the perfused pancreas (Alberti et al., 1973; Curry et al., 1974; Efendic et al., 1974). However, concerning its direct effect on insulin secretion from the pancreatic islets, there have been two controversial results. While Efendic and co-workers (1974) failed to show the inhibitory effect of somatostatin on insulin secretion from the isolated islet, Oliver and Wagle (1975) reported that the inhibition of insulin release from the islet was demonstrated in experiments with incubation media containing

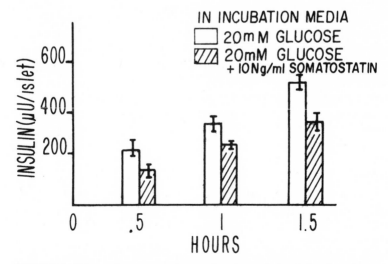

FIGURE 7 Effect of somatostatin on the glucose-induced insulin release from pancreatic islet cells. Adapted from the data reported by Okamoto et al. (1975).

somatostatin concentrations ranging from 0.2 to 100 μg/ml. Okamoto et al. (1975) have recently studied the effect of somatostatin on glucose-induced insulin release by the islets of Langerhans. These results show that somatostatin in concentrations as low as 10 ng/ml inhibited insulin release from the islet and that the somatostatin inhibition of insulin release was completely reversed by increasing the calcium concentration in the incubation medium (Fig. 7). This suggests that the hypothalamic hormone somatostatin exerts a direct action on beta cell insulin release.

Somatostatin is the first agent to be discovered that simultaneously inhibits insulin and glucagon release. When insulin and glucagon secretions are both inhibited by somatostatin, blood glucose concentration falls rather than rises. To ascertain whether somatostatin might act directly by enhancing peripheral glucose uptake, Gerich et al. (1975b) studied its effect *in vitro* on rat hemidiaphragms. Somatostatin had no effect on either basal or insulin-stimulated glucose uptake, thus making it unlikely that the fall in plasma glucose resulted from a direct effect of somatostatin on glucose uptake by peripheral tissues. This has led to the postulation that glucagon may be a vital component in normal glucose balance (Alford et al., 1974; Christensen et al., 1974). The fall in plasma glucose during somatostatin infusion can be ascribed to a concurrent inhibition of glucagon secretion. This provides strong evidence that glucagon normally functions as a glucoregulatory hormone (Gerich et al., 1975a, b).

SUMMARY

The literature cited presents strong support for the hormonal control of metabolic homeostasis. As insulin and glucagon are integral components in the metabolic regulation of glucose balance, it becomes ever more apparent that acute control over carbohydrate metabolism within the body is governed not so much by the absolute concentration of insulin and glucagon, but by the ratio of one hormone, insulin, to another hormone, glucagon. Thus, subtle shifts in the concentration of either hormone through dietary, genetic, or stress manipulation, can elicit drastic changes in the metabolism of carbohydrates.

REFERENCES

Alberti, K., Christensen, M., Hansen, A., Iversen, J., Lundbaek, K., Seyer-Hansen, K. and Orskov, H. 1973. *Lancet* 2:1299.
Alford, F., Bloom, S., Nabarro, J., Hall, R., Besser, G., Coy, D., Kastin, A. and Shally, A. 1974. *Lancet* 2:974.
Anderson, J. and Marks, V. 1973. *Lancet* 1:1962.
Aquilar-Parada, E., Eisentraut, A. M. and Unger, R. H. 1969. *Diabetes* 18:717.
Ariens, E. J. 1966. *Adv. Drug Res.* 3:235.
Berdanier, C. D., Marshall, M. W. and Moser, P. 1971a. *Life Sci.* 10:105.
Berdanier, C. D., Szepesi, B., Moser, P. and Diachenko, S. 1971b. *Proc. Soc. Exp. Med.* 137:668.
Bergman, R. and Bucolo, R. 1974. *Am. J. Physiol.* 227:1314.

Bishop, J., Goldberg, N. and Larner, J. 1971. *Am. J. Physiol.* 220:499.
Bitensky, M. W., Clancy, J. W. and Gomache, E. 1967. *J. Clin. Invest.* 46:1037.
Blazquez, E. and Quijada, C. L. 1968. *J. Endocrinol.* 44:107.
Bruckdorfer, K. R., Khan, I. H. and Yudkin, J. 1972. *Biochem. J.* 129:439.
Brunzell, J. D., Lerner, R. L., Hazzard, W. R., Porter, K., Jr. and Bierman, E. L. 1971. *N. Engl. J. Med.* 284:521.
Buchanan, K. D. and McKiddie, M. T. 1967. *Diabetologia* 3:460.
Butcher, R. W. and Baird, C. E. 1969. In *Drugs affecting lipid metabolism*, ed. C. R. Paoletti, pp. 5–23. New York: Plenum.
Butcher, R. W., Ho, R. J., Meng, H. C. and Sutherland, E. W. 1966. *J. Biol. Chem.* 240:4515.
Caspary, W. F. 1972. In *Na-linked transport of organic solutes,* ed. E. Heinz, pp. 99–110. New York: Springer-Verlag.
Cerasi, E. and Luft, R. 1970. *Horm. Metab. Res.* 2:246.
Chang, M. L. W., Lee, J. A., Schuster, E. M. and Trout, D. L. 1971. *J. Nutr.* 101:323.
Cherrington, A. and Vranic, M. 1974. *Metabolism* 23:729.
Chesney, T. M. C. and Schofield, H. G. 1969. *Diabetes* 18:627.
Christensen, S., Hansen, A., Iverson, J., Lundbaek, K., Orskov, H. and Seyer-Hansen, K. 1974. *Scan. J. Clin. Lab. Invest.* 34:321.
Cohen, A. M., Teitelbaum, A., Balogh, M. and Groen, J. J. 1966. *Am. J. Clin. Nutr.* 19:59.
Conn, J. W. 1940. *Am. J. Med. Sci.* 199:355.
Cook, G. C. and Jacobson, J. 1971. *Br. J. Nutr.* 26:187.
Coore, H. G. and Randle, P. J. 1964. *Biochem. J.* 93:66.
Corbin, J. D., Reiman, E. M., Walsh, D. H. and Krebs, E. G. 1970. *J. Biol. Chem.* 745:4849.
Curnow, R., Rayfield, E., George, D., Zensz, T. and DeRuberts, F. 1975. *Am. J. Physiol.* 228:80.
Curry, D. L., Bennett, L. L. and Grodsky, G. M. 1968. *Endocrinology* 83:572.
Curry, D. L., Curry, K. P. and Gomez, M. 1972. *Endocrinology* 91:1493.
Curry, D. L., Bennett, L. L. and Li, C. H. 1974. *Biochem. Biophys. Res. Commun.* 58:885.
Davidson, M. B. and Berliner, J. B. 1974. *Am. J. Physiol.* 227:79.
Durand, A. M. A., Fisher, M. and Adams, M. 1968. *Arch. Pathol.* 85:318.
Eaton, R. P. and Kipnis, D. M. 1969a. *Am. J. Physiol.* 217:1153.
Eaton, R. P. and Kipnis, D. M. 1969b. *Am. J. Physiol.* 217:1160.
Eaton, R. P., Kipnis, D. M., Karl, I. and Eisenstein, A. B. 1974. *Am. J. Physiol.* 227:101.
Edwards, J. C. and Taylor, K. W. 1970. *Biochim. Biophys. Acta* 215:297.
Edwards, J. C., Taylor, K. W. and Howell, S. L. 1969. *Nature (London)* 224:808.
Edwards, J. C., Hellestrom, C., Peterson, B. and Taylor, B. W. 1972. *Diabetologia* 8:93.
Efendic, S., Luft, R. and Gull, V. 1974. *FEBS Lett.* 42:169.
Eisenstein, A. B. and Strack, I. 1968. *Endocrinology* 83:1337.
Exton, J. H. and Park, C. R. 1968a. *Biochem. Biophys. Res. Commun.* 29:113.
Exton, J. H. and Park, C. R. 1968b. *Adv. Enzyme Reg.* 6:391.
Exton, J. H. and Park, C. R. 1968c. *J. Biol. Chem.* 243:4189.
Exton, J. H. and Park, C. R. 1969. *J. Biol. Chem.* 244:1424.
Exton, J. H., Jefferson, L. S., Butcher, R. W. and Park, C. R. 1966. *Am. J. Med.* 40:704.

Frieden, E. and Lipner, H. 1971. *Biochemical endocrinology of the vertebrates.* Englewood Cliffs, N.J.: Prentice Hall.

Gerich, J. E., Langlois, M., Noacco, C., Karam, J. H. and Forsham, P. H. 1973. *Science* 182:171.

Gerich, J. E., Lorenzi, M. and Schneider, W. 1974a. *N. Engl. J. Med.* 291:544.

Gerich, J. E., Schneider, V., Dippe, S. E., Langlois, M., Noacco, C., Karam, J. H. and Forsham, P. H. 1974b. *J. Clin. Endocrinol. Metab.* 38:77.

Gerich, J. E., Langlois, M., Schneider, V., Karam, J. H. and Noacco, C. 1974c. *J. Clin. Invest.* 53:1284.

Gerich, J. E., Lovinger, R. and Grodsky, G. M. 1974d. Program of the Fifty-Sixth Annual Meeting of the Endocrine Society, Atlanta, June 12–14, p. A-190.

Gerich, J. E., Lorenzi, M., Hane, S., Gustafson, G., Guillemin, R. and Forsham, P. H. 1975a. *Metabolism* 24:175.

Gerich, J. E., Tsalikiam, E., Lorenzi, M., Karam, J. H. and Bier, D. M. 1975b. *J. Clin. Endocrinol. Metab.* 40:526.

Glinsmann, W. H., Hern, E. P. and Lynch, A. 1969. *Am. J. Physiol.* 216:698.

Goodner, C. J. 1975. *N. Engl. J. Med.* 292:1022.

Grodsky, G. M., Karam, J. H., Pavlatos, F. C. and Forsham, P. H. 1965. *Lancet* 1:290.

Haft, D. E. 1967. *Am. J. Physiol.* 213:219.

Hales, C. N. and Kennedy, G. C. 1964. *Biochem. J.* 90:620.

Hers, H. G., DeWulf, H. and VanDenBerger, G. 1969. *Fed. Eur. Biochem. Soc. Symp.* 19:149.

Himsworth, H. P. 1935. *Clin. Sci.* 2:67.

Iverson, J. 1971. *J. Clin. Invest.* 50:2123.

Jefferson, L. S., Exton, J. H., Butcher, R. W., Sutherland, E. W. and Park, C. R. 1968. *J. Biol. Chem.* 242:1031.

Karam, J. H., Grodsky, G. M. and Forsham, P. H. 1963. *Diabetes* 22:197.

Karlson, P. and Serkeris, C. E. 1966. *Acta Endocrinol.* 53:505.

Kaufmann, N. A., Poznanski, R., Blondheim, S. H. and Stein, Y. 1966. *Am. J. Clin. Nutr.* 18:261.

Kelsay, J. L., Behall, K. M., Holden, J. M. and Prather, E. S. 1974. *Am. J. Clin. Nutr.* 27:926.

Koerker, D. J., Goodner, C. J. and Ruch, W. 1974. *N. Engl. J. Med.* 291:262.

Lewis, S. B., Exton, J. H., Ho, R. J. and Park, C. R. 1970. *Fed. Proc.* 29:379. (Abstr.)

Levey, G. S. 1975. *Metabolism* 24:301.

Levey, G. S., Fletcher, M. A., Klein, I., Ruiz, E. and Schenk, A. 1974. *J. Biol. Chem.* 249:2665.

Litwack, G. 1970. *Biochemical actions of hormones.* New York: Academic Press.

Lossow, W. J. and Chaikoff, I. L. 1954. *Arch. Biochem. Biophys.* 57:23.

Lossow, W. J., Brown, G. W. and Chaikoff, I. L. 1956. *J. Biol. Chem.* 220:839.

Luyckx, A. 1972. In *Glucagon, molecular physiology, clinical and therapeutic implications,* ed. P. J. Lefebvre and R. H. Unger, pp. 217–227. Oxford: Pergamon Press Ltd.

Luyckx, A. and Lefebvre, P. J. 1970. *Proc. Soc. Exp. Biol. Med.* 133:524.

Mackrell, D. J. and Sokal, J. E. 1969. *Diabetes* 18:724.

Madison, L. L., Seyffert, W., Unger, R. H. and Barker, B. 1968. *Metabolism* 17:301.

Makman, M. H. and Sutherland, E. W. 1964. *Endocrinology* 75:127.

Malaisse, W., Leclercq-Meyer, V., Malaisse-Lagae, E. and Mahy, M. 1969. *Arch. Int. Physiol. Biochem.* 77:531.

Mallette, L. E., Exton, J. H., Ho, R. J. and Park, C. R. 1969. *J. Biol. Chem.* 244:5713.

McGarry, J. D. and Foster. D. W. 1974. *J. Biol. Chem.* 249:7984.

McGarry, J. D., Wright, P. H. and Foster, D. W. 1975. *J. Clin. Invest.* 55:1209.

Meier, J. M., McGarry, J. D., Faloona, G. R., Unger, R. H. and Foster, D. W. 1972. *J. Lipid Res.* 13:228,

Michaelis, O. E. and Szepesi, B. 1973. *J. Nutr.* 103:697.

Miller, T. B. and Larner, J. 1973. *J. Biol. Chem.* 248:3483.

Mortimore, G. E. and Mondon, C. E. 1970. *J. Biol. Chem.* 245:2375.

Mortimore, C. H., Turnbridge, W. M. G., Carr, D., Yeomann, L., Besser, G. M., Shally, A. V. and Hall, R. 1974. *Lancet* 1:697.

Mueller, P. S., Daugela, M. A. and Heald, F. D. 1965. *Am. J. Clin. Nutr.* 16:256.

Müller, W. A., Faloona, G. R. and Unger, R. H. 1971. *N. Engl. J. Med.* 285:1450.

Newsholme, E. A. and Start, C. 1973. In *Regulation in metabolism,* pp. 252–253. New York: Wiley.

Ohneda, A., Aquilar-Parada, E., Eisentraut, A. M. and Unger, R. H. 1968. *Acta Diabetes Lat.* 1:191.

Okamoto, H., Miyamoto, S., Mabuchi, H. and Takeda, R. 1975. *Biochem. Biophys. Res. Commun.* 59:623.

Oliver, J. R., Wagle, S. R. 1975. *Biochem. Biophys. Res. Commun.* 62:772.

Park, C. R., Lewis, S. B. and Lewis, J. H. 1972. *Diabetes* 21:439.

Parrilla, R., Goodman, M. N. and Toews, C. I. 1974. *Diabetes* 23:725.

Pohl, S. L., Birnbaumer, L. and Rodbell, M. 1969. *Science* 164:566.

Polak, J. M., Pearse, A. G. E., Grimelius, L., Bloom, S. R. and Arimura, A. 1975. *Lancet* 1:1220.

Renold, A. E., Crofford, B. W. and Jeanrenaud, B. 1965. *Diabetologia* 1:4.

Rinard, G. A., Okuma, G., and Hayes, R. C. 1969. *Endocrinology* 84:622.

Robison, G. A., Butcher, R. W. and Sutherland, E. W. 1971a. In *Cyclic AMP,* pp. 232–270. New York: Academic Press.

Robison, G. A., Butcher, R. W. and Sutherland, E. W. 1971b. In *Cyclic AMP,* pp. 298–301. New York: Academic Press.

Rodbell, M., Birnhaumer, L. and Pohl, S. L. 1971. In *The role of adenyl cyclase and cyclic 3′5′-AMP in biological systems,* ed. T. W. Rall and M. Rodbell, pp. 59–103. Washington, D.C.: U.S. Govt. Printing Office.

Ross, B. D., Hems, R. and Krebs, H. A. 1967. *Biochem. J.* 102:942.

Samols, E., Tyler, J. M., Marks, V. and Mialhe, P. 1969. In *Progress in endocrinology,* ed. C. Gaul, p. 184. Amsterdam: Excerpta Medica.

Santeusanio, F., Faloona, G. R., Knochel, J. P. and Unger, R. H. 1973. *J. Lab. Clin. Med.* 81:809.

Siddle, K., Kane-Maguire, B. and Campbell, A. K. 1973. *Biochem. J.* 132:765.

Sokal, J. E. 1966. *Am. J. Med.* 41:331.

Sokal, J. E. and Abdulla, A. 1966. *Am. J. Physiol.* 211:1334.

Sokal, J. E. and Ezdenli, E. Z. 1967. *J. Clin. Invest.* 46:778.

Storm, D. R. and Dolginow, Y. D. 1973. *J. Biol. Chem.* 248:5208.

Swan, D. C., Davidson, P. and Albrink, M. J. 1966. *Lancet* 1:60.

Szanto, S. and Yudkin, J. 1969. *Postgrad. Med. J.* 45:602.

Tata, J. R. 1968. *Nature* 219:331.

Unger, R. H. 1974. *Diabetes* 20:834.

Unger, R. H. and Orci, L. 1975. *Lancet* 1:14.

Unger, R. H., Aquilar-Parada, E. and Müller, W. A. 1970. *J. Clin. Invest.* 49:837.

Unger, R. H., Madison, L. L. and Müller, W. A. 1972. *Diabetes* 21:301.

Vance, J. E., Buchanan, K. D., Challoner, D. R. and Williams, R. H. 1968. *Diabetes* 17:187.

Veech, R., Guynn, R., Lawson, R. and Harris, R. 1973. *Fed. Proc.* 32:935. (Abstr.)

Vrana, A., Slabochova, Z., Kazasova, L. and Fabry, P. 1971. *Nutr. Rep. Intern.* 3:31.

Weinhouse, S. R., Millington, H. and Friedman, B. 1949. *J. Biol. Chem.* 181:489.

Weir, G. C., Knowlton, D. and Martin, D. B. 1974. *J. Clin. Invest.* 54:1403.

Wicks, W. D., Kenney, F. T. and Lee, K. L. 1969. *J. Biol. Chem.* 244:6008.

Yen, S. S. C., Seler, T. M. and DeVane, G. W. 1974. *N. Engl. J. Med.* 290:935.

Chapter 5

METABOLIC CONSEQUENCES OF CARBOHYDRATE-FREE DIETS

Robert W. Boggs

Miami Valley Laboratories
The Procter & Gamble Company
Cincinnati, Ohio

INTRODUCTION

The original carbohydrate-free diet studies were initiated by Donaldson et al. (1957) and Rand et al. (1958), who showed that the growing chick could tolerate high levels of dietary fat. Early unpublished studies by Hill and Renner suggested that triglycerides could completely replace carbohydrate in the diet of the chick without affecting the rate of growth—an observation later confirmed by Renner (1964). In addition, Renner and Elcombe (1964) showed that the removal of glycerol from triglyceride-based, carbohydrate-free diets significantly depressed the growth of chicks. The removal of glycerol from the diet was accomplished by substituting the triglycerides in the diet with free fatty acids.

The term "carbohydrate-free" may have more than one meaning, depending on the reader's point of reference. Diets in which all the nonprotein calories originate from triglycerides have been termed "carbohydrate-free." Diets formulated with fatty acids (devoid of glycerol), thus supplying all the nonprotein calories as fat, are more correctly termed carbohydrate-free diets. High-protein–low-fat diets have also been referred to as carbohydrate-free diets by some investigators. The metabolic consequences of diets composed of triglycerides and fatty acids as sources of nonprotein calories will be discussed in this review. Comparisons to high-protein–low-fat diets will be discussed where the data are relevant to studies using diets composed of triglycerides or fatty acids.

The metabolic consequences of diets devoid of carbohydrate have received limited scientific investigation until recently. This is most probably due to the abundance of commonly used carbohydrate diets. Since the early studies of Renner, similar studies have been conducted in rats (Akrabawi and Hill, 1970; Akrabawi and Salji, 1973; Akrabawi et al., 1974; Goldberg, 1971; Zaragoza-Hermans, 1973).

Carbohydrates have long been thought to be required by the body as a source of energy and for the maintenance of blood glucose. Renner and Elcombe (1964) and Brambila and Hill (1967), both using chickens as experimental animals, have shown that triglycerides could totally replace carbohydrates in the diet without affecting growth or blood glucose. However, replacing a triglyceride-based diet with a fatty acid-based diet results in a marked depression in growth and low blood glucose (hypoglycemia). Supplementing the fatty acid diet with glucose partially reversed the growth depression and hypoglycemia. The results of these studies suggest a specific role for dietary carbohydrates besides that of supplying calories.

The development of carbohydrate-free diets has provided the opportunity to study the effects of chronic carbohydrate insufficiency, ketogenesis, and gluconeogenesis. In other words, carbohydrate-free diets have provided the opportunity to study the metabolic consequences of fasting in an animal that is maintained in the fed state.

Only in the last 10 yr has the scientific community set about to determine whether domestic animals and humans require dietary carbohydrate. Although most current diets (both experimental and practical) contain an abundance of carbohydrate, only recently have experiments been conducted to determine the carbohydrate requirement of domestic animals and humans.

DIETARY STUDIES

A number of different formulations of carbohydrate-free diets have been used to study the metabolic effect of the complete replacement of dietary carbohydrate with fat. Various protein, lipid, and carbohydrate sources have been used in the formulation of these carbohydrate-free diets. The effects of each of these dietary variables will be discussed.

Proteins

The diets used in Renner's (1964) original studies were based on soybean protein isolate. These studies were conducted to determine the role of protein in facilitating the chicken to utilize carbohydrate-free diets where the nonprotein calories were supplied by triglycerides. Renner's diets were formulated to contain 29.0, 24.9, 21.8, 19.3, or 17.4% of the dietary calories as protein. In all dietary studies, fat was substituted isocalorically for the carbohydrate in the diets. In most of the feeding studies cellulose has been added to the carbohydrate-free diets to improve the texture and palatability of the diets. Many investigators have expressed the ratio of nonprotein calories to protein calories differently; Table 1 summarizes the various ratios.

Various diets have been used with differing protein concentrations and caloric densities. The caloric content of all diets fed to chickens has had an energy content of between 3,500 and 4,500 kcal of metabolizable energy per

TABLE 1   Different Means of Expressing the Calories-to-Protein
Ratio Used by Various Investigators Studying
Carbohydrate-Free Diets

Investigator	kcal ME[a]/ kg diet	kcal ME/ g protein	% protein in diet	% calories from protein
Renner	3,720	11.0	33.8	34.8
		13.2	28.2	29.0
		15.4	24.1	24.9
		17.6	21.1	21.8
		19.8	18.8	19.3
		22.0	16.9	17.4
Brambila and Hill	4,029	12.0	33.6	32.0
Evans and Scholz	3,564	15.6	22.9	24.5
Goldberg	4,000	17.0	23.5	25.0
Madappally et al.	3,482	18.4	18.95	21.7
	(carbohydrate diet)			
	4,481	19.0	23.6	21.1
	(high-fat diet)			
Boggs	4,000	17.6	22.6	22.6
		14.9	26.8	26.8
		12.0	30.9	30.9
Brant	4,000	19.9	20.1	21.6
Akrabawi et al.	4,100	19.0	21.7	22.4
	4,095	18.8	21.7	22.7
Allred and Roehrig	4,029	12.0	33.6	32.0

[a]ME, metabolizable energy.

kilogram diet. Renner's (1964) original studies showed that the complete substitution of triglyceride for carbohydrate in the diet of growing chickens resulted in equivalent growth. In addition, Renner demonstrated that neither growth nor nitrogen retention decreased when triglycerides were substituted isocalorically for glucose in diets containing various levels of dietary protein. There was, as would be expected, a decrease in growth as the level of protein was decreased, in either the carbohydrate-free or -containing diet. Using rate of growth as a criterion, Renner concluded from her studies that the protein requirement for chickens fed carbohydrate-free diets was no greater than for chickens fed diets containing carbohydrate. This conclusion was confirmed by Brambila and Hill (1966) who, using a slightly different experimental design and dietary formulation, also found that the chicken utilizes a high-fat diet (soybean oil) as efficiently as a carbohydrate-based (glucose) diet. These conclusions were based on growth and nitrogen retention. As a result of these early observations many investigators (Allred, 1969; Allred and Roehrig, 1970; Boggs, 1970; Brant, 1971; Madappally et al., 1971) have corroborated these findings:

complete substitution of the dietary carbohydrate with triglyceride results in comparable growth for the growing chicken.

Although some studies have been conducted in rats to determine the consequences of replacing the dietary carbohydrate with triglyceride, only Goldberg (1971) and Hill et al. (1973) have reported the effect on growth when dietary carbohydrate is replaced with dietary triglyceride. Their studies show that the effect is similar to that found in the chicken—namely, a very slight reduction in growth when triglyceride is substituted.

Since dietary triglycerides can serve as a partial source of carbohydrate (glycerol), experiments have been directed at formulating a totally carbohydrate-free diet. This was accomplished by substituting the triglyceride-based diet with a fatty acid-based diet. Investigators have formulated such diets using soybean oil fatty acid (SOFA) or other sources of fatty acids such as oleic acid, thereby constructing a totally carbohydrate-free diet.

Many investigators (Allred and Roehrig, 1970; Boggs, 1970; Brambila and Hill, 1966; Brant, 1971; Renner and Elcombe, 1964) have shown that dietary replacement of triglycerides with fatty acids reduces growth considerably. Depending on the level of dietary protein, growth can be reduced by as much as one-half of comparable triglyceride-fed animals. Renner and Elcombe (1967a) compared the effect on growth in chickens fed graded levels of dietary protein in which nonprotein energy was supplied entirely by triglycerides (soybean oil) or fatty acid (SOFA) and showed a marked depression in growth at each protein level when fatty acids were substituted for triglycerides.

Brambila and Hill (1966) reported that young growing chickens fed a fatty acid-based diet had a decreased nitrogen retention after 4 wk of dietary treatment. Nitrogen retention measured after 2 wk of dietary treatment was not different from that recorded for the chickens fed the triglyceride- or glucose-based diets. This lowered nitrogen retention after 4 wk of treatment suggests that a time relationship is required to deplete the chickens' protein reserves before nitrogen retention can be affected.

Only a limited number of studies have been conducted examining the utilization of dietary protein in rats when carbohydrate-free diets are fed. Hill et al. (1973) measured net protein utilization (NPU) in rats fed graded levels of casein protein, from 6 to 30% of the dietary energy. Replacing dietary carbohydrate with triglyceride reduced the NPU by approximately 10%. Substitution of fatty acids for triglycerides resulted in a further lowering of the NPU. The reduction in NPU depends on the level of dietary protein. In addition, these authors suggested that the protein requirement for the rat is increased when rats are fed fatty acid diets compared with those receiving a carbohydrate-containing diet. This observation confirmed Brambila and Hill's (1967) findings that the chickens' requirement for protein is increased when fatty acids are used as the source of nonprotein calories.

Brambila and Hill (1967) added glucose or glycerol to the triglyceride-based diets with no effect on growth or nitrogen retention. To the contrary, adding either glucose or glycerol to the fatty acid-based diets of chickens resulted in a marked improvement in the growth.

Renner and Elcombe (1967a) claimed that the addition of 3% dietary glycerol to a fatty acid diet improves growth, equaling the growth of chickens fed a triglyceride diet. This result is contrary to that reported by Brambila and Hill (1967) who conducted a similar experiment in chickens. Growth was significantly improved by adding glycerol or glucose to the fatty acid diet but did not equal that of the triglyceride diet.

Renner and Elcombe (1964) showed that the growth of chickens fed a fatty acid diet was improved by the addition of 6% dietary glucose. At this level of glucose supplementation the growth of the chickens fed a fatty acid diet approached that of triglyceride-fed chickens. Brambila and Hill (1967) reported that considerably more dietary glucose (between 18 and 30% of the calories) must be added to the fatty acid diets to produce growth equivalent to triglyceride-fed chickens. Both the studies of Renner and Elcombe and those of Brambila and Hill have clearly shown that glucose and glycerol are equally effective in improving the growth of fatty acid-fed chickens.

Glucose Equivalents of Dietary Protein

The effectiveness of dietary protein in promoting growth of chickens and rats fed carbohydrate-free (fatty acid) diets has been investigated. These studies have led to conflicting conclusions regarding the carbohydrate equivalency of dietary proteins. Studies by Wolfberg (1876) predicted that approximately 50% of an average protein can be converted to carbohydrate under appropriate metabolic conditions. Renner and Elcombe (1967a) suggested that soybean protein was 6-19% as effective as glucose in promoting the growth of chickens fed fatty acid diets. These authors concluded that the carbohydrate requirement of the chicken could be met by protein but that protein was much less efficient than glucose in meeting this requirement. In somewhat different studies Boggs (1970) concluded that dietary casein was 56% as effective as glucose in improving the growth of chickens fed a fatty acid diet. This response approaches the theoretical glucose equivalency of casein when the amino acid composition is used to calculate glucose equivalents.

The glucose yield from a protein was determined by calculating a theoretical glucose yield from each amino acid derived from the protein. Glucose yield from each amino acid was based on the number of carbon atoms that could be metabolically converted to glucose. The calculated glucose equivalent for casein is 64.9 g glucose/100 g casein protein. Boggs (1970) fed graded levels of dietary casein (19.2, 22.6, 26.8, and 30.9%) to chickens maintained on fatty acid diets. These diets were formulated so that the essential amino acid requirements of the chicken were met at each protein level. This was accomplished by calculating the amount of essential amino acids provided by the dietary casein and supplementing the diet with an amount of each essential amino acid necessary to meet the chickens' requirement. The graded levels of dietary protein used by Boggs were chosen because each dietary increment of protein was calculated to theoretically yield 3 g glucose from amino acids/100 g diet consumed.

Significant improvement in body weight was produced by each protein increment when glucose was absent from the diet. Addition of glucose to the fatty acid diets produced a significant growth response at the three lowest levels of dietary protein, but no increase in growth was noted when the diet contained 30.0% protein. This result agrees with those of Renner and Elcombe (1967a) who also showed that glucose added to a 34% protein diet produced no increase in growth. Boggs (1970) concluded that the maximum growth response to glucose was obtained when either 19.2 or 22.6% dietary protein as casein was used in the fatty acid diets. In the presence of 3% dietary glucose, no significant improvement in growth could be realized when the protein level was increased above 22.6% of the diet.

Boggs (1970) also calculated a glucose equivalency of 0.56 g of glucose/g protein from dietary casein using growth as the criterion. Lusk (1928), experimenting with phlorizinized dogs, determined the glucose yield from casein was 0.58 g glucose/g protein. Janney (1915) reported a value of 0.48 g glucose/g casein protein. The slight differences between the values reported by Boggs, Lusk, and Janney may be a function of the purity of the casein protein and differences due to the animal models used. In retrospect, the values are surprisingly close considering the diversity of techniques used. The considerably lowered glucose equivalents Renner and Elcombe (1967a) reported for soybean protein (0.6–0.19 g glucose/g protein) most likely is due to the level of protein used and the quality of the protein.

Renner and Elcombe (1967a) used a diet containing 24.9% protein, a level of dietary protein that Boggs (1970) found to result in a very limited response to added dietary glucose. Therefore, the added protein or glucose was possibly in excess of the chickens' requirements for protein, thereby decreasing the full expression of the glucogenic potential of the soybean protein.

Glucose Equivalents of Dietary Amino Acids

Using a carbohydrate-free (fatty acid) diet Boggs and Hill (1971) studied the glucogenic properties of various dietary amino acids. Differences in the rate of production of glucose from amino acids would seem reasonable considering the interplay of enzymes involved in the metabolism of amino acids prior to their entry into the tricarboxylic acid (TCA) cycle and ultimately the metabolism to glucose by means of gluconeogenesis. Boggs and Hill studied nine amino acids, the choice based on the intermediary products through which each amino acid entered the TCA cycle. (The metabolite entry point into the TCA cycle for each amino acid is depicted by enclosure in parentheses.)

Alanine (pyruvate) and valine (propionyl CoA) added to a fatty acid-based diet resulted in body weight gain in chickens equal to those chickens fed an equivalent amount of dietary glucose. L-aspartic (oxalacetate) resulted in an intermediate growth response, not significantly different from the basal (fatty acid) diet. L-histidine (succinate) and L-isoleucine (propionyl CoA) yielded no improvement in growth when compared with the basal diet. Tyrosine (malate) gave a growth response somewhat less than the basal fatty acid-based diet, but not significantly different. L-threonine (propionyl CoA), L-methionine (propionyl-CoA), and L-leucine produced a growth response significantly less than the basal diet. The response to threonine and methionine is unexpected. Threonine has been classified as a glucogenic amino acid by a number of investigators (Butts et al., 1938; Hall et al., 1940; Krebs, 1964). Methionine has been classified as both glucogenic and ketogenic by different authors (Harper, 1969; Krebs, 1964). The reduced growth seen by Boggs and Hill (1971) in the chickens given methionine was probably due to a toxic level of dietary methionine since it was added to the diet at a level of 2.83%.

Akrabawi and Hill (1970) fed rats a 12–15% casein diet and used growth, plasma glucose, and plasma ketone bodies as the criteria to quantitate the glucose equivalency of various dietary amino acids. They found alanine, arginine, glycine, histidine, and isoleucine to be 100–150% as effective as glucose. Phenylalanine, serine, threonine, tryptophan, tyrosine, and valine were between 50 and 90% as effective as glucose; cysteine, cystine, leucine, lysine, and methionine were ineffective and thus nonglucogenic when fed in a carbohydrate-free diet. Renner (1969) quantitated the glucose equivalents of various amino acids added to the diet of chickens fed a carbohydrate-free diet composed of amino acids and triglyceride. These studies showed that the chickens' requirement for glutamic acid was increased when carbohydrate was deleted from the diet. In addition, L-aspartic acid was shown to be as effective as L-glutamic in providing nonessential nitrogen to a carbohydrate-free diet.

Glucose Equivalents of Dietary Carbohydrates

Boggs (1970) measured the growth response of chickens fed graded levels of glucose added to a fatty acid diet. In this study 1.5–30% glucose was added to the fatty acid–casein-based diet. The growth response of the chickens was a linear increase from 0 to 3% added dietary glucose. A second linear increase in growth was noted between 3 and 30% added dietary glucose. Brambila and Hill (1967) conducted a similar study with a higher dietary protein level (33.6% soybean protein) and observed an analogous linear increase in growth as increasing amounts of glucose were added to the diet. Brambila and Hill observed a maximum response at 30% dietary glucose.

Akrabawi et al. (1974) demonstrated a similar response in young growing rats when starch was added in graded levels to a fatty acid-based diet. The maximum growth response to dietary starch was attained when starch composed 1.87% of the diet. Some conflict is in evidence between the data and the conclusions of these authors. One experiment suggests that the maximum growth response to dietary starch is between 15 and 30% while another experiment suggests that 2% produces the maximum response. Akrabawi et al.

have shown that the decreased weight gain resulting from feeding fatty acid diets to rats was due to a reduced food intake. This was shown by pair-feeding experiments in which carbohydrate-containing diets were pair-fed to a fatty acid-based diet. The growth patterns were essentially identical when the intake of the carbohydrate diet equaled that of the fatty acid diet.

EFFECT OF CARBOHYDRATE–FREE DIETS ON METABOLITE CONCENTRATION

Blood Glucose

A number of investigators have fed carbohydrate-free diets and measured the variable responses in blood glucose concentrations in both chickens and rats. Brambila and Hill (1966) concluded that triglyceride-based diets did not decrease blood glucose in chickens samples in the postabsorptive state. Blood glucose was reduced in those chickens fed a fatty acid diet sampled in the postabsorptive state. The addition of a small amount of glucose to the diet restored blood glucose levels to those observed in the chickens fed a triglyceride- or high-carbohydrate-based diet. Unfortunately, the effect of fasting was not studied in these dietary treatments. Previous studies would suggest that the fasting of animals fed a glucose-supplemented, fatty acid-based diet resulted in blood glucose concentrations that parallel animals fed a triglyceride- or carbohydrate-based diet. Brambila and Hill (1967) suggested that chickens fed a fatty acid-based diet increased their blood glucose concentration during fasting, while chickens previously fed a carbohydrate- or triglyceride-based diet decreased their blood glucose concentration when fasted.

The effect of fatty acid diets on the blood glucose concentration of rats maintained in the fed state has produced variable responses. Akrabawi and Hill (1970) reported a hypoglycemia in rats fed fatty acid diets compared with those fed a carbohydrate-containing diet. Akrabawi et al. (1974) confirmed this lowered blood glucose level in response to feeding fatty acid diets. Goldberg (1971) was unable to show a significant difference in blood glucose as a result of feeding fatty acids, triglyceride, or carbohydrate diets. Akrabawi and Salji (1973) also were unable to show a difference in the blood glucose concentration of rats fed either fatty acid diets or triglyceride diets. This lack of difference in blood glucose concentrations between rats fed fatty acid- and triglyceride-based diets is not unusual as Renner and Elcombe (1967b) were also unable to demonstrate a difference in the blood glucose of chickens fed similar diets. The conflicting results regarding the lowering of blood glucose in rats fed fatty acid diets is unexplainable at present. Some authors have attributed the variable blood glucose effect to the level of protein in the diet; however, no consistent trend seems to be apparent at this time.

Renner and Elcombe (1967b) have been unable to show a reduction of blood glucose when feeding a fatty acid diet to chickens. Brambila and Hill

(1967) reported that the blood glucose concentration of chickens fasted 18 hr was similar whether a high carbohydrate, triglyceride, or fatty acid diet had been fed. The blood glucose of chickens fed a high-carbohydrate diet or a triglyceride diet decreased during a fast, while the blood glucose of chickens fed a fatty acid diet increased as a function of fasting. This increase in blood glucose as a result of fasting is in sharp contrast to the usual response to fasting when high-carbohydrate diets are consumed. The important observation resulting from these studies is the lower blood glucose concentration of chickens sampled in the absorptive state and previously fed a fatty acid-based diet, compared with chickens fed a carbohydrate diet. When starved, the fatty acid-fed chickens increase their blood glucose, while the carbohydrate-fed chickens decreased their blood glucose levels.

These observations show that there was an increased glucose demand in the fed state as compared with fasting, which is an inverse relationship vis-à-vis rats fed a normal high carbohydrate diet. Hill et al. (1974) investigated the turnover of glucose in fasting rats previously fed fatty acid diets and concluded that a net synthesis of liver glycogen occurred in the first 24 hr of fasting, with little or no degradation of glycogen occurring during this period. This observation adds to the suggestion that fatty acid-fed animals have a higher glucose demand in the fed state than in the fasting state.

By means of the glucose tolerance technique Goldberg (1971) investigated glucose utilization in rats fed fatty acid-based diets. She concluded that glucose tolerance was impaired and the metabolic state resembled a mild diabetic— namely, increased gluconeogenesis and decreased utilization of glucose. Goldberg (1971) was unable to detect differences in pancreatic insulin-like activity in rats fed carbohydrate-free diets.

In summary, the response of blood glucose to fasting in rats is now confused. Hill et al. (1974) reported an increase in blood glucose as a result of fasting when a fatty acid diet was fed. Akrabawi et al. (1974) showed a decrease in the concentration of blood glucose in both the fatty acid and carbohydrate-fed rats as a consequence of fasting 18 hr. The reason for this conflict seems unexplainable since similar diet formulation and similar sources of protein were used in each of the studies.

The addition of graded levels of glucose to the diet results in a significant increase in postabsorptive blood glucose. Graded additions of dietary protein to fatty acid-based diets increased blood glucose but to a limited extent. Studies by Boggs (1970), using chickens, showed that blood glucose could be increased more efficiently by adding graded levels of glucose to the diet than by increasing the amount of protein in the diet.

Ketone Bodies

A number of investigators have studied the effect of carbohydrate-free diets on ketone body concentrations in the blood and urine of experimental animals (Akrabawi and Hill, 1970; Akrabawi et al., 1974; Allred and Roehrig,

1969; Brambila and Hill, 1966; Boggs, 1970; Boggs and Hill, 1971; Brant, 1971; Renner, 1964; Renner and Elcombe, 1967a, b). Furthermore, some investigators have studied the metabolic pathways involved in ketone body synthesis and oxidation as a result of feeding animals carbohydrate-free diets. As stated previously, Brambila and Hill (1966) initially showed that chickens fed carbohydrate-free diets (fatty acid-based diets) became ketonemic. The degree of ketosis of the chickens fed free fatty acids was much higher than that seen in chickens fed a triglyceride-based diet. These investigators showed that the level of ketone bodies in the blood of chickens fed fatty acid diets increased approximately tenfold above that of the high-carbohydrate diet. The animals fed a triglyceride-based diet had a ketonemia approximately two and one-half times that of the carbohydrate-fed animals. Brambila and Hill (1966) also showed that the severe ketonemia could be prevented when as little as 6% dietary glucose was supplemented to the fatty acid-based diet. Finally, Brambila and Hill (1966) showed that the major ketone body in the chicken was β-hydroxybutyrate. The marked ketosis found in the chicken was contrary to the generally accepted view that the chicken is not susceptible to ketosis. The magnitude of the ketonemia induced by the high-fatty acid diet is comparable to that reported for ketotic cows, ewes, sows (Sampson, 1947), and fasting ducks (Mirsky et al., 1942). Renner and Elcombe (1967b) also noted a similar increase in blood ketone bodies in chickens fed a high-fatty acid-based diet. Their data showed four- to sevenfold increase, rather than a tenfold increase in blood ketone bodies. These differences in absolute blood ketone body concentrations may be caused by the level of dietary protein fed to the animals. Boggs (1970) has shown that increasing the protein content of the diet resulted in a significant reduction in blood ketone body concentration, but had no effect on increasing blood glucose concentration or liver glycogen concentration. These observations suggest that the amino acids from dietary protein may supply substrates (intermediates of the TCA cycle) that enhance the oxidation of ketone bodies but do not yield sufficient carbon intermediates for the synthesis of glucose or liver glycogen. The abolition of ketonemia by dietary glucose supplementation was also shown by Renner and Elcombe (1967b). These workers also studied the metabolic dynamics of blood ketone bodies in chickens fed fatty acid-based diets and showed that total blood ketone bodies of the chicken increased as a function of fasting time. However, the increases in blood ketone bodies brought about by fasting for 24 or 48 hr were much smaller in magnitude than the increases brought about in starved (24–48 hr) chickens fed either a carbohydrate- or triglyceride-based diet. Comparable values for rats fed diets in which the nonprotein energy was supplied by either carbohydrate or triglyceride have been reported by Roberts et al. (1944). In addition, similar results reported by Azar and Bloom (1963) suggest that the blood ketone body concentration of chickens fed a carbo-hydrate diet is higher than rats and humans fed a carbohydrate diet.

Boggs (1970) has shown that supplementing a carbohydrate-free diet with glucose resulted in significant decreases in plasma ketone bodies in chickens. The level of plasma ketone bodies in chickens fed a glucose-free diet was always significantly greater than that in chickens fed glucose supplemented diets. Boggs (1970) concluded that increasing levels of dietary glucose added to any of the protein diets (22.6, 27.8, or 30.9%) produced a progressive decrease in the level of plasma ketone bodies. Interestingly, the plasma glucose followed a more linear response to dietary glucose than did the plasma ketone bodies. The addition of increasing levels of protein without additional glucose resulted in a significant decrease in plasma ketone bodies at each protein level tested. A maximum response was noted between 31 and 35% dietary protein. Adding as little as 3% glucose to the diet reduced the ketone body concentration in the blood so that additions of dietary protein produced no further reduction in ketone body concentration. Boggs (1971) reported that 15% glucose must be added to a fatty acid-based diet to reduce the ketone body concentration to the level observed in chickens fed a high carbohydrate diet.

Akrabawi and Hill (1970) reported a similar finding for blood ketone bodies in rats fed fatty acid-based diets. In these studies rats fed a fatty acid-based diet, with casein as the source of dietary protein, showed a marked ketonemia. These rats responded with a marked reduction in blood ketone bodies when 3–4% glucose was added to the diet. When Akrabawi and Salji (1973) compared the blood ketone body concentration of rats fed either a fatty acid- or triglyceride-based diet, they were unable to show a difference. This is contrary to the results reported by Akrabawi and Hill (1970) and Goldberg (1971). This inconsistency may result from the level of dietary protein used by the different investigators. Akrabawi and Hill (1970) used a 15% casein diet; Akrabawi and Salji (1973) used a 20% casein diet. In a later study with rats Akrabawi et al. (1974) were able to show an increase in plasma ketone bodies when a fatty acid-based dietary treatment was compared with a carbohydrate-based dietary treatment. Although these investigators encountered considerable variability in the plasma ketone body concentrations, they confirmed the observation that a marked ketonemia does occur in rats when a fatty acid-based diet is fed. Akrabawi et al. (1974) have suggested that rats fed a fatty acid-based diet adjust to fasting in a manner similar to that observed in rats fed a carbohydrate-based diet. These adjustments to fasting by rats fed a fatty acid-based diet included increases in the concentration of plasma ketone bodies. Although these increases were significant, the changes in those animals fed the fatty acid-based diets were much less as a result of fasting than were those fed carbohydrate-based diets. Rats fed a carbohydrate-based diet and then fasted, showed a fourfold increase in plasma ketone bodies; by comparison, rats fed a fatty acid-based diet showed a two and one-half times increase in plasma ketone bodies as a result of fasting.

These responses of rats to fasting after having been fed a fatty acid-based diet appear to be in direct contrast to those of the chickens fed similar diets. This observation suggests that further work is needed in rats and chickens fed fatty acid-based diets. It may be informative to determine the effect of starvation on ketone body concentrations and on the β-hydroxybutyrate and acetoacetate ratios.

Allred and Roehrig (1969) have conducted the most extensive study of ketogenesis in chickens fed carbohydrate-free diets. The investigators, studying chickens maintained on a carbohydrate-free (fatty acid) diet measured the concentrations of several metabolites in liver, frozen *in situ* by means of the freeze clamp technique. A general increase in those compounds was found to be associated with ketogenesis and a general decrease in precursors of glucose, including citrate. Feeding fatty acid-based diets resulted in decreased NAD/NADH ratio in liver without a concomitant decrease in oxaloacetate content or a rise in ATP/ADP ratios. In the absence of any significant dietary effect on the specific activity of the acetoacetate synthetic system, citrate synthase, or citrate cleavage enzyme, it is proposed that the utilization of acetyl-CoA shifts from the normal oxidative pathway to the ketogenic pathway when the carbohydrate-free diets are fed. The reasoning for this conclusion is based on the fact that acetyl-CoA is transported out of the mitochondria to the cytoplasm, where acetoacetate synthesis occurs in chicken liver.

That the NAD/NADH ratio decreases in chickens fed carbohydrate-free diets is in disagreement with those metabolic conditions that stimulate gluconeogenesis and ketogenesis in both chickens (Allred and Roehrig, 1969) and rats (Krebs, 1966). The control of the concentration of mitochondrial NADH is undoubtedly very complex because there are several mechanisms whereby electrons are removed from mitochondria. Electrons can be transported to the cytoplasm by the malate-oxalacetate and the α-glycerolphosphate dihydroxy acetone shuttles that decrease the cytoplasmic NAD/NADH ratio. The formation and subsequent diffusion of β-hydroxybutyrate into blood also removes electrons from the mitochondria. Despite increased removal of electrons by these mechanisms, carbohydrate-free diets fed to chickens resulted in a decreased NAD/NADH ratio in mitochondria. From equilibrium considerations a decreased NAD/NADH ratio would be expected to increase ATP/ADP ratios in liver; however, analysis of liver extracts from chickens fed carbohydrate-free diets showed no apparent correlation between redox state and ATP or ADP content. Since diet has been shown to influence oxidative phosphorylation, the possibility was considered by Allred and Roehrig (1970) that feeding carbo-hydrate-free diets may adversely affect either the rate or efficiency of oxidative phosphorylation. The rate of oxidation of NADH and NADH-like substrates, as well as succinate, by mitochondria isolated from the liver of chickens fed either a carbohydrate control diet or diets in which all nonprotein calories are provided by fatty acids were studied. The results of these studies indicate that the shift in NAD/NADH ratio cannot be attributed to a mitochondrial lesion. In these studies Allred and Roehrig showed that feeding carbohydrate-free diets to chickens resulted in an increase in the rate of oxidation of NADH in uncoupled mitochondria. An increase in mitochondria protein in response to feeding a fatty acid diet was also noted.

These studies suggest that chickens fed fatty acid-based diets have an altered mitochondrial metabolism that is worthy of further studies to elucidate the mechanisms of these alterations.

Glycogen

Liver and muscle glycogen have been measured in both chickens and rats fed carbohydrate-free diets. Contrary to expectation, Brambila and Hill (1966) showed a reduced concentration of liver glycogen in postabsorptive chickens fed carbohydrate-free diets, compared with carbohydrate-fed chickens. Addition of dietary glucose to the fatty acid-based diet caused an increase in liver glycogen when assayed in the postabsorptive state. This increase in liver glycogen did not approach that of chickens fed a glucose-based reference diet or a triglyceride-based diet. Feeding a triglyeride-based diet reduced liver glycogen by one-third compared with the carbohydrate diet.

Renner and Elcombe (1967b) also reported a significant reduction in liver glycogen when dietary calories from glucose were replaced by triglyceride calories. The concentration of liver glycogen was reduced still further when glycerol was deleted from the diet by substituting fatty acids for dietary triglyceride. These results suggest that gluconeogenesis in the chicken is not of sufficient magnitude to maintain liver glycogen when a carbohydrate-free diet is fed.

This apparent lack of sufficient gluconeogenesis for the maintenance of liver glycogen in the chicken was confirmed by Boggs (1970) who showed that increasing the level of protein of a fatty acid-based diet from 19 to 31% had no effect on the liver glycogen concentration. On the other hand, adding 3% dietary glucose to the fatty acid diet resulted in significant increase in liver glycogen at each of the protein levels. Brant (1971) has also shown that adding dietary protein to a fatty acid-based diet does not increase liver glycogen at each protein level.

Akrabawi et al. (1974) showed a decrease in liver glycogen as fatty acids were substituted for carbohydrate in the diet of rats. These results are similar to those reported for chickens by other investigators (Boggs, 1970; Brambila and Hill, 1966; Brant, 1971; Renner and Elcombe, 1967b). The effect of fasting on liver glycogen in response to carbohydrate-free diets was also investigated by Akrabawi et al. (1974). Although these rats were fed for only 12 hr daily, vs. an *ad libitum* regime used in the chicken experiments, the rats fed the fatty acid-based diets then fasted 18 hr did not utilize appreciable amounts of liver glycogen. Using a similar feeding regime, rats fed a carbohydrate (starch)-based diet, then fasted (18 hr) had a significant reduction in liver glycogen. These results suggest that the fatty acid-fed rat is already in the fasting state metabolically and thus can adapt more readily to the absence of food than can a rat fed a carbohydrate-based diet.

Boggs (1970) has shown that in chickens fed a fatty acid-based diet, the increase in liver glycogen appears to depend on the level of blood glucose concentration. The concentration of liver glycogen did not increase until the blood glucose levels approached 170 mg/100 ml or greater. When the blood glucose level was below 170 mg/100 ml the liver glycogen level did not increase. Further studies are necessary to delineate this relationship between blood glucose and liver glycogen levels. The use of radio-labeled glucose could be used to follow the metabolic dynamics between the concentration of blood glucose and the synthesis of glycogen by the liver. In contrast to the liver, Renner and Elcombe (1967b) have shown that the glycogen content of chicken muscle is not altered significantly by replacing dietary glucose with either triglyceride or fatty acids. These results indicate that the chicken does not deplete muscle glycogen as a result of a demand for carbohydrate elsewhere in the body. Zinnemann et al. (1966) have made a similar observation in other species.

Free Fatty Acids

The effect of carbohydrate-free diets on free fatty acid concentration has been studied in chickens. Allred and Roehrig (1969) demonstrated that fatty acid diets increase liver free fatty acid levels approximately twofold when compared with chickens fed a carbohydrate-containing diet. This increase in liver free fatty acids was paralleled by a similar twofold increase in acetyl-CoA concentration. Chickens fed a triglyceride-based diet also exhibited an intermediate concentration of liver free fatty acids and acetyl-CoA.

Boggs (1970) studied the plasma free fatty acid concentrations of a mature chicken fed first a carbohydrate-free diet then a carbohydrate-containing diet. He found an increase in plasma free fatty acids when the chicken was fed a carbohydrate-free diet. Replacing the fatty acid-based diet with a glucose-based diet resulted in a lowering of plasma free fatty acids. Allred and Roehrig (1970) were unable to show a difference in plasma free fatty acid concentration as a result of feeding a carbohydrate-free diet. These authors did show an increase in total plasma lipids when a carbohydrate-free diet was fed to young growing chickens.

A limited number of studies have been conducted to ascertain the effect of carbohydrate-free diets on tissue and plasma free fatty acid concentrations. Studies designed to compare the consequences of feeding a carbohydrate-containing with a carbohydrate-free diet on plasma free fatty acids have the potential of delineating the effect of dietary carbohydrate on the metabolism of fatty acids.

Plasma Amino Acids

Boggs (1970) measured the effect of feeding carbohydrate-free diets on plasma amino acids in growing chickens and concluded that adding glucose to these diets resulted in changes in the plasma amino acid profile. Generally, dietary substitution of fatty acids for carbohydrate resulted in a decrease in plasma alanine and glycine and an increase in valine, isoleucine, leucine, proline, aspartic acid, and glutamic acid. Boggs (1970) also noted that the total concentration of amino acids in the plasma was altered by dietary treatment.

Chickens fed a carbohydrate diet had the lowest concentration of total plasma amino acids, while those chickens fed the fatty-acid diet had the highest concentration of total plasma amino acids. Adding graded levels of glucose to the diet resulted in a reduction in the concentration of total plasma amino acids. This effect of dietary carbohydrate on lowering plasma amino acids is similar to that obtained by other investigators.

Lusk (1928) and Munro et al. (1959) experimenting with rats and Zinneman et al. (1966) experimenting with humans showed that dietary carbohydrate stimulated an increase in the uptake of amino acids by the muscle. This stimulation by dietary glucose is most likely due to the well-known response to insulin secretion that induces an equilibration of amino acids from the blood to the muscle. A similar effect, a lowering of total plasma amino acids, was noted in the chickens when glucose (dietary carbohydrate) was added to a carbohydrate-free (fatty acid-based) diet. The lowering of plasma amino acids in animals fed fatty acid-based diets probably is not due to insulin activity since Goldberg (1971) showed that insulin-like activity was not affected by feeding fatty acid-based diets to rats. The reduction in plasma amino acids is most likely due to an increased demand for gluconeogenic substrates and thus the utilization of amino acids as precursors of glucose.

Adding glucose to the diet of the chicken results in an increase in plasma alanine concentration. A decrease in plasma alanine when carbohydrate-free diets are fed to chickens suggests that alanine is being used to maintain body glucose as suggested by Felig et al. (1970). Plasma glycine also decreased when fatty acid-based diets were fed, suggesting that the metabolism of glycine was involved in the maintenance of blood glucose. In chickens, plasma serine also decreased during dietary carbohydrate insufficiency. Since serine can be metabolically interconverted to glycine perhaps such a conversion can explain the decrease in plasma glycine. The increase in plasma concentrations of threonine, glutamic acid, and tyrosine when fatty acid diets were fed may result from two regulatory mechanisms. It appears that tyrosine is not utilized for the maintenance of blood glucose by the chicken (Boggs, 1971), suggesting a limited gluconeogenic potential for tyrosine and thus the increase in plasma when fatty acid diets were fed. The increase in plasma threonine and glutamic acid appear to be due to an effect of dietary lipid rather than a dietary carbohydrate insufficiency, since adding triglyceride to the diet also caused an increase in these two amino acids.

Boggs (1970) found that plasma hydroxypyroline was affected by the presence of glucose in the diet. When carbohydrate was added to the diet of chickens fed a fatty acid-based ration, the concentration of plasma hydroxyproline decreased in alloxan-diabetic rats. Their studies allowed them to conclude that the diabetic rat was unable to hydroxylate proline, suggesting that the maturation of collagen was insulin dependent. The lowered hydroxyproline concentration noted in the plasma of chickens fed a carbohydrate-free diet may be a function of a decreased insulin response resulting from the lack of carbohydrate in the diet. Although Goldberg (1971) showed that fatty acid diets do not lower pancreatic insulin-like activity, the blood insulin concentration may be the more important parameter to measure since dietary carbohydrate induces insulin secretion by the pancreas. Since fatty acid diets are devoid of carbohydrate, stimulation of insulin secretion is probably absent and thereby the concentration of circulating insulin following a meal is low. This suggests that insulin plays a role in the regulation of plasma hydroxyproline in chickens fed fatty acid-based diets. This result suggests the need for further experimentation to determine plasma insulin concentrations in chickens fed carbohydrate-free diets. The hydroxyproline–proline relationship suggested by Brown and Liddy (1970) is further supported by the work of Boggs (1970) who also noted a decrease in plasma proline concentration as carbohydrate is added to the diet.

EFFECT OF CARBOHYDRATE-FREE DIETS ON ENZYMES RELATED TO VARIOUS METABOLIC PATHWAYS

Gluconeogenesis

Animals fed a carbohydrate-free diet would be expected to increase the synthesis of glucose in order to maintain a homeostatic blood glucose concentration. To this end, the liver plays an important role in regulating blood glucose by controlling the enzymes in the gluconeogenic and glycolytic metabolic pathways. Whether the liver removes glucose from the circulation or contributes glucose to blood depends on the relative rates of opposing reactions in the gluconeogenic and glycolytic pathways. The kidney also contributes to the synthesis of glucose by means of the gluconeogenic enzymes. Allred and Roehrig (1970) quantitated hepatic gluconeogenesis and glycolysis in chickens fed carbohydrate-free diets by measuring both enzymic activities and metabolite concentrations. In general, the authors found an increase in activity of the gluconeogenic enzymes and a decrease in activity of the glycolytic enzymes resulting in a net production of glucose by the liver. Allred and Roehrig (1970) also noted differences in the regulation of the gluconeogenic enzymes when triglyceride-based and fatty acid-based diets were fed to chickens. When triglyceride was the source of dietary nonprotein energy, the alterations in enzymic activity and metabolite concentration occurred primarily at the hexose phosphate and triose phosphate levels. Feeding fatty acid diets resulted in additional changes in enzymic activity and metabolite concentration at the phosphoenol-pyruvate levels. Based on metabolite concentrations these investigators suggested that feeding a triglyceride diet resulted in increased gluconeogenesis from glycerol, while feeding fatty acid diets resulted in increased gluconeogenesis from amino acids and lactate.

Allred and Roehrig (1970) also found that hepatic glucose-6-phosphatase played a major role in controlling blood glucose concentrations when carbohydrate-free diets were fed to chickens. They suggested that the activity of this enzyme is directly related to glycerol metabolism. Based on observations of Allred and Roehrig (1970), there appears to be a competition for available carbon sources for glucose and glyceride–glycerol synthesis when fatty acid-based diets are fed to chickens. In addition, since animals fed carbohydrate-free diets have reduced rate of growth when compared with animals fed triglyceride- or carbohydrate-based diets, these enzymic results suggest that the combined glucose and glycerol synthetic processes deplete the available supply of amino acids provided by the diet and thereby limit growth.

Evans and Scholz (1971) have studied the carbohydrate-free state in chickens by using high-protein–normal-fat and high-fat–normal-protein diets. These investigators have demonstrated a marked increase in the activity of the gluconeogenic enzymes located in the liver and kidneys. These increases in the gluconeogenic enzymes (glucose-6-phosphatase and fructose-1, 6-diphosphatase) were noted as early as 24 hr following exposure to the high-protein diet. Evans and Scholz (1973) also suggested that the avian kidney was an important gluconeogenic organ, at least equal in importance to the liver and perhaps contributing more glucose than the liver. The importance of the kidney in gluconeogenesis is magnified since the avian kidney is an important site for the catabolism of amino acids. Evans and Scholz (1973) have further suggested that the kidney required an adaptation period for the gluconeogenic enzyme (PEPCK) to increase in activity when high-fat, carbohydrate-free diets are fed. This adaptation response was not present in the liver, suggesting a different regulatory mechanism involved between the liver and the kidney.

Brant and Hill (1973) have also measured the gluconeogenic enzymes in both the liver and kidneys of chickens fed a carbohydrate-free diet. The diet used by Brant was a fatty acid-based diet; the high-fat diet used by Evans and Scholz was a triglyceride-based diet. As Evans and Scholz had shown with a triglyceride diet, Brant and Hill (1973) concluded that the gluconeogenic enzymes (glucose-6-phosphatase, fructose-1,6-diphosphatase, and phosphoenol-pyruvate carboxykinase) in the liver and kidney were increased when a fatty acid-based diet was fed. Brant (1971) also noted that the glycolytic enzyme (pyruvate kinase) was also increased when carbohydrate-free (fatty acid-based) diets were fed to chickens. This finding suggests that the flow of metabolites in chickens fed a carbohydrate-free (fatty acid-based) diet may be multidirectional. More specifically, metabolites may flow partially through the gluconeogenic pathway then return to the TCA cycle by means of the glycolytic pathway. If such a metabolite flow occurred, an increase in activity of PEPCK and pyruvate kinase would be expected.

Brant and Hill (1973) also found that the gluconeogenic enzymes decreased when glucose was added to the fatty acid-based diet. Each increment of glucose addition to the diet resulted in a further reduction in the activity of the gluconeogenic enzymes.

Brant (1971) has suggested that feeding fatty acid- or triglyceride-based diets to animals may confound the responses measured. This is because the results measured may be due either to a lipid effect or to a carbohydrate deficiency. If a condition occurred in the fatty acid-based diet but not in the triglyceride-based diet, then the response is not a general effect of lipids and is due to the fatty acids per se. The response could also be compounded by an additional carbohydrate deficiency imposed upon the animal by the removal of glycerol, resulting in an increased demand for glycerol that might be met by increased gluconeogenesis.

If adding 3% glucose to the fatty acid-based diet (the amount of glucose that, theoretically, could be produced from the glycerol present in a triglyceride diet) eliminates the effect, then the effect should be classified a carbohydrate deficiency. Therefore, it may be worthwhile to classify responses to fatty acid diets that are reversed by adding glucose as a carbohydrate deficiency and responses to a fatty acid diet that are not reversed by adding glucose to the diet as fatty acid-induced effects.

Brant (1971) concluded that feeding fatty acid-based diets increased the gluconeogenic enzymes in both the liver and kidney and that these increases were not an effect of inanition. This conclusion was based on the finding that chickens fed *ad libitum* a fatty acid-based diet and pair-weighed, carbohydrate-fed chickens had significantly different enzymic activities and organ weight ratios. The chickens fed fatty acid-based diet *ad libitum* had increased gluconeogenic enzymic activities compared with the pair-weighed, carbohydrate-fed chickens.

Brant (1971) also found that chickens fed a triglyceride-based diet did not show an increase in liver phosphoenol-pyruvate carboxykinase activity. Brant found a difference between glucose-6-phosphatase activity in fatty acid-fed chickens compared with triglyceride-fed chickens, while Allred and Roehrig (1970) did not show a significant difference. This discrepancy may be due to the expression of enzymic activity. Brant expressed his enzyme activities on the basis of relative organ size; Allred and Roehrig expressed their activities per gram of tissue. Since Brant showed that organ size (liver and kidney) is affected by the kind of dietary fat or carbohydrate fed to the chicken, it may be meaningful to express enzymic activity relative to the size of the organ. Both liver and kidney weights are increased in chickens fed a fatty acid diet compared with those chickens fed a triglyceride- or carbohydrate-based diet. In Brant's studies this increase in organ size seemed related to the level of tissue gluconeogenesis. This relationship appears reasonable since other studies involving high-protein diets have shown a similar relationship (Freedland and Harper, 1957; Niemeyer et al., 1962; Voight and Matzelt, 1962).

Studies by Akrabawi et al. (1974) showed an increased glucose-6-phosphatase and glucokinase activity in the liver of rats fed a fatty acid-based diet supplemented with various levels of carbohydrate. As expected, the activity of glucose-6-phosphatase decreased with each addition of carbohydrate to a fatty acid-based diet. Conversely, the activity of glucokinase increased with successive additions of carbohydrate to the fatty acid diet. A plateau of the activity of each enzyme was noted when carbohydrate composed 15% or more of the diet.

Goldberg (1971) studied glucose-6-phosphatase and fructose-1,6-diphosphatase activity in the liver of rats fed a fatty acid, a fatty acid plus glucose, or a triglyceride- or carbohydrate-based diet. He showed a marked increase in the glucose-6-phosphatase activity of rats fed both the fatty acid and fatty acid plus glucose diets. Although the activity of fructose-1,6-diphosphatase was also significantly increased, the increase was much less than the increase in glucose-6-phosphatase activity. Glucokinase, to the contrary, was low in the liver taken from those rats fed fatty acid diets and highest in the liver of those fed a carbohydrate diet. Goldberg (1971) also showed that the enzyme that catalyzes the utilization of glutamic acid, glutamic–pyruvate transaminase, increased threefold when a fatty acid-based diet was fed. This enzyme also seemed to reflect the carbohydrate status of the rat because successive addition of glucose to the diet resulted in a decrease in enzyme activity. Allred and Roehrig (1970), using the chicken, investigated the effect of feeding a fatty acid diet on liver glutamic–oxalacetate transaminase and showed no change in enzymic activity. This finding is different than that of Goldberg (1971), who experimented with rats, thus suggesting a species difference.

EFFECT OF CARBOHYDRATE-FREE DIETS ON AMINO ACID METABOLISM

A few enzymes involved in amino acid metabolism have been studied in chickens and rats fed carbohydrate-free diets.

Threonine

Boggs (1970) has shown that the activity of chicken liver threonine dehydrase is increased when chickens are fed fatty acid-based diets. Although the activity of this enzyme is much lower in the chicken than in the rat, the increase in activity was significant. Unfortunately, kidney threonine dehydrase was not investigated, as it has been shown that the avian kidney enzyme is much higher in activity than the liver enzyme. The low threonine dehydrase activity of the chicken liver may account for the decreased ability of dietary threonine to maintain blood glucose in the chicken fed the fatty acid diet vs. rats fed the same diet.

L-Cysteine

Simpson et al. (1974) have reported that L-cysteine is a poor gluconeogenic substrate for rats. Liver perfusion studies suggest that L-cysteine is very slowly converted to glucose by the rat. Studies fractionating the small amount of L-cysteine converted to glucose suggest that approximately one-third the glucose came via the cysteine–sulfinic acid pathway and the other two-thirds via another pathway not involving cysteine–sulfinic acid.

Glutamic and Aspartic Acid

Goldberg (1971) suggested that the transaminases associated with these two amino acids increased in rats fed a carbohydrate-free diet. Conversely, Allred and Roehrig (1970) showed no increase in glutamic–oxalacetate transaminase when chickens were fed a carbohydrate-free diet. This apparent discrepancy may result from species differences or differences in dietary protein levels. These differences suggest that further studies are needed to determine the metabolic pathways involving amino acids and their intermediates. These studies will help define the contribution of each amino acid in the maintenance of glucose in animals fed a carbohydrate-free diet.

EFFECT OF CARBOHYDRATE–FREE DIETS ON ORGAN SIZE

Liver and Kidney

Evans and Scholz (1973) demonstrated that organ weights increase as a result of feeding carbohydrate-free diets. Evans and Scholz defined a carbohydrate-free diet as being high in protein and low in triglyceride, which is different from the fatty acid-based diet used by others. Evans and Scholz also found that the ratios of liver and kidney weight to body weight are increased as a result of feeding a high-protein, carbohydrate-free diet. The increased ratio was greater for the kidneys than for the livers. Histologic examination of the kidneys and the liver revealed a hypertrophy of the cells taken from the respective organs. Soluble protein in the liver and kidney was also increased in chickens fed the high-protein, carbohydrate-free diet.

These observations are similar to those reported by Brant (1971) who showed that the ratio of liver and kidney weight to body weight was increased in chickens fed a fatty acid-based diet. These changes in organ size were reduced when glucose was added to the diet. Apparently, the increased size of the organ was related to the level of gluconeogenesis taking place in that organ. Increases in the relative size of the rat liver have been reported in many metabolic conditions where gluconeogenesis is known to be increased: injection of cortisone into normal (Freedland and Harper, 1957; Niemeyer et al., 1962; Voight and Matzelt, 1962; Weber and Singhal, 1964; Weber et al., 1961) or adrenalectomized rats (Weber et al., 1961, 1965); injection of triacinolone (Blázqner and Quijada, 1968); refeeding of fasted animals (Weber et al., 1962); or exercise (Krebs and Yoshida, 1963). The observation relating a decrease in the size of liver and kidney when glucose is added to the diet, further infers that the increase in organ size when carbohydrate-free diets are fed is in response to the increased demand for glucose and thus the increased gluconeogenesis in these tissues. This response to dietary glucose also suggests that the response is not due to the dietary lipids.

Muscle and Adipose Tissues

Other tissues, such as muscle and adipose tissue, have not been investigated as a result of feeding carbohydrate-free (fatty acid-based) diets. Brambila and Hill (1967) did show an increase in body protein and a decrease in body fat when fatty acids were substituted in the diet for carbohydrate. An increase of $\sim 6\%$ in protein and a decrease of $\sim 6\%$ in fat was noted. Since animals fed fatty acid-based diets are leaner in body composition, one would expect differences in the ratio of muscle and adipose tissue weight to body weight. The controlling factors for these differences remain to be determined.

Adrenals and Pancreas

Since Goldberg (1971) has demonstrated a doubling of serum cortico-steroids as a result of feeding fatty acid-based diets to rats, one might expect the adrenal glands to be enlarged in these animals. Unfortunately, the adreneal weights were not recorded by these investigators. Goldberg (1971) has also shown that feeding fatty acid-based diets to rats does not affect the concentration of insulin in the pancreas. This evidence suggests that the ratio of pancreatic weight to body weight may not change as a result of feeding fatty acid-based carbohydrate-free diets.

MISCELLANEOUS CONSEQUENCES OF CARBOHYDRATE–FREE DIETS

Effect of Carbohydrate-Free Diets on Laying Hens

Roland and Edwards (1972) fed triglyceride-based diets to laying hens and showed a reduction in egg production. In addition to feeding corn oil, linseed oil, and lard, Roland and Edwards (1972) also fed menhaden oil to laying hens. In all cases the hens fed the triglyceride-based diets continued to produce eggs for some period of time (with a discontinuance after 80 days of dietary treatment), although the size of the egg was reduced by those hens fed diets containing either lard or menhaden oil. Eggs from hens fed menhaden and linseed oil as the sole source of nonprotein calories had a reduced hatchability compared with eggs from hens fed corn oil or lard. The progeny from all treatments performed equally well when fed a stock diet.

Meal Feeding

Akrabawi and Salji (1973) have compared the effect of *ad libitum* and meal feeding in rats fed either a triglyceride or fatty acid-based diet. *Ad libitum* feeding resulted in equivalent growth whether the rats were fed a triglyceride- or fatty acid-based diet. Conversely, meal feeding resulted in significantly greater growth in triglyceride-fed vs. fatty acid-fed rats. Food consumption was reduced in those rats meal fed fatty acid-based diet, and this reduction may explain the decreased weight gain of these rats. Both *ad libitum* feeding and meal feeding resulted in a less efficient utilization of the fatty acid-based diet when compared with the triglyceride-based diet. Meal feeding appeared to intensify the effects of the fatty acid diet, as measured by a reduced liver glycogen, decreased plasma glucose, and increased plasma ketone bodies.

REFERENCES

Akrabawi, S. S. and Hill, F. W. 1970. *Fed. Proc.* 29:764.
Akrabawi, S. S. and Salji, J. P. 1973. *Br. J. Nutr.* 30:37.
Akrabawi, S. S., Saegert, M. M. and Salji, J. P. 1974. *Br. J. Nutr.* 32:209.
Allred, J. B. 1969. *J. Nutr.* 99:101.
Allred, J. B. and Roehrig, K. L. 1969. *J. Nutr.* 99:109.
Allred, J. B. and Roehrig, K. L. 1970. *J. Nutr.* 100:615.
Azar, G. J. and Bloom, W. L. 1963. *Arch. Intern. Med.* 112:338.
Blázqner, E. and Quijada, C. Lopez. 1968. *J. Endocrinol.* 42:489.
Boggs, R. W. 1970. Ph.D. thesis, University of California, Davis.
Boggs, R. W. and Hill, F. W. 1971. *Fed. Proc.* 30:401.
Brambila, S. and Hill, F. W. 1966. *J. Nutr.* 88:84.
Brambila, S. and Hill, F. W. 1967. *J. Nutr.* 91:261.
Brant, G. 1971. Ph.D. thesis, University of California, Davis.
Brant, G. and Hill, F. W. 1973. *Fed. Proc.* 32:936.
Brown, R. G. and Liddy, E. P. 1970. *Can. J. Comp. Med.* 34:265.
Butts, J. S., Blunder, H. and Dunn, J. S. 1938. *J. Biol. Chem.* 124:709.
Donaldson, W. E., Combs, G. F., Romoser, G. L. and Supplee, W. D. 1957. *Poult. Sci.* 36:807.
Evans, R. M. and Scholz, R. W. 1971. *J. Nutr.* 101:1127.
Evans, R. M. and Scholz, R. W. 1973. *J. Nutr.* 103:242.
Felig, P., Pozefshy, T., Marliss, E. and Cahill, G. F. 1970. *Science* 167:1003.
Freedland, R. A. and Harper, A. E. 1957. *J. Biol. Chem.* 228:743.
Goldberg, A. 1971. *J. Nutr.* 101:693.
Hall, W. K., Eaton, A. G. and Doty, J. R. 1940. *Am. J. Physiol.* 129:372.
Harper, H. A. 1969. Protein and amino acid metabolism. In *Physiological chemistry,* ch. 15. Los Altos, Calif.: Lange Medical Publ.
Hill, F. W., Akrabawi, S. and Oddoye, E. A. 1973. *Fed. Proc.* 32:936.
Hill, F. W., Rucker, R. B. and Faqih, A. M. 1974. *Fed. Proc.* 33:718.
Janney, N. W. 1915. *J. Biol. Chem.* 20:321.
Krebs, H. A. 1964. *Mammaliary protein metabolism,* ed. H. N. Munro and J. B. Allison, vol. I, ch. 5. New York: Academic Press.
Krebs, H. A. 1966. *Adv. Enzyme Regul.* 5:409.
Krebs, H. A. and Yoshida, J. 1963. *Biochem. Z.* 338:241.
Lusk, G. 1928. *The elements of the science of nutrition,* 4th ed. Philadelphia: Saunders.
Madappally, M. M., Paquet, R. J., Mehlman, M. A. and Tobin, R. B. 1971. *J. Nutr.* 101:755.

Mirsky, I. A., Nelson, N., Grayman, I. and Korenberg, M. 1942. *Am. J. Physiol.* 136:223.

Munro, H. N., Black, J. G. and Thomson, W. S. T. 1959. *Br. J. Nutr.* 13:475.

Niemeyer, H., Clark-Turri, L., Garcés, E. and Vergara, F. E. 1962. *Arch. Biochim. Biophys.* 98:77.

Rand, N. T., Scott, H. M. and Kummerow, F. A. 1958. *Poult. Sci.* 37:1075.

Renner, R. 1964. *J. Nutr.* 84:322.

Renner, R. 1969. *J. Nutr.* 98:297.

Renner, R. and Elcombe, A. M. 1964. *J. Nutr.* 84:327.

Renner, R. and Elcombe, A. M. 1967a. *J. Nutr.* 93:25.

Renner, R. and Elcombe, A. M. 1967b. *J. Nutr.* 93:31.

Roberts, S., Samuels, L. T. and Reinecke, R. M. 1944. *Am. J. Physiol.* 140:639.

Roland, D. A. and Edwards, H. M. 1972. *J. Nutr.* 102:229.

Sampson, J. 1947. *Univ. Ill. Agric. Exp. Stn. Bull.* No. 524, p. 407.

Simpson, R. C., Freedland, R. A. and Hill, F. W. 1974. *Fed. Proc.* 33:681.

Voight, K. D. and Matzelt, D. 1962. *Symposium International Association. Study of liver, 2nd, Munich,* p. 164. Bad Reichenhall.

Weber, G. and Singhal, R. L. 1964. *J. Biol. Chem.* 239:521.

Weber, G., Banerjee, G. and Bronstein, S. B. 1961. *J. Biol. Chem.* 236:3106.

Weber, G., Banerjee, G. and Bronstein, S. B. 1962. *Am. J. Physiol.* 202:137.

Weber, G., Srivastava, S. K. and Singhal, R. L. 1965. *J. Biol. Chem.* 240:750.

Wolfberg, S. 1876. *Z. Biol.* 12:266.

Zaragoza-Hermans, N. M. 1973. *Eur. J. Biochem.* 38:170.

Zinneman, H. H., Nutfall, F. Q. and Goetz, F. C. 1966. *Diabetes* 15:5.

Chapter 6

CARBOHYDRATE NUTRITION AND HYPERALIMENTATION

Carolyn D. Berdanier
Departments of Biochemistry and Medicine
University of Nebraska College of Medicine
and Veterans Administration Hospital
Omaha, Nebraska

Mitchell V. Kaminski
Physical Sciences Division
U.S. Army Medical Research Institute
of Infectious Diseases
Fort Detrick
Frederick, Maryland

INTRODUCTION

Intravenous therapy, particularly intravenous nutritional therapy, has been used for many years to improve the survival of traumatized or diseased patients. As early as 1831 Thomas Latta infused isotonic saline solutions to combat the fluid and salt losses due to the diarrhea of cholera. Later, Claude Bernard (Foster, 1899) infused various solutions, including sugar, albumin, and milk, into experimental animals with some success. In 1873 Edward Hodder treated cholera victims with milk infusions, and in 1891 Rudolph Matas used saline solutions to combat surgical shock. The use of glucose solutions following surgery was pioneered by Kausch in 1911, and in 1914 Henriques and Anderson demonstrated that infused protein hydrolysates had therapeutic value. Murlin and Riche (1915) and Yamakawa (1920) showed that fat emulsions could be infused successfully. While all of these pioneers demonstrated the usefulness of various nutrient solutions, due to the number of complications that arose, the use of parenteral nutritional support was deemed unsafe. With the discovery of the harmful effects of pyrogens (Seibert, 1923) and the procedures devised to overcome these effects, intravenous hyperalimentation began to develop as a safe therapeutic procedure.

Initially, intravenous hyperalimentation was limited to the provision of fluid to replace fluid losses, some electrolytes, small quantities of glucose, and perhaps amino acids. However, adequate intravenous nutrition via the peripheral veins is limited by a number of factors. First, all the nutrients must be water soluble in order to be infused. This technical problem can be overcome through the use of various water-miscible ingredients. In some formulas, lipids are excluded (leading to a possible essential fatty acid deficiency), while other formulas contain lipid emulsions. The second problem, which seemed insurmountable until the work of Dudrick et al. (1967, 1968, 1970; Dudrick and Ruberg, 1971), is the limitation imposed by the use of peripheral veins for infusion. Peripheral veins cannot tolerate hypertonic solutions and if the patient is to receive even a modicum of nutritional support via the parenteral route, large volumes of isotonic solutions must be infused. This places a severe burden on the kidney to excrete the excess water. This need to use isotonic solutions (with a low caloric/nutrient density) when infusing into a peripheral vein naturally sets an upper limit on the absolute amounts of nutrients that can be provided. Dudrick et al. (1967, 1968, 1970; Dudrick and Ruberg, 1971; Long et al., 1971; Wilmore and Dudrick, 1968) have shown that it is possible to infuse hypertonic solutions if the vein chosen for infusion has a sufficient volume of blood flowing through it to dilute the nutrient solution to tolerable tonicity.

Perhaps the most important problem yet to be resolved is identifying the many absolute requirements for nutrients, that is, the requirements for nutrients with no allowance for availability or for gut recycling. In addition, the effect of trauma on these requirements has received little attention. Thus, while intravenous hyperalimentation has been in use for a long time, intravenous nutritional support based on a sound data base of nutrient requirements under these conditions is only now emerging. In spite of our ignorance of the needs of patients for these nutrients, intravenous hyperalimentation has proved to be a valuable adjunct in the treatment of patients with severe burns, anorexia nervosa, severe gastrointestinal disease, or severe trauma. While these patients may be able to eat, their illnesses may interfere with the consumption of enough nutrients to meet their nutritional requirements.

EFFECT OF TRAUMA OR STRESS ON METABOLISM

Before any discussion of the nutrient requirements of patients nourished intravenously can be presented, it is necessary to review the effect trauma or debilitating illness has on metabolism. Almost any deviation from the "normal" state of health and well-being can be considered a stress. However, for the purposes of this discussion, stress or trauma will be restricted to mean a severe or debilitating illness or injury resulting in the hospitalization of the patient for treatment.

Hormonal Responses to Trauma

The capacity of the patient to respond to trauma or stress rests largely with the functional state of the endocrine system. Trauma or physiologic insult in man or experimental animals elicits a fairly predictable cascade of events that result in increases in protein catabolism in the peripheral tissues, in the energy requirement, and usually but not always in body heat production. The hormones that regulate the choice of metabolic fuels, as well as the balance between protein anabolism and catabolism, are important components of this stimulus-neuro-endocrine-metabolic effect set in motion when patients are traumatized.

Upon injury, the adrenal medullary secretion rate is raised approximately 10-fold (Coward and Smith, 1966; Johnston, 1972, 1974; Walker, 1965), and the excretion of urinary catecholamine metabolites is elevated for 3-4 days following injury (Johnston, 1972, 1974). The secretion of norepinephrine appears to be greater than the secretion of epinephrine. In addition, there appears to be a greater responsiveness of the sympathetic nerve tissue to trauma than the cholinergic parasympathetic tissue. This responsiveness augments the adrenal medullary response. Adrenal medullary and sympathetic gangli norepinephrine levels have been found to be markedly reduced in severely traumatized patients, indicating a depletion of the hormone stores (La Brosse and Cowley, 1973). The mechanism whereby trauma induces this depletion of the catecholamines has been described. Hume (1953) has shown that trauma induces the transmission of afferent impulses from the carotid sinus to the medulla oblongata where efferent impulses are released. These impulses, in turn, stimulate the adrenal medulla via the sympathetic outflow. The metabolic effects of this outpouring of epinephrine and norepinephrine are important events in the response to injury. Epinephrine and norepinephrine increase the blood flow through the liver, enhance protein catabolism and lipolysis, and probably contribute to the increased heat production and energy utilization following injury.

Stress has been shown to result in an immediate rise in ACTH (Cooper and Nelson, 1962; Holzbauer, 1964) and in some instances a rise in growth hormone release (Berson and Yalow, 1968; Yalow et al., 1969). This indicates that one of the first endocrine glands to respond to trauma is the pituitary. The rise in ACTH may account for the early (within 24-48 hr) increase in aldosterone and cortisol levels in the sera of traumatized patients (Hayes and Brandt, 1952; Llaurado, 1955; Marks, 1961). In surgical patients, the pattern of aldosterone release follows that of cortisol and is related in time and extent to changes in sodium and potassium excretion (Casey et al., 1957). Aldosterone levels have been shown to remain high for at least 60 days in severely burned patients, while cortisol levels return to nearly normal levels within 4-7 days depending on the severity of the burn (Bane et al., 1974). The elevations in aldosterone in these patients plays a role in the renal conservation of sodium thus maintaining electrolyte balance, which may be distorted due to the loss of fluid and electrolytes through the burn-damaged skin. Recovery from surgical trauma may not involve such a prolonged elevation in aldosterone levels since these patients are not losing significant fluids and electrolytes through the injured body surfaces as are the burned patients.

The close association of the adrenal cortex and medulla suggests that the cortical hormones and the catecholamines may interact during the stress response. Indeed, in experimental animals it has been shown that cortisol participates in the conversion of norepinephrine to epinephrine and that stimuli that enhance cortisol release also enhance catecholamine release (Harrison et al., 1968).

Porte et al. (1966), Efendic et al. (1974), and also Cerasi et al. (1971) have shown that the catecholamines can inhibit glucose-stimulated insulin insulin release. Thus, the trauma-induced glucose intolerance (Howard, 1955; Taylor et al., 1944) may be attributed to a rise in these hormones following injury. Studies of traumatized animals pretreated with α and β blocking agents or whose adrenal medullas were removed demonstrated an inhibitory action of the catecholamines on insulin release and on peripheral tissue uptake (Vigas et al., 1973; Marliss, et al., 1973). However, elevations in catecholamine levels alone cannot account for all of the posttrauma glucose intolerance. Studies by other workers have implicated other hormones as well (Gump et al., 1974; Meguid et al., 1974). Elevation in glucagon secretion due to elevations in the serum levels of catecholamines (Gerich, 1973; Iverson, 1971; Leclerq-Meyer et al., 1971), stimulation of the hypothalamus (Frohman and Bernardis, 1971), or in response to trauma (Lindsey et al., 1974; Meguid et al., 1972, 1973; Wilmore et al., 1974) have been reported. These reports suggest that the trauma-related glucose intolerance is due in part to the effects of the catecholamines on insulin release and of cortisol, and catecholamines, and growth hormone on peripheral tissue sensitivity to insulin and in part to the effects of glucagon and cortisol on hepatic glucose production. Studies of the choice of metabolic fuels following trauma and the accompanying hormonal responses appear to support this suggestion (Meguid et al., 1974).

It has been observed (Woodruff et al., 1973) that corticosteroids administered prior to or immediately after an injury shorten the recovery period. Corticosteroids have been shown to increase glucagon release by the α cells of the pancreas (Marco et al., 1973; Wise et al., 1973) and also to be required for the gluconeogenic action of glucagon (Exton et al., 1970). Thus, it seems that much of the gluconeogenic action of cortisol is mediated by glucagon and that the cortisol response to trauma may be responsible for the trauma-induced rise in serum glucagon with an attendant rise in gluconeogenesis. Trauma-induced rises in serum glucose and free fatty acid levels are consistent with an inhibited insulin release (and low serum insulin levels) and an enhanced glucagon release (and elevated serum glucagon levels). These rises are also consistent with elevations in the levels of catecholamines and glucocorticoids. It seems reasonable to assume that the more severe the trauma, the more exaggerated are the metabolic and hormonal responses. These responses are schematically presented in Fig. 1.

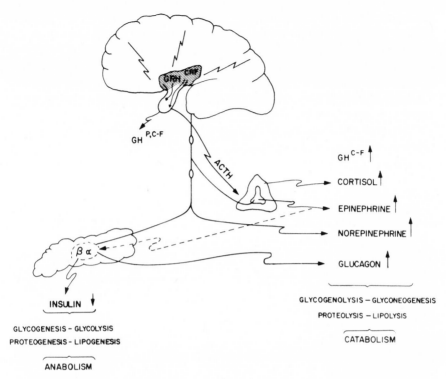

FIGURE 1 Schematic representation of the multiple responses to stress. Multiple etiologies produce shifts in cellular metabolism from those under the control or influence of insulin (anabolic processes) to those under the influence of antiinsulin hormones (catabolic processes). Glycogen and lipid synthesized during the anabolic periods undergo degradation and mobilization by glycogenolysis and lipolysis in the stressed animal. The free amino acids mobilized are converted to glucose in the liver and kidney by gluconeogenesis. These metabolic responses to stress occur simultaneously and are ultimately directed and coordinated by the hypothalamus.

Metabolic Responses to Trauma

The endocrine and metabolic responses to injury are closely related (Fig. 2). Increased production of some hormones and inhibited release of other hormones are integral parts of the body's basic defense mechanism. The primary function of this mechanism is to provide a continuous fuel supply to the central nervous system and the required substrates for the repair of body tissue. While the body may respond to trauma with an increased release of the hormones that regulate metabolism through cAMP, this response, in comparison with the overall metabolic response to injury or illness, is relatively short-lived. It appears, therefore, that the hormonal responses to injury serve as initiators or inducers of metabolic events that must occur if recovery is to proceed. As relief from the stressful events occurs, these hormonal responses recede, and other metabolic

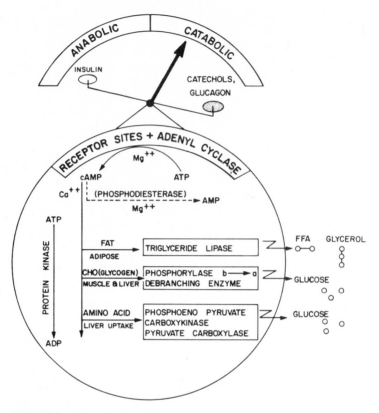

FIGURE 2 Trauma elicits a rise in catecholamines, glucagon, and other hormones that act to shift metabolism from its previous state of balance between anabolism and catabolism to a state of predominant catabolism. This shift is mediated in part by the release of cAMP and is characterized by an increase in lipolysis, glycogenolysis, gluconeogenesis, and proteolysis.

control mechanisms assume command. These, in turn, give way to the normal metabolic control mechanisms as recovery proceeds.

As described, trauma induces glucose intolerance. In humans following a simple stress, the fasting glucose level is higher than normal; after a glucose load, the fall in blood glucose levels is less than normal. In contrast, if fructose is given instead of glucose, no difference in fructose uptake is observed (Drucker et al., 1952, 1961). The uptake of fructose apparently is not affected by stress or trauma; however, when converted to glucose, it is subjected to the same hormonal controls, and at that point its metabolism is affected by stress or trauma. Thus, when fructose is administered to a traumatized patient, a rise in blood glucose is observed. This rise in blood glucose following fructose is greater in the traumatized patient than in the normal subject. The effect of trauma on carbohydrate metabolism appears to extend to those regulatory steps that are insulin or hormone sensitive. Thus, while the assimilation of glucose metabolites such as citrate is not affected, the metabolism of such compounds is altered. Infusion of citrate into a normal person results in a fall in blood glucose levels; citrate infused into a stressed patient results in a rise in blood glucose. Other studies have shown that plasma free fatty acids rise during trauma and recovery despite the presence of hyperglycemia (Allison et al., 1968a, b).

While hyperglycemia may be observed immediately after trauma, a decrease in blood sugar may occur if food is withheld 24 hr preceding the trauma (Mraz et al., 1959; Nemeth et al., 1972). This suggests that even though trauma results in a decrease in serum insulin levels and a decrease in pancreatic insulin release, glucose metabolism particularly by the liver and the central nervous system continues unimpaired. With severe injury, hyperglycemia and glycosuria may continue for many days (Evans and Butterfield, 1951; Rosenberg et al., 1965). As indicated earlier, this hyperglycemia is due to both an increased glycogenolysis and gluconeogenesis and a reduced peripheral uptake of glucose.

With trauma, plasma free fatty acids rise. These increases correlate well with the increases in serum catecholamines and indicate an increased mobilization of adipose tissue lipids. While this mobilization initially occurs in response to increases in epinephrine, the increased lipolysis continues long after the serum epinephrine levels have fallen. This indicates that other factors in addition to the catecholamines influence or regulate plasma free fatty acid levels in the traumatized individual. Concomitant with an increase in plasma free fatty acids is an increase in hepatic triglycerides (Carlson, 1972). In studies using traumatized dogs, it has been shown that the rate of free fatty acid mobilization from the adipose tissue determined the uptake of these fatty acids by the various tissues in the body (Carlson, 1972). Thus, if mobilization is pathologically accelerated, more fatty acids will be released than can be utilized, and deposition in the organs utilizing this fuel will result. Fatty livers have been observed in severely traumatized patients who have died during the early recovery phase.

While glucose tolerance is impaired in the traumatized patient, fat tolerance appears to be enhanced (Carlson, 1972). The mechanism of this increased tolerance is unclear but may be related to the increased activity of the hormone-sensitive lipoprotein lipase as well as to the effects of both catecholamines and cortisol on lipolysis.

In injured or traumatized patients, protein catabolism is accelerated without an increase in protein anabolism (Beisel, 1966, 1972; Cuthbertson, 1930). This results in a net negative nitrogen balance and probably represents the mobilization of tissue protein to provide amino acids for tissue repair and precursors for gluconeogenesis. In normal people there appears to be an upper limit to the activity of the gluconeogenic pathway. In traumatized persons, however, this limit is exceeded and protein catabolism for gluconeogenesis continues unabated. In part, this may be due to the need for glucose metabolites as tissue fat stores are mobilized for energy (Blackburn et al., 1973). In part, the negative nitrogen balance may also be attributable to the decreased food intake by patients who are ill. Nonetheless, this decreased food intake can account for only a fraction of the total body protein lost during illness and subsequent recovery. Obviously, there are a number of other factors that contribute to the accelerated body protein loss. As described, trauma or illness can result in increased endocrine activity with a resulting increased release in the catabolic hormones. While increases in these hormones can account for a portion of the body protein lost, all losses cannot be attributed to these hormones. Wannemacher et al. (1972) has explained the early change in free fatty acid and amino acid levels in the serum as being due to the release of a factor (leukocyte endogenous mediator, LEM) from the leukocytes. This factor appears to enhance hepatic uptake of certain amino acids, zinc, and iron, stimulate RNA and protein synthesis, and enhance the release of extra ceruloplasmin and new α proteins. All these changes appear to reflect the activation of the body's defense mechanisms needed to repel invading pathogens.

With trauma, additional losses of up to 20 g nitrogen (120 g protein) per day have been reported for severely traumatized patients (Cuthbertson, 1930, 1964, 1972). Previous studies of the time sequence of events in the metabolic responses to trauma show that these responses occur in two phases. The early phase (the first 24-48 hr) is characterized by an impairment of glucose utilization and an impairment of the activity of the Krebs cycle (Henderson and Jones, 1974). During this period, it is likely that there is a deficiency of intracellular glucose and Krebs cycle intermediates and an impaired oxidative metabolism. In the second phase, characterized by an increase in nitrogen excretion, secondary metabolic responses to trauma or injury are observed. Responses such as an increased synthesis of hepatic enzymes that catabolize amino acids for energy are observed (Henderson and Jones, 1974). The work of Hinton et al. (1971) has shown that the administration of large doses of insulin to a traumatized patient can suppress this latent protein catabolic response to trauma and also suppress gluconeogenesis.

The total effect of the metabolic responses to trauma or severe illness is to provide the body with carbohydrate intermediates, amino acids, and other elements important to the immunologic response to overriding infection or to the inflammatory response to tissue damage. These responses are characterized by the need to synthesize new proteins appropriate for these responses. The body exchanges the value of immediate energy availability for the disadvantage of a subsequent nitrogen debt similar to the oxygen debt incurred during exercise. Should the catabolic state persist unduly, the total debt may be insupportable and indeed exceed the body's capacity to reverse the trend. In this case, death may result.

EFFECTS OF TRAUMA ON NUTRIENT REQUIREMENTS

Since Cutherbertson (1930) first described the body's disproportionate catabolic response to trauma, physicians, nutritionists, and physiologists alike have accepted this response as an obligatory and necessary response to illness or injury. Recently, however, it has been shown that this loss in body tissue can be minimized and in some cases reversed with the provision of adequate nutritional support (Hallberg et al., 1967; Heller, 1970; Kreiger et al., 1957; Peaston, 1967; Reigel et al., 1947; Wadstrom and Wirklund, 1964; Werner et al., 1951). This implies, then, that the catabolic response to trauma or illness is more a response to inadequate nutrition (i.e., a greatly increased set of nutrient requirements in the face of a decreased nutrient intake) than to trauma per se.

Kinney (1966) has shown that basal energy requirements increase by as much as 200% in traumatized patients. Part of this increase in energy requirements can be attributed to the hypercalorigenic effects of the catabolic hormones that are released in response to injury. In addition, increases in the energy requirement may be due to the energy used to support the synthesis of new proteins needed for the inflammatory and immunologic responses of the body to illness or injury. The synthesis of these proteins usually takes place at the expense of the other body proteins that, in turn, serve as sources of amino acids. The amino acids not used in this synthesis are deaminated and used for fuel. Urea production, which must accompany this deamination, is highly energy dependent. Thus, large increases in both protein synthesis and urinary nitrogen excretion represent an increase in the basal energy requirements as well as an increase in the protein requirement.

The protein catabolic response to injury is nutritionally dependent. If the energy intake of the traumatized patient is inadequate, protein will be catabolized to meet this energy need. Furthermore, it has been shown in experimental animals that the magnitude of the protein catabolic response is proportional to the level of protein intake prior to the injury. Protein-deficient rats lost less nitrogen (since they had proportionately less to lose) than rats fed adequate protein diets prior to injury (Abbott and Albertson, 1963; Cairnie et al., 1957; Munro, 1964, 1974; Munro and Chalmers, 1945; Munro and Cuthbertson, 1943). However, the repletion of these losses was dependent both on the total caloric density of the repletion diet and on the percent dietary protein. The time course of the recovery as well as the survival of animals to severe trauma may also be related to the dietary intakes of these animals both before and after the trauma. This points out the need to separate the effects of "starvation" either prior to or immediately after the trauma from those of trauma per se in determining the nutrient requirements of the ill or traumatized patient.

It may be well to remember that most micronutrient requirements are based on the needs for these micronutrients as cofactors or coenzymes in protein and energy metabolism. Thus, as the energy and protein requirements are increased, the requirements for these nutrients are increased as well. Table 1 summarizes these relationships. Severe tissue damage is frequently followed by losses in sodium, potassium, nitrogen, calcium, phosphorus (Share and Stadler, 1958), and zinc (Touillon et al., 1975). The postoperative loss in nitrogen has been found to be associated with a consistent fall in protein synthesis (O'Keefe

TABLE 1   Effect of Trauma on the Basal
Requirements for Selected Nutrients

Nutrient	Basal requirement[a]	Stress effect
Calories	833 cal/m² body surface	Up to 200% increase
Protein[b]	2 mg N/basal calorie	60–500% increase
Calcium	~ 1% basal protein requirement	Increase[c]
Phosphorus	~ 2% basal protein requirement	Increase[c]
Zinc	5–22 mg/day[d]	Increase[c]
Vitamin A (retinol equivalents)	0.5–1.2 mg/day	Increase[c]
Vitamin C	10 mg/day	Increase[c]
Thiamin	0.2–0.5 mg/1,000 calories	Increase[c]
Riboflavin	0.55–1.1 mg/day	Increase[c]
Niacin equivalents[e]	4.4 mg/1,000 calories	Increase[c]

[a]Requirement is defined as that intake below which deficiency symptoms can occur. The figure makes no allowance for increments due to age, activity, or bioavailability.
[b]Assumes a good quality protein.
[c]Percent increase unknown; research is needed to establish the needs for these and other nutrients in traumatized persons.
[d]Broad range given due to insufficient data (Halsted et al., 1974).
[e]Includes tryptophan, which is available for conversion to niacin.

et al., 1974). As protein catabolism occurs in excess of anabolism, certain intracellular components such as potassium will be lost. As recovery proceeds and protein anabolism overtakes catabolism, the needs for these nutrients will exceed the basal requirement figures. Since riboflavin serves as a cofactor in several steps in biologic oxidations of both carbohydrates and proteins, increases in protein turnover or in the energy requirement will increase the riboflavin requirement. Studies of riboflavin excretion following severe trauma show that excretion is increased in traumatized animals (Andrea et al., 1946).

Factors such as disturbed renal function in the immediate posttrauma period and an increased heat production as in fever will also affect the energy, water, and electrolyte requirements. Wound healing, in addition, imposes special requirements for those nutrients involved in the maintenance of the integrity of the body's outer surface and in the synthesis of skin and collagen. Thus, the requirements for amino acids, vitamin A (Rodriguez and Irwin, 1972), vitamin C (Gerson, 1975), zinc (Halsted et al., 1974), and perhaps other trace minerals can be expected to increase as a result of trauma. As the energy requirement is increased, thiamin, riboflavin, niacin, phosphorus, magnesium, and manganese requirements can also be expected to increase. Unfortunately, the percentage increases in all of the above-mentioned nutrients are unknown. No controlled studies have been performed that can provide the necessary data on the effect of trauma on nutrient requirements. Hence, increases in the needs of traumatized or ill patients can only be surmised based on the knowledge that the requirements of these nutrients are related to each other and are needed for specific functions without which recovery is impossible.

EFFECTS OF INTRAVENOUS HYPERALIMENTATION ON METABOLISM

It is now evident that normal wound healing and recovery from severe trauma or illness in the absence of adequate nutrient intake is only that which can occur in spite of the inadequate nutritional status of the patient. [See Bistrian et al. (1974) for a report on the nutritional status of surgical patients.] As pointed out in the previous section, it is possible through the provision of adequate nutritional support to reduce or reverse the disproportionate catabolic response to trauma. In severely debilitated or traumatized patients, intravenous hyperalimentation is the only means for providing adequate nutritional support. When used carefully, this therapeutic procedure can promote anabolism, improve the chances of survival of the patient, and shorten the recovery time. This has been shown both in experimental animals (Daly et al., 1974; Langlois et al., 1972) and in humans (Anderson et al., 1974; Dudrick and Ruberg, 1971; Hindmarsh and Clark, 1973; Parsa et al., 1972; Wilmore et al., 1973; Yeo et al., 1973; Zohrab et al., 1973) with a variety of illnesses or injuries.

Since the true body requirements (the requirements via the intravenous route without the modulating effect of the gut) for most nutrients are unknown, the formulations of the nutrient solutions for intravenous feeding have been based on the requirements for these nutrients when consumed in the normal fashion. In Table 2 are presented several formulas that have been used. Early formulations made no allowances for the effect of trauma on nutrient requirements or for the protective effect of the gut on the regulation of trace element balances. As problems arose, however, the formulas have been changed as have the procedures used in monitoring the treatment.

When intravenous hyperalimentation consists of the infusion of a fat-free glucose/amino acid/micronutrient formula over a long period of time, essential fatty acid deficiencies have been observed (Collins et al., 1971; Sgoutas and Jones, 1974; Wene et al., 1975; Wretlind, 1972). Burn patients appear to be particularly susceptible to essential fatty acid deficiency (Wilmore et al., 1973). These deficiency symptoms required up to 100 days to develop depending on the age and prior nutritional status of the patient. Essential fatty acid deficiency can be avoided by including essential fatty acids in the formula (Macfadyen et al., 1973). However, the inclusion of essential fatty acids through the use of cottonseed oil emulsions has presented problems. The occurrence of thrombosis, which did not occur when lipid-free formulas were used, has been reported (Lawson, 1965; Levenson et al., 1957; Shuttleworth, 1963; Wilmore et al., 1973; Yeo et al., 1973). Lipid emulsions that utilize a 10% soybean oil–egg yolk phosphatide glycerol emulsion have been infused successfully with none of the

TABLE 2 Examples of Different Formulas in Use
for Intravenous Nutritional Support

Component	Azotemic patients[a]	Adult patients[b]	Infants and children[c]
Volume	750 ml	1000 ml	130 ml/kg
Nitrogen source	13.1g	37 g	2.5 g/kg
Glucose	350 g	212 g	20–30 g/kg
Vitamin A	5000 USP units	d	d
Thiamine HC1	25 mg	d	d
Riboflavin	5 mg	d	d
Pyridoxine HC1	7.5 mg	d	d
Niacinamide	50 mg	d	d
Pantothenol	12.5 mg	d	d
Vitamin C	1.5 mg	d	d
Vitamin D	500 USP units	d	d
α-Tocopherol	2.5 IU	d	d
Calcium	e	4–5 meq	0.25 mmol/kg (as Ca gluconate)
Magnesium	e	4–10 meq	0.125 mmol/kg (as $MgSO_4$)
Phosphate	e	4–5 meq	–
Potassium	e	43–53 meq	2–3 mmol/kg (as KH_2PO_4)
Sodium	e	47–57 meq	3–4 mmol/kg (as NaCl)
Folate	0	0.5–1.5 mg	50–75 μg/day
Vitamin B$_{12}$	0	10–30 μg	250–500 μg/day
Vitamin K	0	5–10 mg	0
Iron	0	2–3 mg	

[a]From Abel et al. (1974).
[b]From Dudrick and Ruberg (1971).
[c]From Heird and Winters (1975).
[d]Added as a multivitamin supplement, composition not stated.
[e]Added as needed according to results of blood monitoring.

problems associated with the earlier cottonseed oil emulsions (Deitel and Kaminsky, 1974; Zohrab et al., 1973).

Other problems associated with the infusion of hypertonic nutrient formulas include glucosuria, electrolyte imbalance, acid–base imbalance, hyperammonemia, and hypophosphotemia. Competent investigators have repeatedly shown that such problems are avoidable in most cases (Dudrick et al., 1972; Kaminski and Stollar, 1974).

The hypercatabolic state is characterized by a shift in nutrients from the intracellular compartment to the extracellular compartment for transport to the appropriate organ for utilization. Shifts in electrolytes can be expected to follow shifts in intracellular components. These shifts in electrolytes can affect the acid–base balance of the body as well. As these shifts in nutrient flow are reversed through hyperalimentation, acid–base and electrolyte imbalances may occur (Doromal and Canter, 1973; Dudrick et al., 1972; Heird et al., 1972a,b; Parsa et al., 1972; Prins et al., 1973; Sand and Pastore, 1973). If the patient was malnourished prior to hyperalimentation, this malnourishment may affect the capacity of the kidney to excrete an acid load (Klahr and Alleyne, 1973). Probably this is attributable to a reduction in the amount of phosphate buffers available. Hypophosphotemia has been reported in several hyperalimented patients (Lichtman et al., 1971; Prins et al., 1973; Sand and Pastore, 1973; Travis et al., 1971) suggesting that a phosphate shift from the intravascular to the intracellular compartment may have occurred when the patient was placed on intravenous hyperalimentation. When extra phosphate (10-15 meq/liter) was added to the infusate, some but not all of the symptoms of hypophosphotemia disappeared. However, if the phosphate is added alone, this can affect the calcium/phosphorous ratio and calcium tetany may result (Dudrick et al., 1972). For this reason it is recommended that both calcium (as calcium gluconate) and phosphate (as potassium phosphate) be added together to the infusate. These electrolytes should be monitored regularly in the hyperalimented patient. It should be noted that imbalances of this sort are unique to intravenous nutrition. In the orally fed patient on a normal diet the absorptive mechanisms of the gut serve to regulate mineral uptake such that optimal ratios of the needed minerals are maintained in the serum. Diseases of various sorts can disrupt this protective action of the gut and points out the need to establish mineral requirements in terms of body stores as well as in terms of optimal tissue and serum levels.

Acid–base imbalance in hyperalimented patients can also be due to the inability of the kidney and liver to synthesize urea in adequate amounts. With the catabolism of tissue proteins or infusate proteins (or amino acids) ammonia is released. This must be converted to urea via the urea cycle for excretion. Protein-depleted subjects have been shown to excrete small amounts of urea and ammonia; when realimented, these individuals exhibit increased levels of blood ammonia (Silvis and Paragas, 1971) probably due to the effect of prior malnutrition on the enzymes of the urea cycle (Schimke, 1962). This can be overcome by first reducing and then gradually increasing the protein or amino acid content of the infusate, thus allowing for the induction of the urea cycle enzymes.

Hyperammonemia may also occur in the hyperalimented patient with liver disease. In this case, the liver rather than the kidney is nonfunctional with respect to the urea cycle. Under these circumstances, it is unlikely that the urea cycle enzymes can be induced. As such, an infusate with a lower amino acid or protein hydrolysate content is recommended.

Protein hydrolysates contain large amounts of ammonia and can severely tax the urea cycle (Ghadimi et al., 1971). Protein hydrolysates, in addition, may contribute excess ammonia if their amino acid composition is "imbalanced" with respect to the amino acid requirements of the hyperalimented patient (Anderson et al., 1974). It has been suggested that the high glutamine content of some protein hydrolysates could possibly lead to brain damage with hyperalimentation (Olney et al., 1973). This has been shown to occur in mice but as yet there is no proof of this occurring in humans.

Infusions of amino acid solutions may result in hyperchloremic metabolic acidosis (Chan et al., 1972; Dudrick et al., 1972). Commercial preparations utilizing crystalline amino acids (precipitated with HCl) have a titratable acidity varying from 50 to 120 meq/liter. These preparations should be buffered (preferably with a bicarbonate buffer) prior to infusion (Chan et al., 1972).

Electrolyte balances play an important role in determining the contribution of the amino acids to metabolic acidosis. Potassium, the major electrolyte in the cell, is excreted by the hypercatabolic patient. When this patient is hyperalimented, potassium must be supplied if the protein catabolic process is to be reversed. Davidson et al. (1968) have reported that elevations in serum amino acids could be reduced by potassium supplements in potassium-depleted subjects. His patients required as much as 300 meq K/day to promote positive nitrogen balance and protein synthesis. The data of Rudman et al. (1975) show that the repletion of body protein and extracellular fluid can be retarded or abolished if nitrogen, potassium, sodium, or phosphorus were missing. Bone mineralization did not occur in the absence of sodium or phosphorus but proceeded in the absence of nitrogen or potassium. Repletion of adipose tissue occurred in the absence of all four elements.

Magnesium deficiency likewise can contribute to electrolyte imbalance and supplements of 2.5-5 meq Mg/liter infusate should be provided to avoid deficiency (Doolas, 1970; Dudrick et al., 1968; Morgan et al., 1970). Copper deficiency has been reported in two patients on intravenous hyperalimentation (Karpel and Peden, 1972; Vilter et al., 1974) as has zinc deficiency in another patient (Greene, 1974).

Disorders of hepatic function and/or structure have been reported in children (Heird et al., 1972a,b; Jacobson et al., 1971) and in experimental animals sustained by parenteral alimentation (Chang and Silvis, 1974). Fatty livers in hyperalimented subjects are probably due to the greatly increased load of glucose that must be metabolized by the body at a time when the peripheral utilization of glucose is impaired. This forces the liver to metabolize more than its normal share of glucose, and what glucose cannot be completely oxidized is converted to lipid and either sent to the periphery for storage or stored in the liver.

Several reports of an initial glucose intolerance in hyperalimented patients have appeared (Parsa et al., 1972; Sanderson and Deitel, 1974). In normal people glucose utilization varies from 0.4 to 1.2 g/kg/hr (Geyer, 1960). Utilization is dependent on the availability of insulin and the sensitivity of the tissues to this hormone. Thus, stress, trauma, sepsis, and diabetes can result in an impairment of glucose utilization. Studies of the insulin responses of patients during the initial period of adaptation to hyperalimentation showed an initial rise in serum insulin followed by a fall in both blood glucose and insulin (Sanderson and Deitel, 1974). In healthy volunteers the drop in serum insulin with continued glucose infusion has been interpreted to mean an increase in the degradation of this hormone (Carlson et al., 1975), whereas in the hyperalimented patient this was interpreted to mean the attainment of a new steady state in the glucose/insulin relationship (Sanderson and Deitel, 1974). A new steady state may not be attained in some patients; rather, metabolic acidosis, glucosuria, and hyperglycemia may result. In severely traumatized patients this can be explained as the effect of trauma on pancreatic insulin release and peripheral insulin sensitivity. This can be overcome by doses of exogenous insulin during the initial hyperalimentation period. Diabetic or prediabetic patients may require exogenous insulin beyond the initial adaptation period. In addition, hyperosmolar nonketotic hyperglycemia may result if the hypertonic glucose solution is administered too rapidly (Dudrick et al., 1972). When the blood glucose levels exceed 200 mg/100 ml for prolonged periods of time, glucosuria accompanied by osmotic diuresis followed by elevations in serum electrolyte levels and urea, progressive lethargy, mental confusion, convulsions, coma, and death results. If detected early enough, this complication can be reversed by slowing the infusion rate and providing additional water and, if necessary, exogenous insulin. The syndrome can be avoided completely by carefully adjusting the glucose infused according to the patient's ability to respond with a rise in serum insulin. Some patients have been shown to have an insulin response to amino acids (Genuth, 1973); thus, hyperinsulinemia followed by hypoglycemia may result. This is a relatively infrequent occurrence (Parsa et al., 1972), however, and careful monitoring of the blood glucose levels will avoid this complication as well. Intravenous administration of lipid emulsions do not evoke an insulin response (Coran and Horwitz, 1972).

Elevated serum lactate levels observed in hyperalimented patients may not be due to inadequate glucose utilization but may be due to some other mechanism such as hypoxia (Nakajima et al., 1973). Elevations in serum lactate levels have been observed in nonhyperalimented patients with a variety of disorders and in each case was related to tissue oxygen deprivation.

Despite the aforementioned avoidable problems, nutritional support through the intravenous administration of hypertonic glucose/amino acid or protein hydrolysate/micronutrient solution does assist markedly in the recovery of some severely ill or traumatized patients. However, the mechanism whereby hyperalimentation reverses the hypercatabolic responses to illness or injury is poorly understood. Some clues to this mechanism can be obtained from the observations of Hinton et al. (1971) who showed that the excessive tissue protein breakdown that occurs in traumatized patients can be suppressed if large doses of insulin are administered within 48 hr of the injury. This indicates a role for insulin in the reversal of trauma-induced hypercatabolism. Since glucose is a potent stimulator of insulin release, it can be deduced that the beneficial effects of hyperalimentation rest with the provision of sufficient glucose to overcome the inhibitory effects of the catecholamines and glucagon on insulin release. Thus, glucose in the hyperalimentation formula serves not only as an energy source but as a pivotal ingredient for the reversal of the hypercatabolic state through its action as a potent secretagogue of insulin. Insulin, in turn, functions as an

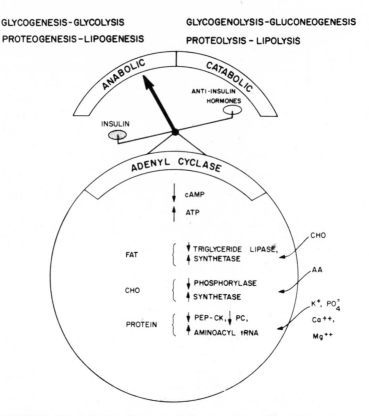

FIGURE 3 The infusion of hypertonic glucose–amino acid solutions serves to stimulate the release of insulin and growth hormone. Through the action of these hormones on adenyl cyclase and cAMP, glycolysis is enhanced as are the synthetic pathways for glycogen, lipid, and protein synthesis. With increased levels of insulin a shift in metabolism from catabolism to anabolism occurs.

anabolic agent promoting lipogenesis, glycolysis, glycogenesis, and protein synthesis (Fig. 3). When bound to the membrane receptor site, insulin results in a decrease in cAMP levels and an increase in ATP. This ATP is then available for the synthesis of a variety of cellular components utilizing available glucose, amino acids, potassium, calcium magnesium, and other micronutrients in the process.

With the infusion of amino acids, growth hormone is released, which with insulin functions to promote protein synthesis from amino acids (Knopf et al., 1966). Arginine is a particularly potent stimulator of growth hormone and stimulates insulin release as well (Knopf et al., 1966; Marliss et al., 1973). Both hormones counteract the effects of the catecholamines, glucagon, and cortisol by an as yet undefined means. The counteraction of glucagon by either insulin or growth may well be related to the competition of these hormones for the same or an overlapping membrane receptor site. However, the counteraction of the catecholamines and cortisol is not so easily explained. The suppression of adenyl cyclase (and lowering of cAMP levels) by insulin may explain this hormone's effect or role in the reversing of the catecholamine induced catabolism (Nakano and Ashida, 1975).

SUMMARY

Parenteral hyperalimentation is a system of intravenous nutritional support for patients unable to consume sufficient nutrients to promote recovery from illness or trauma. This system provides nitrogen, calories, and other micronutrients in quantities that exceed basal requirements. Careful monitoring of the patient is required in order to provide the necessary nutrients without overburdening the patient's capacity to metabolize these nutrients. Much research is needed to establish the parenteral nutritional requirements of patients nourished in this manner. Current knowledge of the mechanism by which parenteral alimentation reverses the hypercatabolic state in severely ill or traumatized patients indicates that glucose serves a unique role in the recovery of the patient due to its action as a potent secretagogue of insulin.

REFERENCES

Abel, R. M., Abbott, W. M., Beck, C. H., Ryan, J. A. and Fischer, J. E. 1974. *Ann. J. Surg.* 128:317.

Abbott, W. E. and Albertsen, K. 1963. *Ann. N.Y. Acad. Sci.* 110:941.

Allison, S. P., Hinton, P. and Chamberlain, M. J. 1968a. *Lancet* 2:1113.

Allison, S. P., Tomlin, P. J. and Chamberlain, M. J. 1968b. *Lancet* 4:1113.

Anderson, G. H., Patel, D. G. and Jeejeebhoy, K. N. 1974. *J. Clin. Invest.* 53:904.

Andrea, W. A., Schenker, V. and Browne, J. S. L. 1946. *Fed. Proc.* 5:3.

Bane, J. W., McCaa, R. E., McCaa, C. S., Read, V. H., Turney, W. H. and Turner, M. D. 1974. *J. Trauma* 14:605.

Beisel, W. R. 1966. *Fed. Proc.* 25:1682.

Beisel, W. R. 1972. *Am. J. Clin. Nutr.* 25:1254.

Berson, S. A. and Yalow, R. S. 1968. *The Harvey Lectures,* Ser. 62, p. 107. New York: Academic Press.

Bistrian, B. R., Blackburn, G. L., Hallowell, E. and Heddle, R. 1974. *J. Am. Med. Assoc.* 230:858.

Blackburn, G. L., Flatt, J. P., Clowes, G. H. A., O'Donnell, T. F. and Hensle, T. E. 1973. *Ann. Surg.* 177:588.

Cairnie, A. B., Campbell, R. M., Pullar, J. D. and Cuthbertson, D. P. 1957. *Br. J. Exp. Pathol.* 38:504.

Carlson, L. A. 1972. In *Intravenous hyperalimentation,* ed. G. Cowan, Jr., and W. Scheetz, p. 55. Philadelphia: Lea and Febiger.

Carlson, L. A., Kaijser, L., Rossner, S., Wahlqvist, M. W. and Wide, L. 1975. *Eur. J. Clin. Invest.* 5:57.

Casey, J. H., Bickel, E. Y. and Zimmerman, B. 1957. *Surg. Gynecol. Obstet.* 105:179.

Cerasi, E., Luft, R. and Efendic, S. 1971. *Acta Med. Scand.* 190:411.

Chan, J. C. M., Asch, M. J., Lin, S. and Hays, D. M. 1972. *J. Am. Med. Assoc.* 220:1700.
Chang, S. and Silvis, S. E. 1974. *Am. J. Gastroenterol.* 62:410.
Collins, F. D., Sinclair, A. J., Royle, J. P., Coats, P. A., Maynard, A. T. and Leonard, R. F. 1971. *Nutr. Metab.* 13:150.
Cooper, C. E. and Nelson, D. H. 1962. *J. Clin. Invest.* 41:1599.
Coran, A. G. and Horwitz, D. L. 1972. *Am. J. Clin. Nutr.* 25:131.
Coward, R. F. and Smith, P. 1966. *Clin. Chem. Acta* 14:832.
Cuthbertson, D. P. 1930. *Biochem. J.* 24:1244.
Cuthbertson, D. P. 1964. In *Mammalian protein metabolism,* ed. H. N. Munro and J. B. Allison, vol. II, p. 373. New York: Academic Press.
Cuthbertson, D. P. 1972. In *Parenteral nutrition,* ed. A. W. Wilkinson, p. 4. London: Churchill.
Daly, J. M., Steiger, E., Vars, H. M. and Dudrick, S. J. 1974. *Ann. Surg.* 180:709.
Davidson, L. A. G., Flear, C. T. G. and Donald, K. W. 1968. *Br. Med. J.* 1:911.
Deitel, M. and Kaminsky, V. 1974. *Can. Med. Assoc. J.* 111:152.
Doolas, A. 1970. *Surg. Clin. N. Am.* 50:103.
Doromal, N. M. and Canter, J. W. 1973. *Surg. Gynecol. Obstet.* 136:729.
Drucker, W. R., Miller, M., Craig, J. W., Jeffries, W., Levey, S. and Abbott, W. E. 1952. *Surg. Forum* 3:548.
Drucker, W. R., Craig, J. W., Kingsbury, B., Hofmann, N. and Woodward, H. 1961. *Surg. Forum* 12:3.
Dudrick, S. J. and Ruberg, R. L. 1971. *Gastroenterology* 61:901.
Dudrick, S. J., Rhoads, J. E. and Vars, H. M. 1967. In *Fortschitte der Parenteralen Ernahrung,* vol. II, p. 16. Locham bei Munchen, West Germany: Pallas Verlag.
Dudrick, S. J., Wilmore, D. W., Vars, H. M. and Rhoads, J. E. 1968. *Surgery* 64:134.
Dudrick, S. J., Wilmore, D. W. and Steiger, E. 1970. *J. Trauma* 10:542.
Dudrick, S. J., Macfadyen, B. V., Van Buren, C. T., Rubert, R. T. and Maynard, A. T. 1972. *Ann. Surg.* 176:259.
Efendic, S., Cerasi, E. and Luft, R. 1974. *Acta Anesth. Scand.* 55:107.
Evans, E. I. and Butterfield, W. J. H. 1951. *Ann. Surg.* 134:558.
Exton, J. H., Mallette, L. E., Jefferson, L. S., Wong, E. H. A., Friedmann, N., Miller, T. B., Jr., and Park, C. R. 1970. *Recent Progr. Horm. Res.* 26:411.
Foster, M. 1899. *Claude Bernard.* New York: Longmans Green Co.
Frohman, L. A. and Bernardis, L. L. 1971. *Am. J. Physiol.* 221:1596.
Genuth, S. 1973. *New Engl. J. Med.* 289:107.
Gerich, J. E. 1973. *Clin. Res.* 37:479.
Gerson, G. D. 1975. *Ann. N.Y. Acad. Sci.* 258:483.
Geyer, R. P. 1960. *Physiol. Rev.* 40:150.
Ghadimi, H., Abaci, F., Kumar, S. and Rathi, M. 1971. *Pediatrics* 48:455.
Greene, H. L. 1974. In *Intravenous nutrition in high risk infants,* ed. R. W. Winters and E. G. Hasselmeyer. New York: Wiley.
Gump, F. E., Long, C. and Killian, J. M. 1974. *J. Trauma* 14:378.
Hallberg, D., Holm, I., Obel, A. L., Schuberth, O. and Wretlind, A. 1967. *Postgrad. Med.* 42:99.
Halsted, J. A., Smith, J. C. and Irwin, M. I. 1974. *J. Nutr.* 104:345.
Harrison, T. S., Chawla, R. C. and Wojtalik, R. S. 1968. *New Engl. J. Med.* 279:136.

Hayes, M. A. and Brandt, R. L. 1952. *Surgery* 32:819.

Heird, W. C. and Winters, R. W. 1975. *J. Pediatr.* 86:2.

Heird, W. C., Dell, R. B., Driscoll, J. M., Grebin, B. and Winters, R. W. 1972a. *New Engl. J. Med.* 287:943.

Heird, W. C., Driscoll, J. M., Jr., Schullinger, J. N., Grebin, B. and Winters, R. W. 1972b. *J. Pediatr.* 80:351.

Heller, L. 1970. In *Parenteral nutrition,* ed. H. C. Meng and D. H. Law. Springfield, Ill.: Charles C Thomas.

Henderson, T. R. and Jones, R. K. 1974. *J. Trauma* 14:317.

Henriques, V. and Anderson, A. C. 1914. *Z. Physiol. Chem.* 92:21.

Hindmarsh, J. T. and Clark, R. G. 1973. *Br. J. Surg.* 60:43.

Hinton, P., Allison, S. P., Littlejohn, S. and Lloyd, J. 1971. *Lancet* 1:767.

Hodder, E. 1873. As cited by I. D. A. Johnston, *Practitioner* 206:103, 1971.

Holzbauer, M. 1964. *J. Physiol. (London)* 172:138.

Howard, J. M. 1955. *Ann. Surg.* 141:321.

Hume, D. M. 1953. *Ann. Surg.* 138:548.

Iverson, J. 1971. *Diabetologia* 7:485.

Jacobson, S., Ericsson, J. L. E. and Obel, A. 1971. *Acta Chir. Scand.* 137:335.

Johnston, I. D. A. 1972. *Adv. Clin. Chem.* 15:255.

Johnston, I. D. A. 1974. In *Parenteral nutrition in acute metabolic illness,* ed. H. A. Lee, p. 211. New York: Academic Press.

Kaminski, M. V., Jr. and Stollar, M. H. 1974. *Am. J. Hosp. Pharm.* 31:228.

Karpel, J. T. and Peden, V. H. 1972. *J. Pediatr.* 80:32.

Kausch, W. 1911. *Beitr. Klin. Chir.* 68:670.

Kinney, J. M. 1966. *Proceedings of a conference on energy metabolism and body fuel utilization.* Cambridge: Harvard University Press.

Klahr, S. and Alleyne, G. A. O. 1973. *Kidney Int.* 3:3.

Knopf, R. F., Conn, J. W., Floyd, J. C., Jr., Fajans, S. S., Rull, J. A., Guntsche, E. M. and Thiffault, C. A. 1966. *Trans. Assoc. Am. Physicians* 129:312.

Kreiger, H., Abbott, W. E., Levey, S. and Holden, W. D. 1957. *Gastroenterology* 33:807.

La Brosse, E. H. and Cowley, R. A. 1973. *J. Trauma* 13:61.

Langlois, P., Williams, H. B. and Gurd, F. N. 1972. *J. Trauma* 12:771.

Latta, T. 1831. *Lancet* 2:243.

Lawson, L. J. 1965. *Br. J. Surg.* 52:795.

Leclerq-Meyer, V., Brisson, G. R. and Malaisse, W. J. 1971. *Nature* 231:249.

Levenson, S. M., Upjohn, H. L. and Sheehy, T. W. 1957. *Metabolism* 6:807.

Lichtman, M. A., Miller, D. R., Cohen, J. and Weinhouse, C. 1971. *Ann. Intern. Med.* 74:562.

Lindsey, C. A., Santensaino, F. and Braaten, J. 1974. *J. Am. Med. Assoc.* 227:757.

Llaurado, J. G. 1955. *Lancet* 1:1295.

Long, J. M., Steiger, E. and Dudrick, S. J. 1971. *Fed. Proc.* 30:300.

MacFadyen, B. V., Dudrick, S. J., Tagudar, E. P., Maynard, A. T., Law, D. K. and Rhoads, J. E. 1973. *Surg. Gynecol. Obstet.* 137:813.

Marco, J., Calle, C., Ramon, D., Diaz-Fierros, M., Villanueva, M. and Valverde, I. 1973. *New Engl. J. Med.* 288:128.

Marks, L. J., Chute, R., O'Sullivan, J. V. I. and Giovannelo, T. J. 1961. *Metab. Clin. Exp.* 10:610.

Marliss, E. B., Giraudier, L., Seydoux, J., Wolheim, C. B., Kanazawa, Y., Orci, L., Renold, A. E. and Porte, D., Jr. 1973. *J. Clin. Invest.* 52:1246.

Matas, R. 1891. *Ann. Surg.* 79:643.

Meguid, M. M., Brennan, M. F. and Muller, W. A. 1972. *Lancet* 2:1145.

Meguid, M. M., Brennan, M. F. and Aoki, T. T. 1973. *Surg. Forum* 24:97.

Meguid, M. M., Brennan, M. F., Aoki, T. T., Muller, W. A., Bull, M. R. and Moore, F. D. 1974. *Arch. Surg.* 109:776.

Morgan, A., Filler, R. and Moore, F. D. 1970. *Med. Clin. N. Am.* 54:1367.

Mraz, M., Triner, L. and Hava, O. 1959. *Arch. Exp. Pathol. Pharmakol.* 236:83.

Munro, H. N. 1964. In *Mammalian protein metabolism*, ed. H. N. Munro and J. D. Allison, vol. I, p. 381. New York: Academic Press.

Munro, H. N. 1974. *Acta Anaesth. Scand. Suppl.* 55:81.

Munro, H. N. and Chalmers, M. I. 1945. *Br. J. Exp. Pathol.* 26:396.

Munro, H. N. and Cutherberton, D. P. 1943. *Biochem. J.* 37:xii.

Murlin, J. R. and Riche, N. 1915. As cited by S. J. Dudrick, *Intravenous hyperalimentation*, ed. G. S. W. Cowan and W. L. Scheetz, p. vi. Philadelphia: Lea and Febiger, 1972.

Nakajima, K., Hirai, Y., Yokoyama, S., Williamson, M. and Hayes, D. M. 1973. *J. Pediatr. Surg.* 8:15.

Nakano, K. and Ashida, K. 1975. *J. Nutr.* 105:906.

Nemeth, S., Vigas, M. and Lichardus, B. 1972. *J. Trauma* 12:891.

O'Keefe, S. J. D., Sender, P. M. and James, W. P. T. 1974. *Lancet* 2:1035.

Olney, J. W., Ho, O. L. and Rhee, V. 1973. *New Engl. J. Med.* 289:391.

Parsa, M. H., Habif, D. V., Ferrer, J. M., Lipton, R. and Yoshimura, N. N. 1972. *Bull. N.Y. Acad. Med.* 48:920.

Peaston, M. J. T. 1967. *Postgrad. Med. J.* 43:317.

Porte, D. Jr., Graber, A. L., Kuzuya, T. and Williams, R. H. 1966. *J. Clin. Invest.* 45:228.

Prins, J. G., Schrijver, H. and Staghowwer, J. H. 1973. *Lancet* 3:1253.

Reigel, C., Koop, C. E., Drew, J., Stevens, L. W. and Rhoads, J. E. 1947. *J. Clin. Invest.* 26:18.

Rodriguez, M. S. and Irwin, M. I. 1972. *J. Nutr.* 102:909.

Rosenberg, S. A., Brief, D. K., Kenney, J. M., Herrera, M. G., Wilson, R. E. and Moore, F. D. 1965. *New Engl. J. Med.* 272:931.

Rudman, D., Millikan, W. J., Richardson, T. J., Bixler, T. J., Stackhouse, W. J. and McGarrity, W. C. 1975. *J. Clin. Invest.* 55:94.

Sand, D. W. and Pastore, R. A. 1973. *Am. J. Dig. Dis.* 18:709.

Sanderson, I. and Deitel, M. 1974. *Ann. Surg.* 179:387.

Schimke, R. T. 1962. *J. Biol. Chem.* 237:459.

Seibert, F. B. 1923. *Am. J. Physiol.* 67:90.

Sgoutas, D. and Jones, R. 1974. *Proc. Soc. Exp. Biol. Med.* 145:614.

Share, L. and Stadler, J. E. 1958. *Endocrinology* 62:119.

Shuttleworth, K. E. D. 1963. *Ann. R. Coll. Surg.* 32:164.

Silvis, S. and Paragas, P. V., Jr. 1971. *J. Lab. Clin. Med.* 78:918.

Taylor, F. H. L., Levenson, S. M. and Adams, M. A. 1944. *New Engl. J. Med.* 231:437.

Touillon, C., Bansillon, V., Vallon, J. J., Badinand, A. and Comtet, J. J. 1975. *Clin. Chem. Acta* 63:115.

Travis, S. F., Sugermann, H. J., Ruberg, R. L., Dudrick, S. J., Papadopoulos, M. D., Miller, L. D. and Oski, L. 1971. *New Engl. J. Med.* 285:768.

Vigas, M., Nemeth, S. and Jurcovitova, J. 1973. *Horm. Metab. Res.* 5:322.

Vilter, R. W., Bozian, R. C., Hess, E. V., Zellner, D. C. and Petering, H. G. 1974. *New Engl. J. Med.* 291:188.

Wadstrom, L. B., and Wirklund, P. E. 1964. *Acta Chir. Scand. Suppl.* 325:50.

Walker, W. F. 1965. *Proc. R. Soc. Med.* 58:1015.

Wannemacher, R. W., Jr., DuPont, H. L., Pekarek, R. S., Powanda, M. C., Schwartz, A., Hornick, R. B. and Beisel, W. R. 1972. *J. Infect. Dis.* 126:77.

Wene, J. D., Connor, W. E. and DenBesten, L. 1975. *J. Clin. Invest.* 56:127.

Werner, W., Habif, D. V., Randle, P. J. and Lockwood, J. 1951. *Surg. Forum* 1:458.

Wilmore, D. W. and Dudrick, S. J. 1968. *J. Am. Med. Assoc.* 203:860.

Wilmore, D. W., Moylan, J. A., Helmkamp, G. M. and Pruitt, B. A. 1973. *Ann. Surg.* 178:503.

Wilmore, D. W., Lindsey, C. A. and Moylan, J. A. 1974. *Lancet* 1:73.

Wise, J. K., Hendler, R. and Felig, P. 1973. *J. Clin. Invest.* 52:2774.

Woodruff, P., Caridis, D., Cuevas, P., Koizumi, S. and Fine, J. 1973. *Arch. Surg.* 107:613.

Wretlind, A. 1972. *Nutr. Metab. Suppl.* 14:1.

Yalow, R. S., Varsano-Aharon, N., Echenmendia, E. and Berson, S. A. 1969. *Horm. Metab. Res.* 1:3.

Yamakawa, S. 1920. *Nippon Naika Gakk. Zasshi.* 17:22.

Yeo, M. T., Gazzaniga, A. B., Bartlett, R. H. and Shobe, J. B. 1973. *Arch. Surg.* 106:792.

Zohrab, W. J., McHattie, J. D. and Jeejeebhoy, K. N. 1973. *Gastroenterology* 64:583.

Chapter 7

EFFECT OF STARVATION AND FOOD RESTRICTION ON CARBOHYDRATE METABOLISM

Bela Szepesi
Carbohydrate Nutrition Laboratory
Agricultural Research Service,
U.S. Department of Agriculture
Beltsville, Maryland

INTRODUCTION

Starvation, caloric restriction, and their aftermath have been a familiar condition of human existence for many years. Part of the reason for past and present interest of nutritional scientists in caloric restriction rests with its being relatively simple, easy to reproduce, and economically cheap. No expensive dietary formulations are necessary to conduct an experiment designed to elucidate some aspect of the effects of starvation. The potential benefits of these studies deal with two principal areas: the most economical use of animal feed and possible health benefits or hazards occurring from overweight and methods used for weight control. In the area of animal husbandry, use of costly feed materials should be minimized, weight gain (useful weight gain) maximized, and the ratio of meat to fat should be optimal from the nutritional and economic point of view. In the area of human nutrition (weight control) it is important that weight loss, when necessary, be accomplished quickly and without injury to the patient. It is not surprising, therefore, that because of these potential economic and health benefits, nutritional scientists have paid a great deal of attention to the biology, physiology, and biochemistry of caloric restriction.

CHANGES OCCURRING DURING CALORIC DEFICIT

Effects of Caloric Restriction

During starvation or caloric deficiency body weight decreases. The rate of weight loss depends on the metabolic rate of the species in question and on the

151

severity of the caloric restriction. During starvation different organs may shrink at different rates (Cameron and Carmichael, 1946; Keys et al., 1950). The organ least effected by starvation is the brain. Two organs that lose weight at a relatively fast rate during the first day of starvation are the liver (Addis et al., 1936; Conrad and Bass, 1957; Gold and Costello, 1974; Harrison, 1953; Munro, 1964) and the intestine (Desai, 1971). Weight loss in the liver is due to the loss of components such as water, glycogen, fat, and protein and is accompanied by a reduction in the number of nuclei (Conrad and Bass, 1957). In severe caloric deficiency, such as starvation, the loss of storage material is first glycogen followed by fat and protein together. During starvation or during the feeding of a fat-free diet the amount of unsaturated fatty acids will decrease in the liver (Allmann and Gibson, 1965; Almann et al., 1965). It has been suggested that the liver may act as a storage organ for essential fatty acids (Allmann and Gibson, 1965; Allmann et al., 1965). The liver also acts as a short-term storage organ of amino acids and some proteins (Munro, 1964). In many respects the liver acts as a buffer between the external environment and the internal environment. This is especially true when considering dietary changes from adequate to inadequate caloric intake.

During starvation the energy and protein needs of the body must be met, even at the expense of the organs themselves. Few if any components will escape catabolism if starvation is severe. For example, besides the expected loss from adipose tissue (Oscai et al., 1972), there is even a loss in heart (Gold and Costello, 1974) and kidney tissues.

Energy use is decreased during starvation (Keys, 1950) 12-17% in humans (Apfelbaum et al., 1971; Keys et al., 1950) and 10-20% in the rat (Quimby et al., 1948). This decrease in energy output is reflected in the decreased oxygen uptake and a general decrease in body activity. The tendency for a decrease in activity is manifested only during prolonged caloric restriction; initially, upon caloric restriction, activity increases. It is important to take this into account in situations where animals are allowed access to an exercise wheel. In such cases the effect of degree of caloric restriction is modified by the resultant increase in activity, which itself may be different from strain to strain (Stern and Johnson, 1975).

It has been noted that caloric intake and water intake are closely correlated (Anon., 1974; Stevenson, 1969). In humans weight loss parallels sodium excretion (Anon., 1974; Bloom, 1962; Weinsier, 1971). Sodium excretion (natriuresis) is heaviest during day 1 of starvation (Bloom and Mitchell, 1960; Boulter et al., 1973), as is the loss of potassium (Barnard et al., 1969). Natriuresis can be decreased by feeding carbohydrate, but not by feeding fat (Anon., 1974). This would suggest an involvement of insulin in the regulation of sodium excretion. It has also been noted that the degree of natriuresis parallels glucagon levels in the blood and can, in fact, be increased by exogenous glucagon (Boulter et al., 1973). During starvation, along with the disturbance in the excretion of sodium and potassium, blood pressure also increases (Bernardis and Brownie, 1965; Brozek et al., 1948; Consolazio et al., 1966; Keys et al., 1950).

Altered Glucose Tolerance

The symptoms of hunger diabetes were first described by Lehmann (1874). These observations were then confirmed and expanded by the eminent French physiologist Claude Barnard in 1877. The term "hunger diabetes" was coined by Hofmeister in 1890. It was later shown by micromethods that starved and refed dogs would exhibit hyperglycemia during refeeding (Bang, 1913; Böe, 1913; Elias and Kolb, 1913). In later years hunger diabetes was ascribed to an impairment in glucose tolerance (Johansson, 1909), and it was suspected that the impairment in glucose tolerance was responsible for the decreased oxygen uptake in starved and refed animals. Glucose tolerance is impaired in man by as little as a 24-hr fast (Anderson and Herman, 1972). In such cases it may require 2-3 days following refeeding before glucose tolerance is again normal. It is apparent, however, that prolonged caloric restriction will result in prolonged alteration in glucose tolerance. Thus, in malnourished children glucose tolerance was found to be impaired 3 months after clinical treatment began (James and Coore, 1970).

It has been variously proposed that impaired glucose tolerance in starvation is due to increased peripheral resistance to insulin (Goodman and Knobil, 1961; Rathgeb et al., 1970) and to alterations in the pancreatic (Unger et al., 1963) and liver response (Hornichter and Brown, 1969; Soskin et al., 1934) or in the function of the pituitary (Hunter et al., 1968; Rathgeb et al., 1970; Soskin et al., 1939). The role of the pituitary in impaired glucose tolerance during starvation has since been virtually ruled out (Buse et al., 1970). For example, glucose tolerance is still impaired in hypophysectomized fasted animals (D'Amour and Keller, 1933), while actinomycin D (Mahler and Szabo, 1969) or glucose (Conway et al., 1969) can prevent the diabetogenic effect of growth hormone with respect to free fatty acid release. Also, growth hormone response to hypoglycemia is not impaired (Tzagournis and Skillman, 1970), while free fatty acid concentration of the blood can be normalized either by nicotinic acid or tolbutamide without normalization of glucose tolerance (Mahler and Szabo, 1970). Thus, since impaired glucose tolerance is not improved either by the absence of growth hormone or by preventing its effects, its involvement in the impairment of glucose tolerance during and following starvation can be ruled out. Even though it is known that gastrointestinal hormones effect insulin release (Assal et al., 1971; Kraegen et al., 1970; Perley and Kipnis 1967; Zunz and LaBarre, 1928), the involvement of the intestine in the glucose intolerance during starvation has not been suggested.

Current work indicates that the impaired glucose tolerance in starvation is due in part to an impairment in insulin release from the pancreas (Ashcroft et al., 1973; Malaisse et al., 1967). The release of insulin is regulated by a number of factors (Porte and Robertson, 1973; Taylor, 1972), including blood glucose, blood amino acids, and other hormones, and nervous stimulation (Misbin et al., 1971; Porte et al., 1973). In the starved animal it has been reported that the release of both glucagon and insulin is impaired (Buchanan et al., 1969). In particular, in fasted animals it is the glucose-stimulated release of insulin that is impaired (Buckman et al., 1973; Grey et al., 1970), while insulin release elicited by alanine is normal (Buckman et al., 1973). This indicates that alanine has an antidiabetogenic role in addition to stimulating insulin release and can thus be ruled out as a potential cause of starvation diabetes. Also, since insulin release involves both endocytosis and exocytosis (Orci et al., 1973; Sharp et al., 1975), it is not clear which of these processes may be altered during fasting. A number of different factors have been examined concerning insulin release in the fasting state. As previously mentioned, alanine-initiated insulin release is not affected by starvation (Buckman et al., 1973). This is further complicated by observations that while the control of insulin and ketone body concentrations in the blood is reciprocal (Cahill et al., 1966), alanine will lower blood ketone bodies even in the diabetic animal (Genuth and Castro, 1974).

This brings us to consider the possible role of amino acids in the impairment of glucose tolerance. It has been reported that in humans plasma levels of leucine, isoleucine, and valine are increased during at least the first week of starvation (Adibi, 1968; Adibi and Drash, 1970; Felig et al., 1969; Pozefsky et al., 1969). The amino acid concentration of plasma can be reduced by feeding a protein-free, high-carbohydrate diet (Bergen and Purser, 1968; Hill and Olsen, 1963; Weller et al., 1969). It has been proposed that different amino acids may initiate insulin release by different mechanisms (Fajans et al., 1967; Lambert et al., 1971). It is also known that amino acids increase the level of plasma glucagon (Assan et al., 1967; Ohneda et al., 1968) and that the control of insulin and glucagon release is reciprocal (Pagliara et al., 1974). However, the action of amino acids on insulin release can be separated from their effect on glucagon release (Pagliara et al., 1974) in part because the amino acid effects on insulin release require glucose. It is doubtful, therefore, that amino acids either directly or indirectly cause impaired glucose tolerance during starvation. Still, the possible involvement of glucagon in the impaired glucose tolerance of starvation should be kept in mind. Glucagon binds to a receptor with a Stokes radius of 42 Å (Giorgio et al., 1974). Glucagon is not destroyed by this receptor when the receptors are isolated (Giorgio et al., 1974), but it is destroyed by the particulate receptor (Rodbell et al., 1971). Glucagon release cannot be suppressed in the diabetic (Müller et al., 1971), indicating that glucagon release or its suppression requires normal alpha cell metabolism. Attempts to implicate plasma glucagon or pancreatic glucagon in the impairment of insulin release during starvation have so far been unsuccessful. It should be kept in mind, however, that glucagon may be involved in the decreased sensitivity of peripheral cells to insulin during starvation. Recent work has shown that glucagon release can be increased by epinephrine and norepinephrine while at the same time insulin secretion is suppressed (Gordon et al., 1974; Lebovitz and Feldman, 1973; Leclercq-Meyer et al., 1971). Even though these effects are demonstrable, it is difficult to perceive that impaired glucose tolerance could be continuously produced by continually elevated levels of epinephrine or norepinephrine, since the concentration of epinephrine and norepinephrine would be expected to fall to normal levels within a relatively short time after refeeding.

Current evidence indicates that the decreased ability of the pancreas to respond to dietary glucose is involved in the impaired glucose tolerance found during starvation. The exact cause of this has not as yet been determined although the impairment in insulin release rather than insulin production is indicated.

In addition to the numerous studies dealing with the ability of the pancreas to respond to insulinogenic stimuli, considerable attention has been paid to the ability of peripheral tissue to respond to insulin. A great deal of progress has been made in this field in recent years. Insulin binds to a receptor on a number of cells, including adipocytes. The receptor protein has a molecular weight of 400,000 and a Stokes radius of 90 Å (Cuatrecasas, 1972). It is known that a smaller molecule in the membrane can be phosphorylated by ATP; under such circumstances the insulin-stimulated transport of glucose is inhibited in the rat (Chang et al., 1974). This type of effect may be involved in the decreased response of some cells to insulin, but the evidence is not sufficient to prove or disprove such hypothesis. This system cannot be found in the guinea pig (Chang et al., 1974). It is known that the insulin sensitivity of larger fat cells is lowered (Livingston et al., 1972; Salans and Dougherty, 1971). This appears to happen without a loss in the number of receptors. The idea that decreased glucose tolerance in starvation is due to both an impaired function of the pancreas and increased peripheral resistance to insulin has recently gained more recognition (Bennett et al., 1972).

Enzyme and Protein Levels during Caloric Deficiency

The role of liver and adipose tissue during starvation. Adipose tissue can produce, store, and release fat. The role of this tissue in caloric oversufficiency is to make and store fat that is then available as an energy source during caloric deficiency. The metabolic role of the liver is unique in the mammalian organism. The liver is the first metabolically active organ to receive nutrients from the gastrointestinal system. The role of maintaining homeostasis rests largely on the liver. This involves such operations as storage, conversion or temporary storage of incoming nutrients, and the production of blood glucose and certain blood proteins. In addition, the liver is constantly called upon to eliminate toxic materials by metabolizing them to nontoxic end products. In some respects the role the liver plays in a higher organism resembles the role played by a single bacterium: that is, the regulation of internal homeostasis. Keeping this in mind it should be easier to perceive the physiological need for the varied and complex regulation of the metabolic pathways of the liver. This is true in the case of amino acid catabolism, and carbohydrate and fat metabolism. In fact, many of the regulatory mechanisms that operate in the liver are necessary to prevent changes in other organs that might be deleterious to the entire organism. Likewise, for those scientists who wish to study regulatory mechanisms and control mechanisms, the liver is the choice of study precisely because it has these control mechanisms. This section, therefore, by necessity will concentrate on the effects of starvation and caloric restriction on the liver.

Decrease in enzyme activity. One of the classic examples of a regulatory mechanism in a higher organism is the control of glycogen synthesis and breakdown in the liver and muscle. This field has been extensively reviewed (Hers et al., 1970; Holzer and Duntze, 1971; Krebs, 1972; Krebs et al., 1964; Larner and Villar-Palasi, 1971; Segal, 1973; Walsh et al., 1968). Although there appears to be a substantial amount of glycogen in the muscle, muscle glycogen per se is not usually involved in the maintenance of blood glucose. The initial requirement for blood glucose after starvation begins seems to come from the breakdown of liver glycogen. The enzyme systems involved in liver glycogen synthesis and breakdown appear to be controlled in a reciprocal fashion. This control is illustrated in Fig. 1. The hormones, epinephrine or glucagon, interact with a receptor in the cell membrane, activating adenyl cyclase, which results in an increased conversion of ATP to cyclic $3',5'$-adenosine monophosphate (cAMP), which in turn interacts with and activates protein kinase (Krebs, 1972). Protein kinase has two subunits: catalytic and regulatory. When the two units are combined in the absence of cAMP, protein kinase is inactive. With large concentrations of cAMP the regulatory subunit of the protein kinase binds cAMP. It then dissociates from the catalytic subunit. Upon dissociation from the regulatory subunit, the catalytic subunit becomes active. Active protein kinase then activates phosphorylase kinase *b*, which activates phosphorylase kinase *a*. Phosphorylase kinase *a* in turn converts phosphorylase *a* to phosphorylase *b*. Phosphorylase *b*, the active form of phosphorylase, catalyzes the

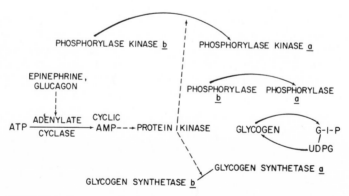

FIGURE 1 The control of glycogen metabolism by cAMP-activated protein kinase. The reciprocal control of glycogen breakdown and synthesis is achieved by the simultaneous activation of phosphorylase and deactivation of glycogen synthetase.

breakdown of glycogen to glucose 1-phosphate. In conjunction with activating the phosphorylase pathway and thus initiating glycogen breakdown, protein kinase converts glycogen synthetase *a* to glycogen synthetase *b,* the inactive form of the enzyme. Thus, by the same mechanism, that is, by the same effector molecule, glycogen synthesis can be shut down and glycogen breakdown initiated. This dual mechanism allows the animal to obtain a relatively quick source of glucose. As starvation becomes more acute, that is to say, goes beyond a number of hours, then other enzyme systems will be activated or induced to begin the production of glucose from other sources.

Another system of control is responsible for the reciprocal control of lipogenesis and lipolysis. In some respects, these controls resemble those regulating glycogenesis and glycolysis. Again, the controlling stimulus appears to be an increase in glucagon and/or epinephrine. These hormones act to inhibit the key lipogenic enzymes acetyl CoA carboxylase and the fatty acid synthetase complex (Collins et al., 1971; Inoue and Lowenstein, 1972; Numa et al., 1965). Acetyl CoA carboxylase was shown to contain phosphorus (Inoue and Lowenstein, 1972) and has since been proven to be present in active or inactive forms (Carlson and Kim, 1974). The control of fatty acid synthetase is quite a mystery at present. To begin with, the enzyme complex is really a very large particle containing either two or five peptides, depending on whether the enzyme complex is isolated from the animal system or from bacteria (Porter et al., 1975). The whole matter is further complicated by the report (Collins et al., 1971) that in starved or diabetic rats a 7-S protein is made that accompanies fatty acid synthetase. Its function is still unknown. Like acetyl CoA carboxylase and fatty acid synthetase, triglyceride lipase is affected by the stress hormones (Khoo et al., 1974; Rizack, 1964). In this case, there is a difference between the enzyme that is isolated from the rat and that which is isolated from humans. The human triglyceride lipase system has an alpha adrenergic receptor, whereby adrenergic stimulation can suppress lipolysis (Khoo et al., 1974). At present, the available evidence does not allow us to conclude that there is a reciprocal control between triglyceride lipase and lipoprotein lipase (Khoo et al., 1974). A reciprocal control of lipoprotein lipase and hormone sensitive lipase in adipose tissue has been suggested (Robinson and Wing, 1970).

The activation by the hormone glucagon of other enzymes, notably fructose diphosphatase, has also been reported (Greene et al., 1974; Taunton et al., 1972). In the same experiments it was reported that glucagon caused a rapid inactivation of pyruvate kinase and phosphofructokinase (Taunton et al., 1972). The effects were observable within 4 min and could be reversed by insulin. The effect of insulin in reversing the glucagon effects was not accompanied by a change in cAMP levels. This observation is very interesting because it was reported that the reversal of the effect of glucagon on the glycogen synthetase and phosphorylase systems in liver by glucose infusion also occurs without a change in cAMP level (Glinsmann et al., 1970). This would indicate that while the effect of glucagon involves cAMP, the reciprocal effect on the same enzymes does not and may be accomplished by the influx of certain substrates such as glucose. This would suggest yet another level of control involved in the regulation of the activity of these enzymes.

The *in vivo* significance of the control exerted over the activities of enzymes involved in glycogen metabolism has been now shown both with respect to glucagon (Krebs, 1972; Segal, 1973) and the stimulation of the nervous system (Shimazu, 1971; Shimazu and Fujimoto, 1971). It was reported that vagal stimulation will increase glycogen synthetase activity and decrease the K_m for UDPG tenfold (Shimazu, 1971). Furthermore it was shown that vagal stimulation is not abolished by pancreatectomy. Splanchnic stimulation, on the other hand, will decrease glycogen synthetase activity (Shimazu, 1971). The amount of glucose exchange in the blood, as well as glucose incorporation into glycogen, was shown to be increased by vagal stimulation (Shimazu and Fujimoto, 1971) and decreased by splanchnic stimulation.

Enzymes increased by starvation. As has been noted the activities of phosphorylase (Segal, 1973), triglyceride lipase (Khoo et al., 1974), and certain gluconeogenic enzymes such as fructose-1,6-diphosphatase and phosphoenol-pyruvate carboxykinase (PEPCK) (Taunton et al., 1972) can be increased by glucagon. These are catabolic enzymes that participate in the breakdown of the body's energy stores to make them available for immediate or delayed energy use. There are other enzymes, notably those involved in amino acid catabolism, that are also increased by starvation (Freedland et al., 1966). The rate of change in the activities of these enzymes, however, is quite variable. Most of the changes in these enzymes, unlike the three enzymes already mentioned (Khoo et al., 1974; Segal, 1973; Taunton et al., 1972), seem to require *de novo* protein synthesis (Freedland et al., 1966). Since the rate at which a new steady state of enzyme activity is achieved depends solely on the half-life of the enzyme rather than on its rate of synthesis, the rate at which the amino acid catabolizing enzymes achieve maximum steady state levels is dependent on their half-lives. As these values are rather variable, ranging from 2–5 hr for tyrosine amino transferase to 2–5 days for arginase, it would appear that the activities of these enzymes reach maximum at different times.

Secondary adaptations arising during starvation can actually decrease or entirely prevent a rise in the activity of some of these amino acid catabolizing enzymes. Because of conflicting needs to produce glucose from amino acids once the glycogen stores are depleted and to conserve amino acids as much as possible, the activities of these enzymes are probably subject to a number of controls geared to respond to the energy state of the animal and to the amount of amino acids and protein that are held in "reserve."

General effect on enzyme levels in starvation. The effect of starvation on the activities of a number of enzymes has been recently reviewed (Freedland et al., 1966). In general, most of the enzyme changes that occur will take place either in the liver or in the adipose tissue although there are some changes in other organs, especially if starvation is prolonged and severe. The responses of

TABLE 1   Rate of Loss of Liver Components
during Starvation[a,b]

Component	Days of starvation			
	1	2	3	4
Body weight	89	86	76	75
Liver weight	64	65	67	51
Liver protein, soluble (mg/100 g body wt)	64	69	75	60
Liver glycogen (mg/100 g body wt)	1	6	6	9
Glucose-6-phosphatase	101	113	95	66
Fructose-1,6-diphosphatase	65	56	61	51
Phosphorylase	77	54	52	30
Phosphoglucomutase	49	52	48	40
Phosphohexose isomerase	77	77	68	44
Pentose phosphate metab. enzyme	79	70	66	54
Glucose-6-phosphate dehydrogenase	44	23	34	11
6-Phosphogluconate dehydrogenase	64	44	46	27
Malic enzyme	36	37	35	16
Succinic dehydrogenase	70	79	75	67
Fumarase	71	79	75	67
Malic dehydrogenase	84	87	84	68

[a]The level before starvation is taken as 100%. All other values
were calculated on that basis. Enzyme levels were calculated on the
basis of prestarvation body weight.
  [b]Data summarized from Freedland (1967).

some key liver enzymes to starvation are illustrated in Table 1. The figures
constitute a summary of data presented by Freedland (1967). The figures bear
out the conclusions of the previous sections: that is, pathways important for
continued survival—such as glycolysis, the tricarboxylic acid cycle, and gluconeogenesis—will be preferentially maintained over the activities of enzymes involved
in "luxury" pathways, such as lipid synthesis. The evenutal drop in phosphorylase activity perhaps reflects the lesser need for phosphorylase as starvation
continues. The activity of PEPCK (not listed in Table 1) not only increases
during starvation (Hanson et al., 1973; Hopgood et al., 1973) but also, when
induced, constitutes some 3% of the total rat liver cytosol protein (Hopgood et
al., 1973). Some other catabolic enzymes such as histidase, and urokinase
(Schirmer and Harper, 1970) and tryptophan pyrrolase (Yuwiler et al., 1969)
have also been reported to increase during starvation. It should be kept in mind
that some of these reports where enzyme increases were noted contain these
conclusions not so much because there is more enzyme present but because of
the way enzyme activity is reported. For example, if enzyme activity is reported
as specific activity then the sharp drop in liver protein seen (see Table 1)
immediately after starvation commences would make it appear that the activity
of the enzyme increased, whereas the actual absolute activity of the enzyme

remained the same. During chronic starvation many amino acid catabolizing enzymes will severely decrease in activity.

The activity of acetyl CoA carboxylase falls not only in the liver but also in the epididymal fat pad during starvation (Barth et al., 1972). Pyruvate kinase (Eggleston and Krebs, 1969), pyruvate dehydrogenase (Patzelt et al., 1973), and cholinesterase activities (Harrison and Brown, 1951) will also decrease. While fatty acid activation enzymes are decreased in the epididymal fat pad, liver, and heart carnitine palmityl transferase is decreased by starvation only in the liver (Aas and Daae, 1971). Some decreases in the activities of lipogenic enzymes can be noted also in brown fat (Hahn and Kirby, 1974). Other investigators have reported relatively small or no changes in the activities of a number of enzymes in the lung (Scholz and Rhodes, 1971), heart, kidney (Gold and Costello, 1974), and muscle (Howarth and Baldwin, 1971b). In the intestine, hexokinase activity (Srivastave et al., 1968; Weiser et al., 1971) has been reported to be decreased but still high (Weiser et al., 1971) along with acid phosphatase, beta-glucuronidase, aryl sulfatase, and cathepsin D (Desai, 1971). Currently, enzyme induction in the pancreas is receiving increasingly greater attention. That some of the changes in pancreatic enzyme levels may have important physiological effects can be deduced from the fact that the glucose-stimulated insulin release in the pancreas can be restored within 24 hr under certain experimental conditions, but this response is blocked if the pancreas is treated with actinomycin D (Grey et al., 1970).

It can be expected that the changes in the liver and the intestine referred to above must be accompanied by greater than normal rates of catabolism. This is indeed the case; the activities of a number of catabolic enzymes in the intestine (Desai, 1971) and liver (Desai, 1969; Filkins, 1970) have been reported to increase during starvation. As can be expected, starvation alters the activity of virtually every enzyme in the liver in every metabolic pathway. Thus, the activity of gulonolactone hydrolase in ascorbate metabolism (Stubbs and Griffin, 1973) and the activities of a number of enzymes involved in steroid metabolism are decreased (Slakey et al., 1972).

Another potentially important system affected by starvation is drug metabolism. Starvation decreases the metabolism of a variety of drugs including aminopyrene and hexabarbitol, while enhancing the metabolism of aniline (Kato and Gilette, 1965). Two other enzymes involved in drug metabolism, dimethylaminoazobenzene reductase (Jervell et al., 1965) and dimethylnitrosamine methylase (Venkatesan et al., 1970), however, are increased by 24 hr of starvation.

In summary, the activities of a number of enzymes in the liver and the adipose tissue are decreased during starvation, while a few are increased. The degree of maintenance of enzyme activity often reflects the physiological role of these enzymes: that is, the physiological need for keeping them active. Thus, enzymes involved in energy production are preferentially maintained, while enzymes involved in lipid synthesis are rapidly degraded. Thus, the shift in enzyme activity during starvation is consistent with the physiologic requirement of maintaining homeostasis and vital functions, so that when realimentation occurs, recovery can be instituted.

Alterations in nucleic acid synthesis and degradation. The rate of protein synthesis per milligram RNA in the liver, muscle, brain, and testes has been shown to vary over a wide range (see Table 2) (Henshaw et al., 1971). It has also been reported that the efficiency of protein synthesis is correlated with the growth rate in liver and muscle but not in brain and testes. This would imply that the brain or the testes would be maintained or would grow at the expense of other organs during caloric deficiency. This maintenance is vital for the survival of the individual, as well as for the survival of the species. Similar conclusions were drawn with respect to starvation (Henshaw et al., 1971). During starvation the amount of RNA, in particular the amount of ribosomal RNA, is drastically reduced in the liver (Hirsch and Hiatt, 1966; Norman et al., 1973). This is reflected in a fast rate of degradation of the rough endoplastic reticulum during starvation (Tomi, 1961). It was reported that the yield of ribosomes is decreased with progressive starvation (over 48 hr), representing a slow and early loss of mRNA and later an alteration in ribosomal function (Shlossberg and Hollenberg, 1970). The loss of ribosomes does not seem to be accompanied by an impairment of function of the remaining polysomes, although the number of polysomes was decreased and the resultant single ribosomes were degraded (Blobel and Potter, 1967; Norman et al., 1973). The mRNA function was not found to be related to RNAse activity (Shlossberg and Hollenberg, 1970). This is in accordance with the relatively long half-life of mRNA in the cytosol (Murphy and Attardi, 1973). DNA and RNA levels can be reduced by prolonged caloric restriction (Howarth and Baldwin, 1971a) and normalized upon restoration of ad libitum feeding even without normalization of total protein synthesis.

The change in RNA metabolism during starvation is not well understood, but it is known that RNAse activity during starvation is increased (Sheppard et al., 1970). However, the increase in RNAse activity was attributed not to an

TABLE 2 Protein Synthetic Capacity of Various Organs[a]

Organ	nmol lysine incorporated/ mg RNA/min
Liver	2.4–9.1
Muscle	1.1–3.9
Brain	0.8–5.6
Testes	0.4–2.7

[a]Data were taken from Henshaw et al. (1971).

increase in RNAse but to the disappearance of an inhibitor (Sheppard et al., 1970). Ribosomal RNA function is impaired and the number of ribosomes decreased in growth hormone deficiency (Florini and Breuer, 1966; Korner, 1959, 1968) and insulin deficiency (Wool and Cavicchi, 1967). Upon insuliniza-tion RNA synthesis increases within 3 hr, reaching a maximum in 6 hr; both nucleolar and nucleoplasmic RNA are synthesized (Pilkis and Salaman, 1972). These authors concluded that insulinization would affect RNA synthesis not by increasing RNA synthesis per se but by inhibiting RNAse activity. In other experiments it was found that upon refeeding nuclear, ribosomal, and transfer RNA reach normal levels per total cell DNA in 24 hr (Onishi, 1970). The bulk of the change in RNA in the refed rats was in ribosomal RNA (Onishi, 1970).

It appears, therefore, that during starvation or caloric deficiency RNA synthesis is decreased and RNA degradation is increased. Most of the changes in RNA levels appear to involve ribosomal RNA. Upon realimentation to an *ad libitum* regimen, normal or even higher than normal rates of RNA synthesis and RNA levels can be noted and decreased degradation allows normalization of RNA levels. This would indicate that the synthetic machinery for RNA is preserved and is not damaged beyond repair by starvation.

Alterations in polysome aggregation. From the previous section it can be discerned that during starvation nucleic acid metabolism undergoes large changes. These changes result in less total RNA and less active RNA that is in a form capable of synthesizing protein. There is quite a controversy concerning the control of protein synthesis, the aggregation and disaggregation of polysomes, and exactly what controls are exerted over these processes during starvation. A number of investigators have shown that during starvation or under a condition of tryptophan deficiency, polysomes can be disaggregated (Arora and DeLamirande, 1971; Sidransky et al., 1968, 1971; Sidransky and Verney, 1971; Staehelin et al., 1967). The controversy arises because other authors have shown that polysomes in the starved animal can be reaggregated by feeding a diet devoid of protein (Webb et al., 1966; Wittman et al., 1969). This would indicate that tryptophan might be a regulating factor, but only when it becomes a limiting amino acid.

The hormonal control of polysomal aggregation and disaggregation is also somewhat unclear at present. The hormone glucagon does not affect the polysome profile (Ayuso-Parrilla and Parrilla, 1973). There is ample evidence, however, that would implicate both glucose and insulin in the control of the rate of polysome aggregation and the rate of protein synthesis (Permutt, 1974; Wittman et al., 1969; Wool, 1972). For example, in previously starved rats, refeeding glucose initiates a reaggregation of heavier polysomes, whereas refeeding a high-fat diet does not (Wittman et al., 1969). In the diabetic animal, insulin alone or with glucose can stimulate hepatic protein synthesis in normal or hypophysectomized rats (Wittman et al., 1969). This would indicate that in the starved rat the critical component factor is glucose, since insulin is available to the animal. However, in the diabetic animal insulin as well as glucose must be provided.

It has been shown that starvation decreases the incorporation of radioactive leucine into protein while increasing leucine oxidation (Ryan et al., 1974). The stress hormones epinephrine and norepinephrine also reduce amino acid incorporation into the diaphragm (Wool, 1960). Recent work designed to elucidate the precise mechanism whereby both glucose and insulin affect the rate of protein synthesis has shown that glucose appears to be involved at initiation (Permutt, 1974) and insulin is involved in altering initiation by altering one of the ribosomal particles (Wool, 1972).

It has also been shown that while insulin can increase protein synthesis in muscle from starved animals it does not do so in muscle from fed animals (Wool et al., 1968). This would indicate that insulin is necessary for the restoration of normal rates of protein synthesis. Since it is now generally accepted that insulin does not get into either the muscle cell or the adipocyte, it is a matter of conjecture as to how a hormone that acts at the cell membrane would have its effect on the competence of a ribosomal particle inside the cytosol.

Protein turnover and its control during caloric restriction. As mentioned, liver protein decreases during starvation (Table 1). It has been estimated that the fractional catabolic rate in the liver of a rat fed *ad libitum* is 14–16% (Enwonwu et al., 1971). During the first hour of starvation this is increased by 50%. During the first day of starvation protein synthesis is also increased somewhat (Enwonwu et al., 1971). After 48 hr of starvation the catabolic rate is still up to 10% but the fractional synthetic rate is less than 10%. Polysomes dissociate, which, of course, would lead to a general and slow disappearance of liver protein. It has been suggested that the rate of degradation of liver protein is proportional to the molecular size of the protein involved (Dehlinger and Schimke, 1970). There seems to be some doubt, however, concerning this proposal.

Since liver protein generally decreases during starvation, it would be expected that most if not all species of liver protein would eventually decrease. As was shown above, this appears to be the case. As can be expected the breakdown of different proteins would be controlled in different ways, resulting in different rates of disappearance of various enzymes and proteins.

The rates of disappearance of many lipogenic enzymes are also altered by starvation. There is evidence indicating that during starvation hepatic malic enzyme (NADP-linked) activity is decreased, not only by a decrease in the rate of synthesis (Murphy and Walker, 1972; Silpananta and Goodridge, 1971) but also by an increase in the rate of degradation. For example, in chick liver the half-life of malic enzyme is decreased from 55 hr in the *ad libitum*-fed animal to 28 hr in the starved animal (Silpananta and Goodridge, 1971). The half-life of acetyl CoA carboxylase ranges from 48–59 hr in the *ad libitum*-fed rat to 18–30 hr in the starved rat (Nakanishi and Numa, 1970). The turnover of fatty acid synthetase, however, does not appear to be altered during starvation (Hayes and Larrabee, 1971).

In another study the rates of degradation of various intestinal enzymes were investigated (Jones and Mayer, 1973). The enzymes studied were hexokinase, 6-phosphogluconate dehydrogenase (6PGD), lactic dehydrogenase, pyruvate kinase, glucose-6-phosphate dehydrogenase (G6PD), phosphoglycerate kinase, and aldolase. It was found that the lifetime of the epithelial cells varied from 1 to 3 days in the fed rat and was actually increased during starvation. On the other hand, the activities of the enzymes studied decreased and reached new steady-state levels after 48 hr. This would indicate that a complex relationship may exist in the priority in which proteins are preserved in the intestine during starvation.

The process of studying protein turnover is complicated by using radioactive precipitation specific for the active enzyme. For example, in studying the degradation of PEPCK, Ballard and Hopgood (1974) were not able to find any radioactive products of enzyme degradation. When biphosphatase from rabbit liver was studied, it was found that the purified enzyme was a peptide shorter than the unpurified enzyme (Pontremoli et al., 1973). At present it is not certain, therefore, whether the breakdown of an enzyme proceeds in one single, well-coordinated event or if it is stepwise and systematic.

The hormonal control of protein degradation in rat liver is well coordinated with the physiological requirements of the body during starvation. For example, protein degradation in general is accelerated by glucagon and decreased by insulin and amino acids (Mortimore et al., 1973). This is particularly important physiologically, since a considerable amount of amino acids is absorbed in the liver during starvation and converted to glucose. In rabbit liver, lysosomes during starvation have been reported to become increasingly fragile, and the activity of enzymes from lysosomes is known to increase (Filkins, 1970; Pontremoli et al., 1973).

A scheme for the control of protein degradation in the liver is illustrated in Fig. 2. ATP has been implicated as a required factor in protein degradation (Umaña, 1970, 1971a; Umaña and Feldman, 1971). It has been suggested that this role of ATP involves the production of aspartyl adenylate (Umaña, 1970). Aspartyl AMP reportedly activates the endopeptidase inhibitor which inhibitor peptide will be broken down and the endopeptidase will become active (Umaña, 1971b). Protein degradation, therefore, may be regulated by glutamic oxalacetic transaminase in the liver. Since the endopeptidase is inhibited by some of the end products of protein degradation, aspartyl AMP would be required in greater amounts during increased protein breakdown. This would necessitate a continuous resynthesis of aspartyl AMP. Since the activity of glutamic oxalacetic transaminase is relatively high in the liver during starvation, the proposal could explain the mechanism of continuous protein breakdown in liver and its regulation. At present, however, further clarification and confirmation is needed to ascertain which of these points are valid under physiological conditions.

Summary. It is apparent that the biochemical changes that take place can for the most part be deduced from the physiological requirement of the organism: (1) to obtain the necessary energy for body maintenance and (2) to preserve vital functions for the time when realimentation becomes possible. The

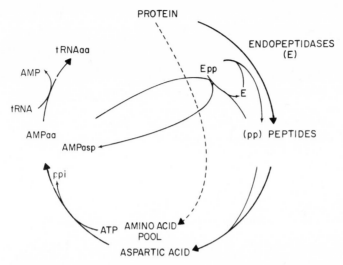

FIGURE 2 The proposed regulation of protein breakdown in the
mammalian cell. The figure is taken from Umaña (1971b), courtesy of
Proceedings of the Society of Experimental Biology and Medicine.

biochemical changes that occur during starvation seem to be geared to
accomplish just these ends. Thus, storage compounds such as glycogen and fat
are catabolized during starvation to provide both blood glucose and a source of
energy. The breakdown of body components is geared in such a way that organs
vital to maintaining life and to the preservation and propagation of the species
are most protected. Within organs that undergo large changes, such as the liver
and adipose tissue, the order of maintenance again follows similar patterns;
components vital for survival are preferentially maintained over components that
are not. These types of adaptations allow animals to undergo caloric restriction
or starvation for long periods of time. Also, during realimentation a return to
normalcy can occur.

Meal Feeding: A Special Case of Caloric Restriction

Meal feeding is a special feeding regimen where food is provided to the
experimental animal or subject within a well-defined and relatively short period
during the day. The subject has been recently reviewed (Fábry, 1967; Fábry and
Tepperman, 1970). This type of feeding regimen calls for adaptive mechanisms
to store the influx of food within a relatively short time and to release the stored
material over a longer period of time. It has been found that meal-fed rats have
higher respiratory quotients than do *ad libitum*-fed animals (Tepperman et al.,
1943a,b). This would indicate that when the respiratory quotient was
determined, there was very little lipolysis and considerable lipogenesis. There is
quite a controversy concerning the effect of meal feeding with respect to body
weight gain and body fat accumulation. Part of the controversy is probably due

to the different approaches used, the different age of the animals studied, and the different lengths of adaptation used in meal feeding. For example, in 90-day-old rats, meal feeding did not affect body composition, while in young adult males, meal feeding increased carcass fat and decreased the percent of carcass protein (Wardlaw et al., 1969). It has also been shown that the time at which lipogenesis is determined may be an important determinant in the comparison between meal-fed and *ad libitum*-fed rats (Sullivan et al., 1971). While lipogenesis was generally found to be inversely proportional to body weight, maximum lipogenesis was recorded 5–9 days after meal feeding began (Sullivan et al., 1971). In meal-fed rats the maximum lipogenesis after a meal was shown to occur about 5 hr after the meal (Sullivan et al., 1971), while 24 hr after the meal the rate of lipogenesis *in vivo* was only 3% of the maximal rate whereas *in vitro* it was 18–25% (Sullivan et al., 1971).

It appears that meal-fed rats are better able to respond to a glucose load than are *ad libitum*-fed rats (Cohn and Joseph, 1970). This was confirmed by other investigators.

Among the types of adaptation to meal feeding are an increase in glucose absorption and utilization in the intestine and general lengthening of the gastrointestinal tract (Leveille and Chakrabarty, 1968). In some instances at least, meal feeding seems to elevate body fat content (Cohn and Joseph, 1960; Fábry, 1967; Fábry and Tepperman, 1970). In the chicken, however, two or even five 1-hr meals per day either did not affect body composition or actually decreased the percent body fat (Griminger et al., 1969). The inability of the chicken to respond like the rat to meal feeding may reflect a greater metabolic rate of *ad libitum*-fed chickens than that of rats. Therefore, one major adaptation to meal feeding (that is, a speedup of storage of incoming food) is not appreciable in meal-fed chickens.

Lipogenesis in meal-fed animals is elevated as compared with *ad libitum*-fed animals, especially right after a meal (Leveille, 1967). The increase in fatty acid synthesis precedes the increase in enzyme activity (Leveille, 1966). Fatty acid synthesis either from glucose or acetate is elevated (Patel and Mistry, 1969). The increases in rate of fatty acid synthesis both in the liver and the adipose tissue are accompanied by increased activities of enzymes involved directly or peripherally in fatty acid synthesis (Chakrabarty and Leveille, 1968, 1969; Wiley and Leveille, 1970).

The adaptation to meal feeding can be deduced from the physiological requirement; the animal system changes in such a way as to use and store incoming food during and after a meal, which can be released slowly. In the meal-fed rat some enzymes undergo diurnal variation, some of which is due to the diurnal variation induced by the light schedule (Freedland et al., 1966); other enzymes are definitely induced by the time of feeding. This type of adaptation—that is, an enzymic periodicity induced by eating—has been termed "fress-urnal variation" in enzyme activity.

It has been reported that when meal-fed rats are allowed to consume as much or more food as *ad libitum*-fed rats, they deposit more body fat (Fábry, 1967; Fábry and Tepperman, 1970). In most instances, however, meal-fed rats and chickens are not able to consume as much food during the short period of time allotted for them to eat as do *ad libitum*-fed rats, which eat either during the dark or during the entire day. The problem is further complicated by the fact that when rats are restricted in their food intake, they eventually become meal eaters (Schnakenberg et al., 1971). To finally resolve the question as to whether meal-fed rats store more body fat than do *ad libitum*-fed rats, experiments were performed where rats were provided pellets by a machine at prescribed times of the day. It was found that when meal-fed and *ad libitum*-fed rats ate the same amount of food they exhibited comparable body parameters, including body fat (Aysel et al., 1975). It would appear, therefore, that meal feeding in a number of cases would reduce body weight because rats would eat less food. It should also be kept in mind that when rats are pair fed and if the caloric restriction is relatively severe, such as 80% of the *ad libitum* intake or less, the possibility that the meal feeding pattern is established is real and should be considered.

Physiological and Biochemical Adaptation to Caloric Deficiency

Overall change in metabolism. During starvation several events take place to preserve homeostasis. A primary drive in maintaining homeostasis is to maintain adequate blood glucose levels. This is necessary since the central nervous system is unable to substitute for the majority of its glucose requirement. As blood glucose falls, body stores of glycogen will be mobilized to maintain adequate levels of blood glucose. This event is shortly followed by the mobilization of available amino acids, which are then converted to glucose. Simultaneously, body stores of fat are broken down (Gilbertson, 1969) and used for energy through the TCA cycle and/or converted to ketone bodies. Lipogenesis from carbohydrate virtually comes to a halt, as does the production of liver glycogen. If starvation is acute and prolonged, however, the overall response of increased gluconeogenesis may lead to somewhat increased glycogenesis in the liver. In short, most of the organs, especially the liver, must change their metabolism to either produce or conserve glucose as much as possible. Along with the drastic change in carbohydrate metabolism during starvation, the ion balance in the urine and the function of the kidney also change. Some of these changes will be discussed in greater detail later.

It has been shown that hypoglycemia causes an increase in glucagon release (Unger et al., 1962). A fall in plasma triglyceride or free fatty acid concentration (Luyckx and Lefebvre, 1970) or inhibition of glucose utilization in the pancreas (Edwards and Taylor, 1970) can also increase glucagon secretion. There is no evidence that insulin breakdown is accelerated (Varandani, 1973). During starvation cAMP has been shown to increase in the liver, kidney, muscle, and adipose tissue (Selawary et al., 1973). In addition to the enzymes mentioned above, glycogenolysis is increased during starvation (Hanson, 1974). One must be careful, however, to keep in mind the species differences encountered both in glycolysis and gluconeogenesis. In the ruminant, such as the sheep (Ballard et al., 1969), the major source of glucose is propionic and butyric acid. In the monogastric animal the major source of glucose during gluconeogenic conditions, such as starvation, is amino acids. Another complicating factor is that while in the rat PEPCK is located exclusively in the cytosol, in rabbit, cow, and man, this enzyme is distributed between the mitochondria and the cytosol (Hanson, 1974). This difference in enzyme location means that those controls in the rat based on the location of PEPCK are not operative in such species as rabbit, bovine, and man.

Glycolysis and lipolysis are regulated not only by glucagon but also by the sympathetic and parasympathetic nervous systems (Lockwood et al., 1971). Thus, it has been suggested that lipolysis is primarily increased in adipose tissue as a result of increased sympathetic discharge (Cantu et al., 1963; Fröberg et al., 1964). Adrenergic receptors have been located in human adipose tissue (Burns and Langley, 1970). Glucose levels were found to be unrelated to growth hormone, free fatty acid, or glucagon levels in the baboon; thus participation of the central nervous system in the regulation of blood glucose in this species was suggested (Koerker et al., 1974). There appears to be little doubt that the regulation of glycolysis and gluconeogenesis involves various factors (Weber et al., 1968) in the various organs (Villar-Palasi and Larner, 1968; Weber et al., 1968). It is now known that as a response to an increased demand for more glucose, gluconeogenesis from alanine is increased (Sladek and Snarr, 1974). However, gluconeogenesis is decreased when insulin is administered (Sladek and Snarr, 1974). During starvation, therefore, when insulin levels are low, gluconeogenesis from amino acids would be expected to increase. As a reflection of the increased amino acid catabolism during starvation, branched chain amino acids in blood are increased (Adibi and Drash, 1970). It has also been shown that branched chain amino acids can be increased in the blood by catecholamines (Buse et al., 1973).

It would appear that in the monogastric animal the increased demand for blood glucose production is met primarily by the liver rather than by the kidney (Bowman, 1970). However, under such conditions as a high-protein diet, the kidney's contribution to gluconeogenesis may be significant. This is reflected by the report that kidney gluconeogenesis is not altered by hormones (Bowman, 1970).

One of the adaptive mechanisms operating during starvation appears to be a decrease in glycolysis. One point at which glycolysis can be inhibited is at the rate-limiting reaction catalyzed by hexokinase (Rolleston, 1972). Another important control point in the glycolytic pathway is the reaction catalyzed by phosphofructokinase (Gumaa and McLean, 1971; Rolleston, 1972). The inhibition of hexokinase primarily involves a change in the V_{max}, whereas the regulation of phosphofructokinase involves a change in the K_m of the enzyme (Rolleston, 1972). The regulation of phosphofructokinase is rather complex, involving ATP and citrate as inhibitors and cAMP, AMP, phosphate, fructose 6-phosphate, and fructose diphosphate as activators. The complexity of this regulation is illustrated by the fact that the inhibition of phosphofructokinase by ATP can be reversed by AMP and P_i but not by fructose 6-phosphate (Gumaa and McLean, 1971). On the other hand, fructose 6-phosphate raises the K_i for citrate (Gumaa and McLean, 1971). It has been reported that glycolysis can effectively be blocked without affecting insulin release (Matschinsky and Ellerman, 1973), suggesting that the participation of substrate-level inhibitors are involved. In the report cited above it was suggested that glycolysis was strongly coupled to the "sodium pump" and that a complex relation, therefore, may exist between sodium output and inhibition of glycolysis (Matschinsky and Ellerman, 1973). The increased sodium excretion during starvation, especially during the first day of starvation, would not be incompatible with this suggestion; however, a mechanism linking sodium pumping in the kidney with a blockage of glycolysis in the liver and muscle is somewhat difficult to envision.

Another possible point of regulation arises from the fact that, at least in rat liver, both glycolysis and gluconeogenesis take place in the same intracellular compartment (Kramer and Freedland, 1971). The operation of pairs of enzymes that are working in opposing fashion such as hexokinase and glucose-6-phosphatase, PEPCK, and pyruvate kinase, provide the basis for the existence of futile cycles (Newsholme and Gevers, 1967; Scrutton and Utter, 1968). That is, by simultaneously phosphorylating and dephosphorylating substrates and using up high energy phosphate bonds in the process, a considerable amount of energy can be wasted. Such a mechanism may be useful during caloric over sufficiency or at times when increased heat production is required, but it would be quite deleterious during starvation when the body must conserve energy. Futile cycles have been shown to operate in *Bombus affinis* (M. G. Clark et al., 1973a) halothane-poisoned pigs (M. G. Clark et al., 1973b), and elsewhere (Hue and Hers, 1974a). The existence of a functional futile cycle at the level of glucose and glucose 6-phosphate has been suggested (Rognstad et al., 1973) and has been shown to operate between 15 and 25% of the time (D. G. Clark et al., 1973). There has been no confirmatory evidence that in rat liver futile cycles might operate at the level of fructose diphosphate or phosphoenolpyruvate (Hue and Hers, 1974b).

The major casualty of starvation with respect to metabolic pathways to be inhibited is lipogenesis. Fatty acid synthesis has been reported to be inhibited as much as 90% 2 hr after starvation commences (Yeh and Leveille, 1970). Fatty acid synthesis is inhibited in virtually every tissue that can synthesize fatty acids, for example, pig adipose tissue (O'Hea and Leveille, 1969) and chicken liver (Yeh and Leveille, 1971). Along with the inhibition of fatty acid synthesis, cholesterol synthesis is also blocked (Bucher et al., 1959; Linn, 1967; Tomkins and Chaikoff, 1952). Lipogenesis from carbohydrate and leucine (Meikle and

Klain, 1972) is inhibited during starvation. Inasmuch as a considerable amount of the reducing potential (NADPH) for lipogenesis is provided by the operation of the pentose phosphate shunt (Patel et al., 1971), it is no surprise that in fat cells the operation of the pentose phosphate shunt is decreased from 8% of the total glucose catabolism in *ad libitum*-fed rats to 1% in starved rats (Kather et al., 1972). This is confirmed by studies in isolated fat cells (Baquer et al., 1973), where the total amount of glucose utilized via the pentose phosphate shunt in the *ad libitum*-fed rat is 16%. The differences in the findings of these laboratories is not easy to explain, although there is indication that for the maintenance of the ultrastructure of the isolated fat cell insulin may be necessary (Wagle et al., 1973). It would appear, therefore, that the figure from the isolated fat cells may be open to some degree of criticism.

Starvation may decrease lipogenesis by the inhibition of acetyl CoA carboxylase and fatty acid synthetase. This may even be augmented by an inhibition of pyruvate carboxylase by acetoacetyl CoA (Scrutton, 1971). It has also been reported that citrate transport out of the mitochondria is inhibited by palmityl CoA (Schiller et al., 1974) and increased by insulin. Because acetyl CoA must be produced from citrate for cytosolic lipogenesis, inhibition of citrate transport would inhibit lipogenesis. Because the interchange of malate between mitochondria and cytosol is relatively rapid (Rognstad and Katz, 1973), the carbon atoms of the TCA cycle may leak out of the mitochondria into the cytosol where malate would then be converted to oxalacetate and thus participate (both carbon atoms and reducing power NADH) in gluconeogenesis rather than in lipogenesis. The shortcircuiting of the TCA cycle at malate would decrease citrate availability and would thus be expected to decrease cytosolic lipogenesis even further.

Relatively early during starvation lipolysis will increase and begin to supply a major source of energy during caloric deficiency. This is accomplished by both a decrease in fatty acid reesterification in adipose tissue and liver and by a breakdown of triglyceride stores in adipose tissue (Jourdan et al., 1974). The turnover of triglycerides depends on adipocytes (Jourdan et al., 1974). Current work indicates that there may be two pools of stored fat: one that can be mobilized relatively quickly and one that is mobilized more slowly (Zinder et al., 1973). Starvation in man is accompanied by a fall in circulating triglyceride levels and a simultaneous increase in free fatty acid turnover (Nestel et al., 1970). This reflects the increased utilization of depot fat. There appears to be some interaction between lipolysis and gluconeogenesis, although the interaction and its mechanism are not clearly understood. It is well known that during starvation growth hormone release is increased in man (Roth, 1963) and that growth hormone administration can increase fasting blood glucose, ammonium, and potassium loss (Felig et al., 1971). On the other hand, gluconeogenesis can be stimulated by free fatty acids (Söling et al., 1968; Struck et al., 1965), as well as by oleic acid (Teufel et al., 1967). The fact that gluconeogenesis can be increased by glucagon without altering cAMP levels

(Wagle, 1974) coupled with the previous effects enumerated above suggests that gluconeogenesis may be stimulated by increased availability of energy-rich compounds such as fatty acids. This would presumably occur by increasing the throughput of the TCA cycle. It should be noted that in the monogastric animal, unlike in the ruminant, net glucose production is not possible from two carbon units derived from fatty acids. However, the two carbon units derived from fatty acids can provide energy and thus spare glucose.

Another adaptation that takes place during starvation is the utilization of ketone bodies as a source of metabolic fuel. It has been shown that adipose tissue (Hanson and Ziporin, 1966) and brain (Owen et al., 1967; Thaler, 1972) can utilize ketone bodies. Ketone bodies will increase significantly in the cerebral spinal fluid 24 hr after starvation (Owen et al., 1974). The role of ketone bodies is twofold: to provide a source of energy and to achieve neutrality of the urine (Owen et al., 1969). The production of ketone bodies is proportional to the plasma concentration of ketone bodies (Balasse and Harvel, 1971; Bergman and Kon, 1964; Krebs, 1966; Nelson et al., 1941; Wick and Drury, 1941). It is assumed that ketone body production is accelerated by free fatty acids, particularly oleate (McGarry et al., 1973; McGarry and Foster, 1974). However, albumin-bound oleic acid does not seem to have this effect (Schimmel and Knobil, 1969). The possible interaction between gluconeogenesis and ketone body production is evidenced by reports that fructose, a gluconeogenic sugar, also increases ketone body production (Sestoff, 1974; Söling et al., 1970) and that tryptophan (Sakurai et al., 1974), as well as insulin (Bieberdorf et al., 1970), decreases ketogenesis. The importance of ketogenesis and ketone bodies can be realized by the fact that in man the maximum ketone body production has been estimated to be 150 g per day during starvation (Reichard, 1974).

Ion balance and long-term adaptation to fasting. During the first 24 hr of starvation, the number of sodium ions in the urine increases (Anon., 1974). As starvation progresses, sodium excretion decreases and the excretion of ammonium ions, which are derived primarily from amino acids, increases (Owen et al., 1969). Ketone body excretion in the urine rises slowly during the first 1-3 days of fasting, markedly during the third to tenth days of fasting, and reaches maximum at 24 days (Owen et al., 1969). However, severe ketonuria is avoided by an increase in the reabsorption of acetoacetate and beta-hydroxybutyrate from the kidney (Sapir and Owen, 1975). The reabsorption of acetoacetate is increased three times, while the reabsorption of beta-hydroxybutyrate is increased two and one half times by the kidney during starvation. If starvation is prolonged 5 or 6 wk, amino acid conservation can be accomplished by decreasing ketone body excretion; at that point the pH neutrality of the urine would have to be maintained by increased excretion of ammonium ions derived from amino acids (Aoki et al., 1974).

Blood glucose (Owen et al., 1969) and blood glucagon (Aoki et al., 1974) reach minimum and maximum levels at about 3 and 5 days, respectively, after starvation. Since glucagon is known to increase urea nitrogen and gluconeo-genesis (Marliss et al., 1970), a decrease in glucagon output would be a physiologically important mechanism to spare body proteins by saving body nitrogen. Possible nitrogen-sparing effects of ketone bodies have been suggested by observations that the nitrogen-sparing effect induced by ketone analogs of amino acids is greater than would be expected from the caloric content of these keto analogs (Sapir, 1974). This would indicate that the keto acids themselves may have some degree of regulatory effect on nitrogen excretion itself.

Adaptation to fasting seems to be an acquired process that may persist for a considerable length of time. For example, it has been reported that during a second episode of starvation, removed from the first episode by at least a week, nitrogen and ketone loss is decreased (Vaughan et al., 1959).

In summary, control mechanisms act during starvation to break down expendable body components relatively easy to replace and relatively unneces-sary to the maintenance of body function. These adaptive mechanisms are accomplished by decreasing enzyme levels in certain synthetic pathways, maintaining, preferentially, those enzymes involved in catabolic pathways, altering the levels of the effectory hormones, and changing the substrate-level activation and inhibition.

Current emphasis of the effect of hormones, cAMP, substrate activation and inactivation and deemphasis of the effect of enzyme levels probably reflect current preoccupation with cAMP and substrate-level activation and inhibition. Since the flux through a metabolic pathway is determined not only by the amount of substrate available to that enzyme but also by the enzyme amount, the importance of substrate levels and enzyme levels should be put into the proper perspective. This is all the more so, because in one of the most thoroughgoing studies the levels of "fashionable" intermediates (long-chain fatty acyl CoA, citrate and glycerol 1-phosphate) and triglyceride and fatty acid synthesis were not as well correlated as the pentose phosphate shunt flux and the 6PGD/G6PD ratio (Saggerson and Greenbaum, 1970).

Weight Loss Therapy in Humans

Inasmuch as overweight and obesity are common conditions among humans, the treatment of these conditions has been a major concern of both nutritionists and physicians. In all responsible dietary regimens designed to reduce weight the following goals should be sought: (1) reduction in body weight; (2) maintenance of muscle protein; (3) preservation of the patient in a state of health good enough to carry on everyday life; and (4) minimum damage to the body.

The first of these goals is relatively easy to meet, since no matter how the body attempts to conserve energy, at some level of caloric restriction weight loss will commence. The preservation of muscle protein, however, is more difficult. A good review of this subject was recently published by Flatt and Blackburn (1974). A consensus of current opinion in this field would indicate that an increase in amino acid intake during caloric restriction will decrease protein loss perhaps more than expected from the simple caloric value of the amino acids ingested (Blackburn et al., 1973; Flatt and Blackburn, 1974). Repeated episodes of fasting were also reported to improve maintenance of blood sugar levels and decrease the level of nitrogen loss and ketone loss in the urine (Taylor, 1945).

Improved protein retention as a result of amino acid supplementation during caloric restriction may be explained by some of the principles of metabolic control already described. The increase in amino acids would be expected to increase insulin levels, a factor known to promote protein anabolism. Also, the body's need to excrete cations during caloric deficiency (while saving sodium and especially potassium ions) is met in part by the excretion of ammonium ions derived from amino acids. By providing the precursor for ammonium ions, exogenous amino acids decrease the need for internal protein breakdown. Amino acid therapy during caloric restriction has been reported to preserve internal protein (Blackburn et al., 1973; Flatt and Blackburn, 1974).

Another important aspect of weight reduction concerns the nature of the fuel to be burned during caloric deficiency. The desired metabolic balance is to achieve starvation ketosis, a partial adaptation of muscle and neural tissue to burn at least some ketone bodies, and the maintenance of adequate blood insulin to prevent substantial internal loss of protein (Flatt and Blackburn, 1974). How is such a metabolic balance to be achieved? The first dietary requirement is to decrease caloric intake, while maintaining or increasing normal protein intake. The second requirement is to carefully adjust the carbohydrate/fat ratio so that amino acids and glucose maintain adequate insulin levels, but carbohydrate intake is low enough so as not to suppress starvation ketosis (Flatt and Blackburn, 1974). Such a dietary regimen may result in slower weight loss than can be obtained by complete starvation, but the maintenance of internal proteins should allow the individual to maintain a considerable capacity to work.

The question of minimizing damage to the body by caloric restriction remains an area of conflicting data and interpretation. There are strong indications that caloric restriction may cause circulatory problems; on the other hand, reduced caloric intake may have beneficial long-term effects. Inasmuch as weight reduction regimens are necessitated as a result of previous overnutrition and are often followed by overnutrition again, the long-term treatment of overweight by periodic dieting should be thoroughly examined. In any case, it would appear more beneficial to control appetite, but this is little more than a mere wish at present and some of the "cures" (such as amphetamines) may be worse than the disease.

CHANGES DURING REALIMENTATION

Glucose Tolerances, Growth, Food Intake, and Body Composition

It has been recounted that during starvation or caloric restriction glucose tolerance is impaired. How long glucose tolerance is impaired following realimentation depends on the severity and length of caloric restriction. In some instances glucose tolerance may become normal after 24 hr of realimentation (Grey et al., 1970), while it may persist for several days (Anderson and Herman, 1972) or weeks after severe and lengthy caloric restriction (James and Coore, 1970).

A considerable amount of work has been conducted on the effect of caloric restriction on growth. It has been reported that growth can be retarded in the rat for a considerable length of time; upon *ad libitum* realimentation the animals will recover and growth will be resumed (McCay et al., 1943). A comprehensive review of the literature concerning growth retardation and its aftermath was presented by Wilson and Osbourn (1960).

One response to *ad libitum* realimentation following caloric restriction or starvation is an increase in food intake (Szepesi and Freedland, 1969; Tepperman and Tepperman, 1958a; Wilson and Osbourn, 1960). Increased food intake increases the rate of weight gain. This increased growth rate has been referred to as "compensatory growth" (Bohman, 1955; Wilson and Osbourn, 1960), a principle that has been demonstrated in numerous species. A number of examples will suffice to illustrate the type of phenomena involved. Rats restricted to 50% *ad libitum* caloric intake for 3 wk and then realimentated to an *ad libitum* regimen will exceed their *ad libitum* counterpart in body weight in 9 wk (Clarke and Smith, 1938). Whether rats completely catch up with their *ad libitum* counterparts, overcompensate, or are unable to catch up with the *ad libitum*-fed rats appears to depend on the time during the life cycle at which caloric restriction is applied (Widdowson and McCance, 1963). Rats restricted very shortly after weaning will not catch up; rats restricted 9 weeks after weaning will actually overshoot their *ad libitum* counterparts, while rats restricted 16–18 wk after weaning will only catch up to their *ad libitum* counterparts (Widdowson and McCance, 1963). In cattle it was demonstrated that the most severely restricted animals will undergo the greatest rate of weight gain after realimentation, but that the least severely restricted animals eventually achieve the greatest weight (Hogan, 1929). Among animals subjected to an equal degree of restriction, those restricted for the shortest period of time will reach the greatest amount of body weight upon realimentation (Hogan, 1929). In young children previously subjected to malnutrition, body weight increased nine times faster than in normal children of comparable age and four times faster than in children of comparable height or weight (Stearns and Moore, 1931). In another study, similar results were found; children rehabilitated after malnourishment grew 15 times faster than did normal children of the same age and five times faster than did normal children of the same height and weight (Ashworth, 1969). It was found that on reaching what the experimenters considered a weight comparable to that of normal children, the rehabilitated children decreased food intake to roughly the level consumed by normal children (Ashworth, 1969). However, it was estimated in this case that rehabilitated children had become obese by storing excess fat (Ashworth, 1969; Graham and

MacLean, 1975). The principle that compensatory growth will result in excess deposition of body fat has been demonstrated (McMeekan, 1941; Meyer and Clawson, 1964; Quimby, 1948; Stewart, 1974; Wilson, 1960). In restricted-realimentated beef cattle there is a subsequent increase in the deposition of subcutaneous fat and a resultant improvement in the quality of meat (McMeekan, 1941). In sheep, however, body fat has been reported to be decreased by restriction and refeeding (Burton et al., 1974; McManus et al., 1972; Reid, 1968). The degree of adiposity achieved after refeeding, however, depends on experimental conditions. Under some circumstances, restricted and realimentated mice contain less body fat than do *ad libitum*-fed mice (Robinson and Lambourne, 1970).

It has been suggested by Tanner (1963) that growth is a target-seeking phenomenon. In other words, the animal is genetically programmed to reach a particular maximum weight or to approach a hypothetical maximal weight. Caloric restriction followed by realimentation might change this theoretical maximum weight. In a series of experiments rats were restricted to 70% of *ad libitum* caloric intake for 21 or 28 days (Meyer et al., 1956) on the basis of metabolic body size (i.e., body weight to the 0.75 power) were then allowed to eat as much as *ad libitum*-fed rats would eat. The restricted–refed rats consumed the allotted regimen in a shorter period of time than did the *ad libitum*-fed rats (Meyer et al., 1956). The restricted–released rats had also greater percent body fat at the end of the experiment. However, if the vitamin, protein, and fat intake during restriction were increased to the level taken in by the rats fed *ad libitum,* the percent body fat at the end of realimentation was similar to that found in *ad libitum*-fed rats (Meyer et al., 1956). In the author's own experiments attempts to normalize restricted–realimentated rats by changing the fat content of the diet during *ad libitum* realimentation were not successful (Szepesi and Vojnik, 1975).

It appears then that in a number of species caloric restriction or starvation is followed by a faster than normal rate of growth—the so-called compensatory growth. Depending on when caloric restriction takes place, the length of caloric restriction, and the time of the life cycle of the animal when caloric restriction is applied, the resultant compensatory growth may lead to increased adiposity. The nature and control of overeating and compensatory growth following caloric restriction is not at all clear now. It appears that this phenomenon, observable in animals, may have a counterpart in humans subjected to caloric restriction, such as in undernourished children or habitual dieters.

Changes in Metabolism

Alteration in nucleic acid metabolism. Caloric restriction has been shown to cause a decrease in the accumulation of DNA, RNA, and protein (Howarth and Baldwin, 1971a; Roeder, 1973). Upon realimentation to *ad libitum* feeding, DNA and RNA levels reach normal in 24 hr (Howarth and Baldwin, 1971a). Protein synthesis returns to normal in approximately the same time (Howarth

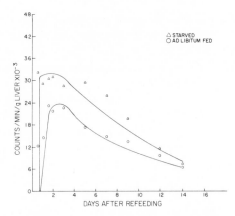

FIGURE 3 Incorporation of [³H] orotic acid into rat liver RNA. The figure is taken from Pfeifer and Szepesi (1974), courtesy of *Journal of Nutrition.* Rats were fed either *ad libitum* or starved and refed a 65% glucose, 25% casein, and 5% fat diet containing adequate vitamins and minerals. [³H] orotic acid was injected intraperitoneally beginning 24 hr after refeeding. Three hours later the rats were killed and the incorporation of label into liver RNA was determined.

and Baldwin, 1971a). In the starved–refed rat nuclear RNA, ribosomal RNA, and transfer RNA were found to be normal 24 hr after refeeding (Onishi, 1970). Template activity of isolated pieces of DNA was found to be slightly higher in the restricted–realimentated rat than in rats fed *ad libitum* (Onishi, 1970). In adipose tissue fasting has been found to reduce the stainable RNA (Fábry et al., 1970), while nucleoli from refed rats were found to be enlarged and very high in stainable RNA (Fábry et al., 1970). The possible significane of alterations in nucleic acid metabolism will be emphasized later.

   In another series of experiments, total liver RNA was found to be reduced by starvation and increased to approximately normal about 24 hr after refeeding (Pfeifer and Szepesi, 1974). The rate of orotate accumulation in RNA was higher in the starved–refed rats than in the *ad libitum*-fed rats (Fig. 3). This was true whether orotate was injected before the rats were refed or 24 hr after refeeding. These findings indicate that there is increased incorporation of orotate into some species of RNA during refeeding and that this increase persists for a considerable length of time. The rate of incorporation of orotate into liver RNA was also higher in starved–refed rats than in *ad libitum*-fed rats (Pfeifer and Szepesi, 1974). Since the total amount of RNA in *ad libitum*-fed vs. starved–refed rats appears to be approximately the same, it was concluded that a substantial amount of the orotic acid incorporated may have been incorporated into a species of RNA that comprises a relatively small fraction of the total RNA, or a species of RNA with a relatively fast turnover rate. Clearly, messenger RNA might fit these requirements.

The dependence of enzyme induction on *de novo* RNA synthesis is a point of interest in many enzyme studies. In microorganisms a large number of antiobiotics have been found to affect protein synthesis at different sites. However, there are difficulties in using these antibiotics with animals. Part of the difficulty arises from animal cells, such as liver cells, often not being permeable to antibiotics. Another difficulty is that many of the antibiotics are toxic and either cause death of the animal within a short time or, at the very least, result in a reduced food intake. Because of these considerations the number of antibiotics used in animal experiments has been limited, or experiments of relatively short duration have been performed. The antibiotic 8-azaguanine, however, has been used rather extensively. 8-Azaguanine is sufficiently similar to guanine to be incorporated into RNA, but the RNA so formed is nonfunctional (Kwan and Webb, 1967; Zimmerman and Greenberg, 1965). 8-Azaguanine is particularly useful for animal studies since it does not decrease food intake substantially (Szepesi and Freedland, 1969), is incorporated intact into RNA and does not decrease the incorporation of orotic acid into RNA (Pfeifer et al., 1974).

In a limited number of cases it has been possible to test the dependence of enzyme induction on *de novo* RNA synthesis by using either actinomycin D or 8-azaguanine. In adipose tissue (Benjamin and Gellhorn, 1966; Kazdová et al., 1968) enzyme induction upon realimentation appears to depend on *de novo* RNA synthesis. Somewhat similar findings were made in liver (Johnson and Sassoon, 1967). Work with azaguanine will be reviewed in a later section.

Actinomycin D is known to interfere with messenger RNA synthesis (Hiroshi et al., 1971) by interacting with the DNA helix at the poly dG site (Schwochau and Hadwiger, 1969) and presumably preventing RNA polymerase from functioning. Unfortunately, there are a number of side reactions[1] when actinomycin D is used, including a decrease in stomach-emptying rates (Yatvin, 1971).

In starved–refed animals some of the enzymes will be increased upon refeeding but some, notably the gluconeogenic enzymes, will be decreased. Among those decreased is PEPCK (Ballard et al., 1974). It has been suggested that PEPCK is deinduced upon refeeding, its synthesis blocked, and the messenger RNA coding for it degraded.

The mechanism and control of RNA synthesis is somewhat obscure. For instance while it is known that insulin (Turkington and Riddle, 1969) and cortisone (Turkington, 1970) promote increased RNA synthesis in rat mammary gland (Turkington and Riddle, 1969), it is not certain just what role insulin plays in the restricted–refed rat. In rats starved and refed a diet containing a large amount of fat, the characteristic rebound in RNA in adipocytes cannot be

---

[1] A number of these side reactions have been reviewed by Freedland et al. (1966).

seen even if the feeding of the high-fat diet is accompanied by the administration of insulin (Fábry et al., 1970). This observation indicates either that insulin is not a major signal for the synthesis of RNA or that the effect of insulin can be obliterated by a high fat-diet. The production of ribose during realimentation appears to be unrelated for the most part to the control of RNA synthesis (De La Garza et al., 1970).

Current evidence indicates that during refeeding following an episode of caloric restriction or starvation, some new species of RNA is synthesized that codes for the enzymes that increase upon refeeding. It would be tempting to conclude that this species of RNA is messenger RNA, but currently available evidence does not allow such an unequivocal conclusion.

Glycogen metabolism, gluconeogenesis, and lipogenesis. Upon realimentation to an *ad libitum* regimen following starvation, animals usually overeat. The excess food intake is channeled into liver glycogen (Miller and Larner, 1973; Szepesi and Freedland, 1970; Tepperman and Tepperman, 1958a) and lipid (Tepperman and Tepperman, 1958a). In general, lipogenesis and gluconeogenesis are controlled in a reciprocal fashion (Tepperman and Tepperman, 1970). Upon refeeding lipogenesis is substantially increased (Halperin, 1970; Hicks et al., 1965; Mirski, 1942; Tepperman and Tepperman, 1958a; Tuerkisher and Wertheimer, 1942). Lipogenesis can be activated by glucose alone before any change in enzyme activity occurs (Baker and Huebotter, 1972, 1973; Jansen et al., 1966). Continued high rates of lipogenesis eventually result in fat accumulation, which will then subside by about 7 days after refeeding (Severson et al., 1973).

One of the most active areas of nutritional biochemistry today concerns attempts to elucidate the control of fatty acid synthesis. As mentioned above, upon realimentation fatty acid synthesis can be increased immediately or almost immediately without an increase in enzyme levels (Baker and Huebotter, 1972, 1973; Schimmel and Knobil, 1970; Tepperman and Tepperman, 1961). However, the overall accumulation of fat in rat liver is very closely related to the overall activity of two accessory enzymes of lipogenesis—G6PD and malic enzyme (Fig. 4). This would at least indicate that a relationship exists between enzyme activity and the lipogenic capacity; however, some scientists believe that it is the flow through the pathway that controls the enzyme activity rather than the other way around.

Fatty acid synthesis can be inhibited by actinomycin D and cycloheximide (Hicks et al., 1965). This inhibition indicates a requirement for *de novo* protein synthesis, although because of possible side reactions caused by these antibiotics, the interpretation of the results is not clear. Lipogenesis can also be inhibited by corn oil (Jansen et al., 1966, 1968) and in the fat pads by dietary fatty acids (Cahill et al., 1960; Korchack and Masoro, 1964). Fatty acids of increasing chain length and unsaturation were found to have an increasing inhibitory effect on lipogenesis (Reiser et al., 1963). Fatty acid synthesis was inhibited by fatty acyl CoA in isolated hepatocytes (Goodridge, 1973). Alpha linoleate (Allmann et al., 1965; Muto and Gibson, 1970) and fatty acids other

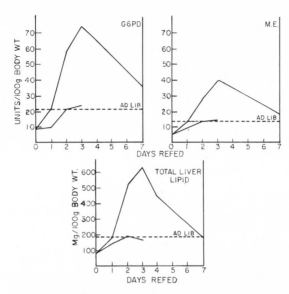

FIGURE 4 The lipogenic response of rat liver to starvation–refeeding. The diet fed contained 65% glucose, 25% casein, 5% corn oil, and adequate minerals and vitamins. Glucose-6-phosphate dehydrogenase (G6PD), malic enzyme (M.E.), and total liver lipid levels rose above *ad libitum*-fed levels. When 8-azaguanine was injected intraperitoneally, the overshoot of *ad libitum*-fed values was prevented (lower response curve in each group).

than linoleate (Hill et al., 1958, 1960) have also been found to inhibit fatty acid synthesis. The inhibition of fatty acid synthesis was shown also in tissue culture (Howard et al., 1974). In this case removal of fat from the tissue culture caused increased lipogenesis that could not be prevented by actinomycin D or cycloheximide (Howard et al., 1974). It appears then that lipogenesis in the liver and the adipose tissue is regulated at least in part by the availability and amount of lipids that reach these tissues. The physiological importance of lipids in the control of lipogenesis was shown by the demonstration that very-low-density lipoproteins, low-density lipoproteins, and high-density lipoproteins were all able to inhibit lipogenesis in tissue culture (Cooper and Margolis, 1971).

One of the areas of current interest is elucidation of the primary control of lipogenesis. Current developments in this area indicate that the major controlling enzymes for fatty acid synthesis appear to be acetyl CoA carboxylase and the fatty acid synthetase complex. Steroid biosynthesis is regulated primarily by hydroxymethyl glutaryl CoA reductase (Howard et al., 1974). There is no general agreement, however, concerning the primary role of enzymes or substrates in regulating the rate of lipogenesis.

Recently, the role of linoleic acid in the control of lipogenesis has been questioned (Gozukara et al., 1972). In experiments where rats were starved and refed diets containing 18% linoleic acid it was found that linoleic acid prevented large elevations in certain enzyme activities and lipogenesis by decreasing the food intake (Gozukara et al., 1972). However, since large concentrations of free fatty acids in the food might have a detergent effect on the digestive tract, therefore leading to decreased food intake, this demonstration of the role of linoleic acid is not conclusive. In the author's laboratory it was found that rats starved and refed diets containing 24% trilinolein had depressed liver glucose-6-phosphate dehydrogenase, malic enzyme, and total liver lipid levels but not food intake (Slayton and Szepesi, 1974).

One important point of control in lipogenesis is the rate at which malonyl CoA is formed from acetyl CoA (Guynn et al., 1973). Since acetyl CoA carboxylase has been shown to be regulated by activation and deactivation and is responsive to hormones, a quick on and off control of lipogenesis can be achieved by controlling the activity of acetyl CoA carboxylase and the rate of malonyl CoA formation. Although the control of acetyl CoA carboxylase can explain the on/off nature of the control of lipogenesis, as well as account for a good share of the phenomena that are observable during lipogenesis, it does not appear by itself to explain all the controls that are needed to maintain certain levels of lipogenesis *in vivo*. In some very thorough studies it was found that one of the factors to which lipogenesis is related in rat liver is the 6PGD to G6PD ratio (Sapag-Hagar et al., 1973). In this case it was found that NADPH would inhibit 6PGD even more than it inhibits G6PD (Sapag-Hagar et al., 1973). Lately, it has been suggested that the NADPH inhibition of G6PD may in itself be subject to a number of control mechanisms not well understood at present (Eggleston and Krebs, 1974). In rodents lipogenesis can be increased by insulin and decreased by glucagon (Jungas, 1971). Regulation of blood glucose, insulin, and lipogenesis are closely related and controlled. However, in the ruminant the control of insulin release is much different since in this case propionic and butyric acid are major products of microorganism metabolism in the multiple stomachs and it is these that give rise to an increase in insulin levels (Trenkle, 1970). Therefore, in such species the relationship among blood glucose, insulin, and lipogenesis is different.

In spite of the relative success of explaining the control of lipogenesis in terms of the on and off switch at the malonyl CoA production site (Guynn et al., 1973), the long-term channeling of excess carbohydrate during *ad libitum* realimentation with a high-carbohydrate diet following caloric deficiency remains to be determined. It is important to note that the channeling of carbohydrate *in vivo* during the first day of refeeding is largely toward liver glycogen and toward liver fat only during the second day of refeeding (Table 3). Although *in vitro* assays or even some *in vivo* assays of lipogenesis indicate that near-maximum lipogenesis can occur in day 1 of refeeding, lipogenesis may not operate at maximum levels until day 2 of refeeding (Table 3). Thus, replenishment of energy stores in the liver occurs in the same order in which they are broken down during starvation, i.e., first glycogen, then lipid. The

TABLE 3 Amount of Radioactivity Incorporated into Liver Glycogen
and Liver Lipids from Dietary [^{14}C-U] Sucrose in Groups
of Rats Fasted 2 Days and Refed for 1 or 2 Days[a]

	Refed 1 day	Refed 2 days		
	G_1 (+)[b] (4)[c]	G_2 (+,+) (8)	G_3 (+,−) (8)	G_4 (−,+) (8)
Liver glycogen				
dpm/mg	620 ± 38[d]	505 ± 33	396 ± 30	40 ± 10
dpm/g liver (× 10^{-3})	67.0 ± 5.7	10.2 ± 2.0	7.7 ± 1.7	0.6 ± 0.2
dpm/100 g body wt (× 10^{-3})	388 ± 25	44 ± 10	36 ± 8.1	3 ± 1
Total liver lipids				
dpm/mg	353 ± 26	730 ± 17	216 ± 10	494 ± 34
dpm/g liver (× 10^{-3})	17.4 ± 1.9	98.6 ± 7.0	33.6 ± 3.1	70.8 ± 7.6
dpm/100 g body wt (× 10^{-3})	85.5 ± 10.5	455.9 ± 38.7	156.5 ± 14.9	364.6 ± 29.9

[a]Data from Chang and Johnson (1975).

[b]The plus and minus signs in the parentheses are designated as follows: (+) = [^{14}C-U]-sucrose in the diet; (−) = nonlabeled sucrose in the diet. The first sign represents the diet refed between 0 and 24 hr. For example (−,+) rats were fed unlabeled sucrose during 0–24 hr and labeled sucrose during 24–48 hr.

[c]The number in parentheses indicates the number of rats.

[d]Mean ±SE.

physiological significance of preferential replacement of glycogen is clear; once liver glycogen is replenished, the animal is again capable of maintaining short-term blood glucose level regulation by breaking down liver and muscle glycogen.

Enzyme Changes

Various pathways and control points. The activities of a number of enzymes return to normal upon refeeding (Freedland et al., 1966), while some reach higher levels than are found in the *ad libitum*-fed animal. This latter type of enzyme response is commonly referred to as the "enzyme overshoot."

One of the first enzymes to increase in activity upon realimentation is glycogen synthetase. The activity of this enzyme can be increased by glucose (DeWulf and Hers, 1968) and acetylcholine (Akpan et al., 1974), without altering insulin levels. Cyclic AMP (Miller and Larner, 1973) and insulin (Blatt and Kim, 1971; Miller and Larner, 1973) can also alter glycogen synthetase activity; cAMP decreases and insulin increases enzyme activity. In intact cells, the activation of glycogen synthetase by insulin can occur even if insulin is bound to Sepharose (Blatt and Kim, 1971). However, neither insulin nor insulin bound to Sepharose has an effect on the enzyme in a broken cell suspension. These observations indicate that the effect of hormones on glycogen synthetase activity requires an intact cell membrane and perhaps a functional sequence of activating events. Glycogen synthesis is correlated both with glycogen synthetase and glycogen transferase activity (Hornbrook and Lyon, 1970).

Another enzyme increased very early during realimentation is acetyl CoA carboxylase (Gibson et al., 1966; Halestrap and Denton, 1973, 1974; Majerus and Kilburn, 1969). The increase in enzyme activity reflects a five- to tenfold increase in the rate of synthesis and a decrease to one-half in the rate of degradation (Majerus and Kilburn, 1969). Acetyl CoA carboxylase activity is increased by citrate (Halestrap and Denton, 1973, 1974) and decreased by fatty acyl CoA compounds (Goodridge, 1972; Halestrap and Denton, 1973, 1974). Even albumin-bound acyl CoA compounds may play a physiological role in the control of this enzyme. Thus, during starvation or feeding of a high-fat diet the expected rise in acyl CoA levels acts to limit lipogenesis.

The activity of fatty acid synthetase is also increased upon realimentation (Burton et al., 1969; Craig and Porter, 1973; Craig et al., 1972b; Gibson et al., 1966; Lakshmanan et al., 1972; Murphy and Steiner, 1972; Rosenfeld, 1973). The change in activity of fatty acid synthetase is paralleled by the change in the rate of fatty acid synthesis (Murphy and Steiner, 1972; Rosenfeld, 1973). Newly made enzyme needs $4'$-phosphopantotheine (Yu and Burton, 1974). Pancreatic secretion is altered upon refeeding (Snook, 1971). There is some indication that enzyme changes in the pancreas may be important in the organ's endocrine function (Grey et al., 1970). Varying the carbohydrate-to-fat ratio was identical in effect to varying the carbohydrate-to-protein ratio (Snook, 1971).

Enzymes unique to gluconeogenesis, such as PEPCK, are increased in the kidney and liver by starvation (Tepperman and Tepperman, 1970), while pyruvate carboxylase, PEPCK, fructose-1,6-diphosphatase, and serine dehydrase are decreased by perfusing the liver with glucose (Wilmurst and Manchester, 1973). These changes in enzyme levels by perfusion were achieved with the high (nonphysiological) levels of glucose, whereas physiological levels of glucose had no effect (Wilmurst and Manchester, 1973).

Steroid synthesis is also increased during realimentation. This is made possible in part by the increase in β-hydroxy-β-methylglutaryl CoA synthetase activity (Higgins et al., 1971). The change in the activity of this enzyme is due to the synthesis of new protein, rather than the activation of an inactive enzyme (Higgins et al., 1971). The inhibition of steroid synthesis by cAMP, however, may involve another site of control (Bloxham and Akhtar, 1971). In addition, there is evidence that liver G6PD is altered in the cytosol but not in the particulate fraction (Baquer et al., 1972).

Malic enzyme (NADP-linked) and citrate cleavage enzyme, two accessory enzymes of lipogenesis, undergo large increases during realimentation (Gibson, 1972). The change in enzyme levels is due to the synthesis of new protein (Gibson, 1972). No evidence of activation could be shown. Pyruvate kinase activity is also increased by insulin (Freedland et al., 1966); in tissue culture this enzyme can be increased either by glucose or insulin (Gerschenson and Andersson, 1971).

The enzyme overshoot in rat liver is prevented by feeding a diet containing a substantial amount of fat (Novello et al., 1969; Tepperman and Tepperman, 1965). Tepperman and Tepperman (1965) suggested that saturated dietary fats may be relatively less effective in decreasing enzyme induction than are unsaturated fats. They suggested that the induction of these enzymes (notably G6PD and malic enzyme) was due to an increased demand for NADPH for the desaturation of palmitic acid to oleic acid (Tepperman and Tepperman, 1965). No evidence has ever been produced to substantiate this.

Acetyl CoA carboxylase is inhibited by exogenous fatty acids (Bortz and Lynen, 1963; Ganguly, 1960), while β-hydroxy-β-methylglutaryl CoA synthetase is inhibited by 2% dietary cholesterol (Craig et al., 1972a). Dietary cholesterol, however, does not inhibit acetyl CoA carboxylase or fatty acid synthetase (Craig et al., 1972a). It appears, therefore, that enzymes accessory to lipogenesis are inhibited by the end product of the pathway in which they function. This pattern of inhibition suggests that the enzyme activity may be related to the rate of flow through the pathway; that is, the enzymes and the rate of flow are controlled in a concerted manner. This relationship is shown by the fact that when the induction of G6PD and malic enzyme is inhibited the accumulation of excess liver lipid is also inhibited (author's unpublished data).

Fatty acid synthetase was found to be inhibited by dietary corn oil but not by dietary cholesterol (Allmann and Gibson, 1965). Glucose-6-phosphate dehydrogenase is reduced by a high-fat diet (Cheng et al., 1969; Tepperman and Tepperman, 1963), particularly by unsaturated fat (Century, 1972). Different unsaturated fats had different degrees of effectiveness in reducing liver G6PD (Century, 1972). Alpha-linoleate decreased the activities of G6PD, 6PGD, fatty acid synthetase, malic enzyme, and citrate cleavage enzyme (Musch et al., 1974b). Alpha-linoleate was found to be more effective than oleate in reducing G6PD and the activities of the above enzymes (Musch et al., 1974a); a high-fat diet was shown to be effective in reducing the activity of malic enzyme and citrate cleavage enzyme in brown adipose tissue (Hahn and Kirby, 1974). In another study it was found that unsaturated fats decreased fatty acid synthetase, G6PD, malic enzyme, and citrate cleavage enzyme activity and that the effect was especially noticeable with safflower oil (Bartley and Abraham, 1972b). In our work we have found that depending on the type of enzyme induction studied trilinolein and trilinolenin were effective in preventing the induction of G6PD and malic enzyme, whereas tristearin, tripalmitin, and triolein were not (C. S. Nace and B. Szepesi, unpublished data).

The overwhelming evidence shows that dietary fat can alter both the induction of enzymes involved in lipogenesis and the rate of lipogenesis itself. The exact manner in which the control of lipogenesis is established is not perfectly elucidated, at least to the satisfaction of the author, because there still appear to be some discrepancies between the way lipogenesis is assayed and the way lipids accumulate in the liver. Thus, while almost everyone agrees that assayable lipogenesis is virtually maximal, shortly upon realimentation the isotope incorporation data cited in Table 3 indicate that lipogenesis and lipid accumulation in the liver is less than maximal during day 1 of refeeding when the activities of the accessory enzymes of lipogenesis are still low and that the incorporation of label into liver fat increases to an even greater level during day 2 of refeeding when the activities of the accessory enzymes of lipogenesis are much higher. These observations would suggest, if not a causal relationship, then at least a common controlling factor regulating both lipogenesis and the activities of enzymes involved in NADPH production.

Nature of enzyme changes during realimentation. Relatively few enzymes remain constant in activity during caloric restriction. The activities of most enzymes decrease during caloric restriction and then increase upon realimentation. Another group of enzymes, as previously discussed, will decrease in activity upon realimentation. Of those enzymes that increase during realimentation, interest has been focused on those that control lipogenesis or are accessory to lipogenesis.

Of the enzymes important for the control of lipogenesis acetyl CoA carboxylase has been shown to be present in both the active and inactive form (Carlson and Kim, 1974); also it has been found that during enzyme induction actually more protein is being made (Majerus and Kilburn, 1969). Another enzyme important in the control of fatty acid synthesis is the fatty acid synthetase complex. During realimentation this enzyme is also induced and the induction is accompanied by increased synthesis of protein (Craig et al., 1972b).

An enzyme accessory to lipogenesis in the liver is the malic enzyme. Malic enzyme was first isolated by Ochoa et al. (1948) and later purified by Hsu and Lardy (1967). Malic enzymes can be induced by thyroxine (Glock and McLean, 1955; Huggins and Yao, 1959; Lockwood et al., 1970; Saito et al., 1971) and by starvation-refeeding. It has been found that the activity of malic enzyme is proportional to the amount of titratable protein (Li et al., 1975; Murphy and Walker, 1974; Saito et al., 1971). Another enzyme that is accessory to lipogenesis, G6PD, is also induced by starvation-refeeding. Its activity has been found to be proportional to the enzyme protein (Holten, 1972; Matsuda and Yugari, 1967; Watanabe and Taketa, 1973). This is true not only in the liver but also in adipose tissue (Geisler and Hansen, 1972). Recently, an equivalence between G6PD activity and enzyme protein amount has been questioned by Hizi and Yagil (1974a, 1974b) and by Kelly et al. (1975).

Because of the success of finding specific isoenzymes of G6PD in red blood cells in certain deficiencies or among some ethnic groups, a search has been made for isoenzymes of G6PD and other enzymes in rat liver. In the liver, however, the search has run into some unexpected problems. In one study a tryptic digest of liver gave "isoenzymes," which were enzymically active and resembled in their electrophoretic behavior the isoenzymes found in rat liver (Hori and Noda, 1971). Generally, there appears to be agreement that in rat liver there can be shown three isoenzymes of G6PD (Holten, 1972; Schmukler, 1970; Taketa and Watanabe, 1971), excluding reports that the enzyme can form dimers, trimers, tetramers, and even high polymers of quaternary structure. A conversion of liver G6PD isoenzymes by $HgCl_2$ and mercaptoethanol has been reported to cause no loss in activity (Taketa and Watanabe, 1971). Isoenzymes in the particulate fraction, such as mitochondria and nuclei, appear to be different from the isoenzymes in the cytosol (Hizi and Yagil, 1974a; Taketa and Watanabe, 1971). Finally Ozols and Hilf reported the induction of "G6PD-1" isoenzyme when testosterone is given to castrated male rats (Ozols and Hilf, 1973).

It now appears certain that of the isoenzymes of G6PD only the cytosolic species are induced, whereas the particulate isoenzymes are not. It would be tempting to envision a control system in liver by which one or more cytosolic isoenzymes of G6PD and perhaps malic enzyme might respond to one set of stimuli, whereas another isoenzyme may respond to another dietary and hormonal stimuli. However, there does not appear to be sufficient evidence that the cytosolic isoenzymes are separately induced.

Proposed control of protein synthesis and enzyme induction. To put the induction of a number of enzymes upon realimentation into the proper perspective, the theories constructed to account for the induction or control of synthesis of a number of protein systems will be reviewed. Several models of protein synthesis have been developed in recent years. Of these perhaps the best known and most explored is the "Jacob and Monod hypothesis" concerning the control of the lactose operon in *E. coli.* The control of the lactose operon in *E. coli* is shown in Fig. 5. The figure is a summary of the model as it is currently presented (Dickson and Abelson, 1975). The operon consists of the structural genes that code for enzymes, the *o* (operator), *p* (promoter), and *i* genes. The operator gene combines with the aporepressor, which prevents transcription. RNA polymerase binds to that portion of the promoter adjacent to the *o* gene. Another part of the promoter binds the cAMP receptor protein (Nakanishi et al., 1973). The *i* gene codes for the repressor. Transcription is initiated by the aporepressor combining with the corepressor (lactose) and dissociating from the

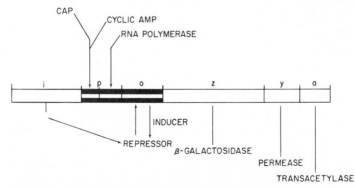

FIGURE 5 Schematic representation of the *lac* operon of *E. coli* as now understood. The size relationship of the *o, p,* and *i* genes has been distorted.

o gene. Binding RNA polymerase to the promoter can then proceed and the structural genes are then transcribed. Messenger RNA production is 10 times greater in the presence of cAMP (Nissley et al., 1971). It has been suggested that binding the cAMP receptor protein interferes with the binding of the aporepressor.

In bacteria there are two malic enzymes; one is NAD dependent, the other NADP dependent (Murai et al., 1971). The NAD-linked isoenzyme is induced by malate and is repressed by glucose. Its function is to increase pyruvate levels for acetyl CoA synthesis by decarboxylating malate. The second isoenzyme has the function of catabolizing malate. It is repressed by glucose, glycerol, lactate, acetate, and even malate. In the animal system there appears to be only one isoenzyme of malic enzyme, and this is NADP-dependent. Its function appears to be to produce NADPH for reductive synthesis, including fatty acid synthesis.

Another model of control of protein synthesis has been proposed to describe the synthesis of hemoglobin (Hb) in higher animals. Hemoglobin messenger RNA was isolated and purified, and it was shown that the product of translation of this messenger RNA was the mouse Hb chain (Lockard and Lingrel, 1971). This model of control of protein synthesis in a higher organism postulates the existence of a translational repressor or inhibitor. An earlier version of this model envisioned a proinhibitor bound to hemin that would be converted to the proinhibitor reversibly then to a reversible inhibitor and finally to an irreversible inhibitor (Gross and Rabinovitz, 1972). A more recent version of this model postulates that there are three stages of the inhibitor: a reversible inhibitor, which is antagonized by hemin; an intermediate inhibitor that can bind hemin but is still antagonized by hemin; and an irreversible inhibitor that is not inhibited by hemin. The inhibitor at the first two stages can inhibit Hb synthesis transiently (Gross, 1974). The partially purified Hb repressor has been isolated, and its molecular weight is estimated to be 4×10^5 (Gross and Rabinovitz, 1973). It was found that one inhibitor (repressor) can inhibit one thousand ribosomes; therefore, a cascade effect of inhibition is being proposed (Gross and Rabinovitz, 1973). This inhibitor then functions by preventing the synthesis of hemoglobin at the translational level. The inhibitor itself is deactivated by hemin. Therefore, when there is sufficient amount of hemin, the Hb protein will be synthesized. When hemin concentration is low, the production of the Hb protein is also slowed down. In this way porphyrin and hemoglobin synthesis can be coordinately controlled.

Another model of protein synthesis was developed to account for the induction and control of tyrosine aminotransferase (Fig. 6) (Tomkins et al., 1969). In this model a repressor is proposed that combines with the messenger RNA coding for tyrosine aminotransferase; this then leads to an increased degradation of the messenger RNA. It is proposed that cortisol can increase the amount of messenger RNA by deactivating the repressor (Tomkins et al., 1969). To account for the fact that tyrosine aminotransferase is superinduced by actinomycin D (Garren et al., 1964) and 8-azaguanine (Levitan and Webb,

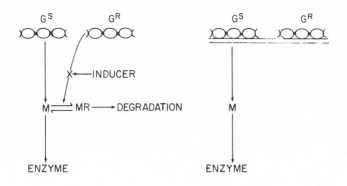

INDUCIBLE PHASE   NONINDUCIBLE PHASE

FIGURE 6 The control of tyrosine aminotransferase, as described by Tomkins et al. (1969). S^s = structural gene that codes for the enzyme; G^R = regulatory gene that codes for the translational repressor; R = the translational repressor; and M = messenger for the enzyme.

1969), it was postulated that the turnover of the messenger RNA, which codes for the repressor as well as the turnover of the repressor itself, is very fast in comparison to the turnover of the messenger RNA for the transaminase (Tomkins et al., 1969). When actinomycin D or 8-azaguanine is administered, the synthesis of the repressor is stopped and the amount of messenger RNA coding for tyrosine aminotransferase will increase for a time. As the effect of actinomycin D or 8-azaguanine becomes noticeable on the synthesis of the messenger for tyrosine aminotransferase, the synthesis of enzyme will also decrease. This model is relatively successful in accounting for the superinduction of tyrosine aminotransferase, an admittedly difficult task. Previous suggestions that the superinduction of tyrosine aminotransferase by actinomycin D or cycloheximide were due to stopping the degradation of the enzyme are not valid since in the system where the model was finally tested (tissue culture), actinomycin D did not change the rate of enzyme degradation (Tomkins, 1972).

Another enzyme that has been extensively studied with respect to the control of its induction is serine dehydrase. This enzyme is induced by dietary protein, some amino acids, and cortisol (Sudilovsky and Pitot, 1973). Serine dehydrase induction is repressed by glucose at the level of translation (Pitot et al., 1971). Two different isoenzymes were found in rat liver, one of which is induced to a different extent under different conditions (Pitot et al., 1971). Interestingly, cAMP-dependent processes were not altered during glucose repression, nor were cAMP receptors (Sudilovsky and Pitot, 1973). The mechanism of glucose repression of serine dehydrase *in vivo* is not now understood, except that it is suspected that enzyme elongation, rather than initiation or termination, is prevented.

Perhaps one of the most thoroughly studied systems of enzyme control in the animal system has been the induction of G6PD in rat liver. It has been noted by the Teppermans (1958b) that there was a good correlation between lipogenesis in liver slices and the amount of liver glycogen at the time incubation of liver slices began. It was suggested later that glycogen that accumulates during the first day of refeeding is later broken down and that the rapid breakdown of liver glycogen is the triggering mechanism that supplies the signal for the induction of G6PD (Sassoon et al., 1973). At present there is no indication that this is so.

In studying the induction of various other enzymes related to carbohydrate metabolism (glucokinase, hexokinase, phosphofructokinase, pyruvate carboxylase), it was suggested that the induction of these enzymes was due to an increase in the level of glucose metabolites (Gunn and Taylor, 1973). Because the study of metabolite levels became fashionable, it was suggested at some meetings that perhaps the signal for the induction of G6PD in the liver is a rise in breakdown products of glucose, in particular the phosphorylated intermediates of the Embden-Meyerhof pathway. This mechanism was suggested for the induction of glucokinase and hexokinase (Pilkis, 1970). However, when the dietary carbohydrate is changed from glucose to fructose, which also induces G6PD activity, the phosphorylated intermediate levels are not noticeably changed (Zakim et al., 1967). In any case, one would have a great deal of difficulty envisioning the mechanism by which phosphorylated intermediates in the cytosol might increase the induction of these enzymes, particularly, if the induction required *de novo* RNA synthesis; if such were the case, the phosphorylated intermediates would need to cross the nuclear membrane, a process not normally accomplished by phosphorylated intermediates.

Another possible signal for the control of G6PD induction was sought in hypothalamic excretions. It was found that in hypophysectomized animals the enzyme overshoot on starvation–refeeding was not noted (Tepperman and Tepperman, 1962), whereas the overshoot could be restored by the administration of three hormones removed by hypophysectomy. A difficulty with these findings, however, is that hypophysectomized animals experience a large decrease in food intake, and it is, therefore, not clear whether hypophysectomy abolishes the enzyme overshoot by removal of the hormones *per se* or by decreasing food intake. Another suggestion that the flow through a pathway triggers enzyme induction directly (Goodridge, 1975) also is without supporting evidence at the present time.

The time course of G6PD and malic enzyme activity on realimentation are shown in Fig. 4. Enzyme activity begins to increase very shortly after the animal is given food and continues to increase to 3–4 days when it reaches maximum. The activities of these enzymes then decrease and reach normal levels anywhere from 14 to 20 days after the original realimentation. It was noted earlier that the time course of the total liver lipid accumulation in the liver is very similar to the time course of changes in G6PD and malic enzyme activities (Fig. 4). In an effort

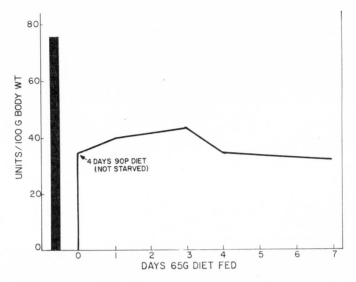

FIGURE 7   The derepression of glucose-6-phosphate dehydrogenase by starvation. The bar on the left represents the level of enzyme in rats starved 2 days, fed a 90% casein, 0% carbohydrate diet for 4 days and fed a 65% glucose, 25% casein diet for 3 days. It is evident that the enzyme overshoot occurs only with previous starvation and will be expressed even after the interposition of the 90% casein diet (which does not allow the enzyme overshoot to take place). All diets contained 5% corn oil, 1% vitamins, and 4% salt mix.

to establish the role of starvation in the subsequent induction of G6PD, an experiment was performed where a high-protein diet was interposed between starvation and feeding the inducer diet (Jomain et al., 1970; Szepesi and Moser, 1971). It was found that the enzyme overshoot could be seen if the rats were subjected to a prior starvation even if the feeding of the inducer diet was delayed by feeding the high-protein diet up to one week. However, no enzyme overshoot was observed when rats adapted to the high protein diet (but without prior starvation) were fed the inducer diet (Jomain et al., 1970; Szepesi and Moser, 1971). These results are illustrated in Fig. 7. It was also shown that the effect of starvation could not be duplicated by the omission of dietary protein, carbohydrate, or fat for 2 days (Szepesi, 1973). Inasmuch as the processes that rendered G6PD inducible by starvation give results analogous to the result of bacterial derepression, this process has been termed derepression. It has been shown that while the enzyme induction (overshoot) can be prevented by 8-azaguanine given during refeeding (Szepesi and Freedland, 1969; Szepesi, 1974), the enzyme overshoot is not abolished if 8-azaguanine is given during starvation (Szepesi, 1974b). These results indicate that while the enzyme induction process is dependent on *de novo* RNA synthesis, the process of derepression is not. It should be mentioned that there appear to be two separate processes with respect to the changes in G6PD levels that occur during realimentation. One of these processes acts to restore the activity of G6PD to "normal" levels (i.e., the level that is found in rats fed the inducer diet *ad libitum*) and another process that will result in enzyme levels in excess of those found in *ad libitum*-fed rats. It is this latter process that appears to be dependent on *de novo* RNA synthesis. This can be discerned by examining Fig. 4, where it is shown that even with azaguanine the enzyme level returns to "normal" after refeeding.

There is evidence that the process that produces the enzyme overshoot is separated from the process that returns enzyme activity to normal levels not only mechanistically but also in terms of time course. Thus, the enzyme overshoot can be prevented by the injection of 8-azaguanine up to 24 hr after refeeding (Szepesi and Freedland, 1970). The interpretation that the enzyme overshoot requires *de novo* RNA synthesis must be amended such that this *de novo* RNA synthesis has to occur after 24 hr of refeeding. There is some evidence (Onishi, 1970) that in starved–refed rats template activity is increased; this would be consistent with the existence of derepression produced by starvation and the maintenance of the state of derepression during refeeding.

The enzyme overshoot of G6PD upon starvation–refeeding requires both dietary protein (McDonald and Johnson, 1965; Niemeyer et al., 1962; Potter and Ono, 1961; Taketa et al., 1972; Vaughan and Winders, 1964) and dietary carbohydrate (Tepperman et al., 1968; Taketa et al., 1972). The enzyme overshoot can be prevented if the diet refed contains at least 20% dietary fat (Szepesi, 1974a). This inhibition of the overshoot by a high-fat diet does not require *de novo* RNA synthesis and can be produced even if the rats are treated with 8-azaguanine (Szepesi et al., 1974b). There is evidence that can be interpreted to mean that a high-fat diet can cause both translational and transcriptional rerepression (Szepesi et al., 1974b).

It has been shown that a second episode of starvation–refeeding will cause an even greater enzyme induction than what is obtained from one starvation–refeeding episode (Szepesi et al., 1972), even if protein or glucose is omitted from the diet during the first refeeding (Szepesi et al., 1973). This induction increment can also be produced if during the first refeeding, the rats are treated with 8-azaguanine (author's unpublished data). However, if during the first refeeding the rats are given a high-fat diet, the induction increment during the second refeeding is no longer produced although the effect of the high-fat diet during the first feeding can be prevented by the action of 8-azaguanine (Szepesi et al., 1972). Further experiments have shown that the effect of fat fed during the first refeeding in abolishing the induction increment during the second refeeding is effective only if dietary fat is provided during the second day of refeeding (Szepesi et al., 1974b). The role of the high-fat diet in transcriptional rerepression is postulated to be a passive one to simply provide dietary fat as a precursor for the synthesis of a lipid corepressor (Slayton and Szepesi, 1973). The process of rerepression is dependent on *de novo* RNA synthesis (i.e., it can be prevented by 8-azaguanine and requires dietary protein but not dietary carbohydrate) (Slayton and Szepesi, 1973).

The previously enumerated facts are summarized in Fig. 8. This model of enzyme induction envisions a gene for G6PD that is repressed by a repressor consisting of a protein aporepressor and a lipid corepressor. During stress such as starvation or caloric restriction, the corepressor and aporepressor separate, the corepressor is destroyed, and the gene becomes derepressed. Upon refeeding a high-carbohydrate, low-fat, and adequate protein diet, enzyme activity is returned to normal by processing the messenger RNA already present. During day 2 of refeeding the RNA necessary for the production of the overshoot is made, probably *de novo*. During this time RNA is produced, which will code not only for G6PD but also for the aporepressor, or enzymes to produce the corepressor, or both. Therefore, if a suitable precursor of the lipid corepressor is provided in the diet, the complete repressor will be made, and the enzyme overshoot will not occur. From the current work in the author's laboratory it appears that while translational rerepression of G6PD can be accomplished by trilionlein or trilinolenin, the transcriptional rerepression of G6PD may also require exogenous triolein (C. S. Nace and B. Szepesi, unpublished data). The active form of linoleate is not known at present. A second episode of starvation causes further derepression perhaps of cells that were previously not derepressed or other copies of genes that code for G6PD that have a higher threshold of caloric restriction for derepression. If during the first refeeding this system is rerepressed, then a second episode of starvation–refeeding will produce an enzyme overshoot that is commensurate with one starvation–refeeding episode. However, if rerepression during refeeding is prevented by 8-azaguanine, the second starvation–refeeding will produce the induction increment.

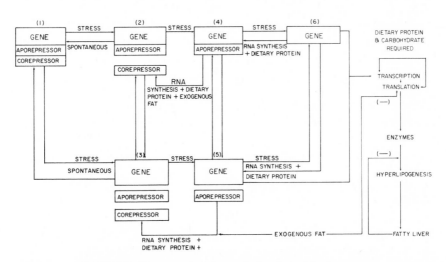

FIGURE 8 The control of glucose-6-phosphate dehydrogenase.

The model presented from the author's laboratory is consistent with all the experimental data available through mid-1974. At that time some excellent work was published by Israeli scientists claiming that G6PD could be induced without increased rate of synthesis or alteration in the rate of degradation (Yagil et al., 1974). These scientists found that antiserum specific for G6PD protein was proportional to enzyme activity. When the antiserum was precipitated with an anti-IgG serum, the amount of precipitate or radioactivity found from G6PD was equal in the uninduced and the induced treatments. The authors account for this difference between these results and the results obtained by precipitation techniques by suggesting that whereas the precipitation of the active enzyme requires one type of antibody, the precipitation of inactive enzymes is due to the presence of other antibodies (Yagil et al., 1974). Thus, when only the active enzyme is precipitated, the enzyme activity is found to be proportional to the antibody that has to be added. Conversely, when the total enzyme is precipitated, the total enzyme protein precipitable is no longer proportional to enzyme activity. Unfortunately in the experiments where the enzyme precipitated by the anti-IgG serum were subjected to SDS electrophoresis, it was found that almost half of the total precipitated and labeled protein was found outside the G6PD peak, suggesting that much of the protein precipitated by the anti-IgG serum is not G6PD (Yagil et al., 1974). They suggested that G6PD is convertible from an active to an inactive form under conditions then being studied. They reported that the total amount of G6PD protein remained relatively constant and that the level of enzyme activity is determined by the proportion of active to inactive protein. At present, the only logical interpretation of Yagil et al.'s data (1974) from their standpoint is that in the induced rat (fed a fat-free diet) the enzyme produced is in the active form, whereas in the noninduced rat (rats fed the high-fat diet) the enzyme that is produced is in the inactive form. According to this explanation, there is no conversion of active to inactive enzyme, and the system produces either the active or the inactive enzyme.

A similar hypothesis has been advanced by Kelly et al. (1975). Their evidence is based on an Ouchterlony plate in which the precipitates are washed with 0.9 M sodium chloride and then stained with a stain that is specific for enzyme activity. In this case it was found that enzyme samples from starved rats or rats fed a high-fat diet have no activity, whereas enzyme samples from rats starved and refed a high-carbohydrate diet that contains a little fat have stainable activity. This sort of evidence is very dubious, since we would expect that on the Ouchterlony plate once the enzymes are precipitated by the antibody they lose activity.

It is not possible at present to resolve this controversy as to whether liver G6PD is induced or whether the changes in enzyme activity reflect an activation or deactivation process. The author believes that some of the data from his own laboratory and some of the data from the laboratories of other scientists can be explained only if it is assumed that there is an enzyme induction that requires *de novo* RNA synthesis. There is no logical explanation that the effect of starvation could be discernible days after it occurred, unless we invoke the concept of derepression. On the other hand, the author's own data indicate that dietary fat has a translational effect that is a translational *repressive* effect that cannot be obliterated by preventing *de novo* RNA synthesis. It is quite possible, therefore, that both the induction and the activation/deactivation processes may go on simultaneously. It can certainly be expected that this field will continue to be one of intense activity in the years to come.

Another area of intense research concerns the signal that initiates the overshoot of G6PD in rat liver. It has been found that enzyme activity can be increased by cortisol in conjunction with insulin (Freedland et al., 1966). Dihydroepiandrosterone (Willmer and Foster, 1965; Tepperman et al., 1968) is known to decrease G6PD activity in the liver. It is known that the induction of fatty acid synthetase, acetyl CoA carboxylase, citrate cleavage enzyme, malic enzyme, and G6PD require insulin (Gibson, 1972; Nepekroeff et al., 1974) while the induction of the same enzymes can be prevented by glucagon (Nepekroeff et al., 1974). Glucagon and cAMP are known to prevent the overshoot of G6PD (Rudack and Holten, 1972; Rudack et al., 1971). Because of the reciprocal action of glucagon and insulin on enzyme induction, it has been suggested that the above enzymes are induced coordinately (Gibson, 1972). However, the demonstration that the lack of insulin results in poorly functioning or nonfunctioning ribosomes (Wool, 1972) should make us cautious lest we consider a general effect to be a signal for a specific effect. In cases where insulin dependence on G6PD induction has been tested, it was found that insulin is not able to produce enzyme induction when the induction is prevented by a high-fat diet (Fábry et al., 1970; Szepesi and Berdanier, 1971) or in cases where enzyme induction is prevented by a lack of carbohydrate (Szepesi and Berdanier, 1971). The inability to find a role for insulin in the induction of G6PD does not rule out the possibility that insulin is necessary as a part of a signal to initiate the enzyme overshoot process.

The involvement of RNA in these processes appears to be indicated, but the type of RNA or the process involved cannot be determined at present. It is indicated that some steps in initiation enhanced by GTP (Wettenhall et al., 1971) may be altered. It is also a question of importance whether inhibitors like actinomycin D alter messenger RNA function or messenger RNA degradation. It has been suggested that messenger RNA stability and degradation are indeed altered by actinomycin D (Lee et al., 1970) and cycloheximide (Endo et al., 1973). It is difficult, therefore, to evaluate experiments where actinomycin D has been used, because some of the effects may be complicated by an effect of actinomycin D on messenger RNA degradation.

Even though the initiation step in protein synthesis seems to be involved with insulin insufficiency (Wool, 1972), there are other possibilities worth investigating. For example, in the rabbit (Kerwar et al., 1970) and guinea pig (Caskey et al., 1967) two transfer RNAs are involved in the incorporation of methionine into protein. It has been suggested that in the rabbit Met-tRNA$_f$ and

Met-tRNA$_m$ can both transfer methionine. The former transfers methionine into terminal location; the latter transfers methionine into an interior location in the polypeptide (Chatterjee et al., 1971). It has been suggested that it is Met-tRNA$_f$ that is responsible for putting on formylated methionine in the initation step of protein synthesis (Culp et al., 1970). At present there is little evidence to support whether there is any alteration in the amount or ability to function of these or other transfer RNAs involved in protein synthesis. The possible role of processing of messenger RNA in enzyme induction is an area that is also beginning to receive increasing attention (Latorre and Perry, 1973).

In the model presented on the control of G6PD induction in rat liver, it is postulated that the corepressor is a lipid molecule. In a recent report it was shown that DNA transcription has been inhibited by phospholipase treatment of DNA (Menon, 1972). Adenyl cyclase activity and ATPase activity in cell membranes are also changed by lipid extraction (Réthy et al., 1971). An interaction between lipid and DNA has been suggested by other work (Manzoli, 1974). It appears possible, therefore, that some lipids under some circumstances may interact with DNA. It is freely admitted by the author, however, that proof of lipoprotein repressor requires a great deal more evidence than is now available.

Concerning other aspects of the model, it might be useful to add that DNA modification and other processes during development have been proposed (Holliday and Pugh, 1975), and it is generally indicated that a number of genes are turned off in the normal animal. Another important fact that has been uncovered is that autotransplants of liver can adapt to a fat-free diet without blood supply (Bartley and Abraham, 1972a). Just how the signal toward increased G6PD levels travels is not known.

Concerning the identity of the signal to set off the development of the overshoot and some other aspects of this process, it might be helpful to briefly review the findings obtained by using oviducts from hens. It has been found that progesterone will bind to a receptor protein in bird oviduct that will then promote the synthesis of ovalbumin (Steggles et al., 1971). The receptor protein is specific to this organ and will not bind in other organs (Steggles et al., 1971). G6PD is also induced in uterus by NADP (Moulton and Barker, 1974). The induction is inhibited by 8-azaguanine (Moulton and Barker, 1974). Ovalbumin messenger RNA has recently been isolated and purified and it has been estimated to contain between 16,070 and 17,040 nucleotides (Haines et al., 1974). The ovalbumin molecule needs only 1,161 nucleotides to produce the complete sequence (Haines et al., 1974). What is the function of the rest of the messenger RNA? It needs to be determined. It is reasonable then to look for some receptor proteins in rat liver that would be involved in the nuclei either during derepression or rerepression of G6PD.

In summary, it appears that in the mammal there may be a number of different mechanisms by which protein synthesis is regulated. The diversity of these mechanisms is not surprising considering that the process of regulation is complicated by the organization of enzymes and proteins, not only within a cell where their control needs to be regulated only with respect to function, but also by distance and the functional cooperation involved among the organs. Certain enzymes that have one function in the liver may have different functions in other organs. Therefore, enzymes from different organs require different types of regulatory mechanisms to regulate their synthesis and breakdown. There are a number of common conditions, such as caloric restriction, that might demand a relatively uniform type of control all over the animal body. In such instances it might be expected that stress hormones or nerve secretions might be involved as a general signal toward decreasing enzyme activity. Such a picture is indeed emerging from the findings that have been discussed.

Another question of considerable importance is whether enzyme induction occurs in the animal system as it does in bacteria. Current indications using antibodies are that it does. The claims of Hizi and Yagil (1974a,b), however, would point in the direction that the precipitation of the active enzyme might not be an adequate way to determine the total amount of enzyme protein present. Indeed, their hypothesis is given credibility by the fact that in most instances the breakdown products of enzymes cannot be found. It seems difficult to reconcile with this hypothesis, however, that in many instances the enzyme induction has been shown to be dependent on *de novo* RNA synthesis either by the use of actinomycin D or azaguanine or other inhibitors.

BIOLOGICAL IMPORTANCE OF PHENOMENA RESULTING FROM CALORIC RESTRICTION

Effect on Growth and Development

One of the fastest growing areas of biology today is the study of development, growth, and aging. The organism appears to be genetically programmed with respect to maximum life-span, development, and growth (Wolpert and Lewis, 1975). Cells remember "when" they are in their program not "where" (Wolpert and Lewis, 1975). Numerous factors can alter the unrolling of the developmental program, including nutritional factors. There are different theories of development and aging: genetic error, redundant message, codon restriction, and transcriptional event (Hayflick, 1975). Depending on which theory or what aspects of each theory are accepted, the effect of nutritional events may alter development at different points of control.

Inasmuch as differentiation continues throughout life as genetic information unfolds (Holliday and Pugh, 1975), different types of interactions may be possible between one aspect of the external environment (food) and the internal environment. It should be kept in mind that much of the biological controls that determine organ identity and function require contact with similar cells; therefore, early effects on the phenotype may be long "remembered" and may even be passed on to succeeding generations. Thus, it is possible to alter the genetic expression without altering the genes themselves (that is, without altering the nucleotide sequence in the genes).

Caloric restriction appears to affect growth and development. The magnitude of the effect depends on the stage of development during which the restriction is applied, the severity of caloric restriction, and the type of caloric restriction. The effects of caloric restriction appear to be most severe if applied during pregnancy or lactation. Restriction during pregnancy results in offspring that are smaller (Chow and Lee, 1964), have less RNA and DNA (Roeder, 1973; Zamenhof et al., 1973), more cathepsin (Roeder, 1973), oxidize more proline (Hsu and Chow, 1973), and age faster (Roeder, 1973). Brain weight of offspring from restricted mothers is smaller (Zamenhof et al., 1973). Chronic underfeeding after birth is reported to delay adipocyte hyperplasia (Hubbard and Matthew, 1971). Food restriction has been reported to cause slower (Stewart, 1973) or faster (Roeder, 1973) than normal rates of growth after birth, but in both cases (Roeder, 1973; Stewart, 1973) mature weight was less than in normal animals. Protein restriction during pregnancy appeared more harmful for the young than did caloric restriction (Baird et al., 1973; Rider and Simonson, 1973). The effect of caloric restriction during lactation (Hsueh et al., 1973; Knittle, 1972) also decreases growth rate, and rehabilitation requires weeks (Knittle, 1972). In general, it can be said that body size may be greatly influenced by restriction during lactation and pregnancy, while behavior is altered by nutritional factors during pregnancy (Hsueh et al., 1973).

Early malnutrition, whether during pregnancy (Rider and Simonson, 1973; Simonson et al., 1973) or after birth (Barnes et al., 1970; Franková and Barnes, 1968), has been reported to cause behavioral abnormalities. Some aspects of undernutrition were improved after administering growth hormone (Stephan et al., 1971), growth hormone and insulin (Lee, 1970), or pituitary extract (Simonson et al., 1973). These results from animal studies have raised the possibility that malnourishment of pregnant women may result in not only smaller babies but emotionally disturbed and mentally less capable babies, or that malnourishment in early childhood may lead to some form of retardation in mental development. Caloric supplementation of expectant mothers has been reported to produce heavier babies and better infant survival (Habicht et al., 1973). In studies in Peru, rehabilitation of malnourished children was reported to normalize growth but not IQ levels (Graham and Adrianzen, 1972). The effect of malnutrition on human intelligence, however, has been and continues to be a controversial subject (Frisch, 1970). There appears to be a general belief that human IQ development is inherited and modified by the intellectual, not the nutritional, environment, barring extremely severe and rather unlikely deficiencies.

The effect of caloric restriction on subsequent growth and development does not appear to depend on the amount or type of carbohydrate intake. Some recent work indicates that sucrose consumption in early life will alter responses of later nutritional stimuli (Berdanier, 1975; Moser and Berdanier, 1974), but the effect of different carbohydrates along with caloric restriction has not been studied.

Caloric Restriction and Longevity

Longevity has been reported to be increased by caloric restriction (Berg and Simms, 1960; McCay et al., 1935), periodic fasting (Carlson and Hoelzel, 1946), or meal feeding (Leveille, 1972). Inasmuch as food-restricted rats tend to become meal eaters (McCay et al., 1935), all these effects could be attributable to reduced food intake. A dissenting view reporting impaired longevity in restricted rats (Widdowson and Kennedy, 1962) may have been influenced by an unusually large amount of lung infection. It is known that during caloric restriction rats become more susceptible to respiratory diseases.

Caloric restriction has been reported to decrease the incidence of spontaneous tumors in rats and mice (Berg and Simms, 1960, 1961; Ross and Bras, 1965; Saxton et al., 1948; Tannenbaum, 1947) and chromophobe adenomas in rat anterior pituitary (Ross et al., 1970). Rats subjected to intermittent fasting also had reduced tumors (Carlson and Hoelzel, 1946). No change in tumorigenesis was reported in GG rats subjected to food restriction (Gilbert et al., 1958) The development of diabetes in spontaneously diabetic mice was alleviated by food restriction (Chick and Like, 1971). Caloric restriction was reported to reduce both hyperglycemia and hyperinsulinemia (Chick and Like, 1971). Infertility was reportedly reduced in older rats from caloric restricted groups (Berg, 1960).

Not all effects of caloric restriction are beneficial. For example, prematurely weaned rats (which starve for 1 or 2 days before they eat) have altered spermatogenesis (Hahn and Koldovsky, 1966) and higher blood cholesterol (Hahn and Kirby, 1973). Myocardial degeneration was also increased by caloric restriction (Berg and Simms, 1960). Blood pressure is increased in starvation (Consolazio et al., 1966) and starvation–refeeding (Wilhelmj et al., 1951, 1956), especially when the diet refed contains high levels of carbohydrate (Wilhelmj et al., 1957). Starvation–refeeding has been reported to cause alterations in the arterial walls in swine (Hermbrough and Link, 1968) and rat (Hermbrough and Riedesel, 1970). The effect in swine was more severe with a high-carbohydrate diet (Smith, 1964). It is possible that the alteration caused in lipid metabolism by starvation–refeeding may alter the physical structure of arterial lipids to promote cholesterol deposition (Shipley, 1974).

It appears, therefore, that caloric restriction may alter longevity by altering the appearance, rate of development, and severity of some diseases. Depending on conditions, caloric restriction may or may not increase longevity. Reports that circulatory diseases are increased by stress (Bassett et al., 1969a, b) should be a warning that the control of stress or our physiological response to stress may be important vectors in disease management. Caloric stress followed by overfeeding may be even more harmful than slight overweight.

REFERENCES

Aas, M. and Daae, L. N. 1971. *Biochim. Biophys. Acta* 239:208.
Addis, T., Poo, L. J. and Lew, W. 1936. *J. Biol. Chem.* 115:117.
Adibi, S. A. 1968. *J. Appl. Physiol.* 25:52.
Adibi, S. A. and Drash, A. L. 1970. *J. Lab. Clin. Med.* 76:722.
Akpan, J. O., Gardner, R. and Wagle, S. R. 1974. *Biochem. Biophys. Res. Commun.* 61:222.
Allmann, D. W. and Gibson, D. M. 1965. *J. Lipid Res.* 6:52.
Allmann, D. W., Hubbard, D. D. and Gibson, D. M. 1965. *J. Lipid Res.* 6:63.
Anderson, J. W. and Herman, R. H. 1972. *Am. J. Clin. Nutr.* 25:41.
Anonymous. 1974. *Nutr. Rev.* 32:78.
Aoki, T. T., Müller, W. A., Murray, F. B. and Cahill, G. F., Jr. 1974. *Metabolism* 23:805.
Apfelbaum, M., Bostsarron, J. and Lacatis, D. 1971. *Am. J. Clin. Nutr.* 24:1405.
Arora, D. J. S. and DeLamirande, G. 1971. *Can. J. Biochem.* 49:1150.
Ashcroft, S. J. H., Chatra, L., Weerasinghe, C. and Randle, P. J. 1973. *Biochem. J.* 132:223.
Ashworth, A. 1969. *Br. J. Nutr.* 23:835.
Assal, J. P., Levrat, R., Stauffacher, W. and Renold, A. E. 1971. *Metabolism* 20:850.
Assan, R., Rosselin, G. and Dolais, J. 1967. *J. Annul. Diabetol. l'Hotel-Dieu* 7:25.
Aysel, F. 1975. *Fed. Proc.* 34(3):889.
Ayuso-Parrilla, M. S. and Parrilla, R. 1973. *Biochem. Biophys. Res. Commun.* 52:582.
Baird, A., Widdowson, E. M. and Cowley, J. J. 1971. *Br. J. Nutr.* 25:391.
Baker, N. and Huebotter, R. J. 1972. *J. Lipid Res.* 13:329.
Baker, N. and Huebotter, R. J. 1973. *J. Lipid Res.* 14:95.
Balasse, O. E. and Harvel, R. J. 1971. *J. Clin. Invest.* 50:801.
Ballard, F. J. and Hopgood, M. F. 1974. *Biochem. J.* 140:531.
Ballard, F. J., Hanson, R. W. and Kronfeld, D. S. 1969. *Fed. Proc.* 28:218.
Ballard, F. J., Hopgood, M. F., Reshef, L., Tilghman, S. and Hanson, R. W. 1974. *Biochem. J.* 144:199.
Bang, I. 1913. *Wiesbaden* 8:162.
Baquer, N. Z., Sochor, M. and McLean, P. 1972. *Biochem. Biophys. Res. Commun.* 47:218
Baquer, N. Z., Cascales, M., Teo, B. C. and McLean, P. 1973. *Biochem. Biophys. Res. Commun.* 52:263.
Barnard, D. L., Ford, J., Garnett, E. S., Mardell, R. J. and Whyman, A. E. 1969. *Metabolism* 18:564.
Barnes, R. H., Moore, A. U. and Pond, W. G. 1970. *J. Nutr.* 100:149.
Barth, C., Sladek, M. and Decker, K. 1972. *Biochim. Biophys. Acta* 260:1.
Bartley, J. C. and Abraham, S. 1972a. *Biochim. Biophys. Acta* 260:169.
Bartley, J. C. and Abraham, S. 1972b. *Biochim. Biophys. Acta* 280:258.
Bassett, D. R., Abel, M., Moellering, R. C., Jr., Rosenblatt, G. and Stokes, J., III. 1969a. *Am. J. Clin. Nutr.* 22:1483.
Bassett, D. R., Abel, M., Moellering, R. C., Jr., Rosenblatt, G. and Stokes, J., III. 1969b. *Am. J. Clin. Nutr.* 22:1504.
Benjamin, W. and Gellhorn, A. 1966. *J. Lipid Res.* 7:285.
Bennett, G. Vann, and Cuatrecasas, P. 1972. *Science* 176:805.

Berdanier, C. D. 1975. *Am. J. Clin. Nutr.* 12:1416.
Berg, B. N. 1960. *J. Nutr.* 71:242.
Berg, B. N. and Simms, H. S. 1960. *J. Nutr.* 71:255.
Berg, B. N. and Simms, H. S. 1961. *J. Nutr.* 74:23.
Bergen, W. G. and Purser, D. B. 1968. *J. Nutr.* 95:333.
Bergman, E. N. and Kon, K. 1964. *Am. J. Physiol.* 206:449.
Bernard, C. 1877. *Cours méd. Coll. France, Paris* 8:576.
Bernardis, L. L. and Brownie, A. C. 1965. *Proc. Soc. Exp. Biol. Med.* 120:146.
Bieberdorf, F. A., Chernick, S. S. and Scow, R. O. 1970. *J. Clin. Invest.* 49:1685.
Blackburn, G. L., Flatt, J. P., Clowes, G. H. A., Jr., O'Donnel, T. F. and Hensle, T. E. 1973. *Ann. Surg.* 177:588.
Blatt, L. M. and Kim, K. H. 1971. *J. Biol. Chem.* 246:4895.
Blobel, G. and Potter, V. R. 1967. *J. Mol. Biol.* 26:293.
Bloom, W. L. 1962. *Arch. Int. Med.* 109:26.
Bloom, W. L. and Mitchell, W., Jr. 1960. *Arch. Int. Med.* 106:321.
Bloxham, D. P. and Akhtar, M. 1971. *Biochem. J.* 123:275.
Böe, G. 1913. *Biochem. Z. (Berlin)* 58:106.
Bohman, V. R. 1955. *J. Anim. Sci.* 14:249.
Bortz, W. M. and Lynen, F. 1963. *Biochem. Z.* 337:505.
Boulter, P. R., Hoffman, R. S. and Arky, R. A. 1973. *Metabolism* 22:675.
Bowman, R. H. 1970. *J. Biol. Chem.* 245:1604.
Brozek, J., Chapman, C. B. and Keep, A. 1948. *Am. Med. Assoc. J.* 137:1569.
Buchanan, K. D., Vance, J. E. and Williams, R. H. 1969. *Metabolism* 18:155.
Bucher, N. L. R., McGarrahan, K., Gould, E. and Loud, A. V. 1959. *J. Biol. Chem.* 234:262.
Buckman, M. T., Conway, M. J., Seibel, J. A. and Eaton, R. P. 1973. *Metabolism* 10:1253.
Burns, T. W. and Langley, P. E. 1970. *J. Lab. Clin. Med.* 75:983.
Burton, D. N., Collins, J. M., Kennan, A. L. and Porter, J. W. 1969. *J. Biol. Chem.* 244:4510.
Burton, J. H., Anderson, M. and Reid, J. T. 1974. *Br. J. Nutr.* 32:515.
Buse, M. G., Johnson, A. H., Kuperminc, D. and Buse, J. F. 1970. *Metabolism* 19:219.
Buse, M. G., Biggers, J. F., Drier, C. and Buse, J. F. 1973. *J. Biol. Chem.* 248:697.
Cahill, G. F., Jr., Lebouef, B. and Flin, R. B. 1960. *J. Biol. Chem.* 235:1246.
Cahill, G. F., Jr., Herrera, M. G. and Morgan, A. P. 1966. *J. Clin. Invest.* 45:1751.
Cameron, R. T. and Carmichael, J. 1946. *Can. J. Res.* 24:37.
Cantu, R. C., Wise, B. S., Goldfien, A., Gullixson, K. S., Fischer, N. and Ganong, W. F. 1963. *Proc. Soc. Exp. Biol. Med.* 114:10.
Carlson, A. J. and Hoelzel, F. 1946. *J. Nutr.* 31:363.
Carlson, C. A. and Kim, Ki-Han. 1974. *Arch. Biochem. Biophys.* 164:478.
Caskey, C. T., Redfield, B. and Weissbach, H. 1967. *Arch. Biochem. Biophys.* 120:119.
Century, B. 1972. *J. Nutr.* 102:1067.
Chakrabarty, K. and Leveille, G. A. 1968. *J. Nutr.* 96:76.
Chakrabarty, K. and Leveille, G. A. 1969. *Proc. Soc. Exp. Biol. Med.* 131:1051.
Chang, K. J., Marcus, N. A. and Cuatrecasas, P. 1974. *J. Biol. Chem.* 249:6854.

Chang, M. L. W. and Johnson, M. A. 1975. *Fed. Proc.* 34:910.

Chatterjee, N. K., Bose, K. K., Woodley, C. L., and Gupta, N. K. 1971. *Biochem. Biophys. Res. Commun.* 43:771.

Cheng, C. H., Koch, M. and Shank, R. E. 1969. *J. Nutr.* 98:64.

Chick, W. L. and Like, A. A. 1971. *Am. J. Physiol.* 221:202.

Chow, B. F. and Lee, C. J. 1964. *J. Nutr.* 82:10.

Clark, D. G., Rognstad, R. and Katz, J. 1973. *Biochem. Biophys. Res. Commun.* 54:1141.

Clark, M. G., Bloxham, D. P., Holland, P. C. and Lardy, H. A. 1973a. *Biochem. J.* 134:589.

Clark, M. G., Williams, C. H., Pfeifer, W. F., Bloxham, D. P., Holland, P. C., Taylor, C. A. and Lardy, H. A. 1973b. *Nature* 245:99.

Clarke, M. F. and Smith, A. H. 1938. *Br. J. Nutr.* 15:245.

Cohn, C. and Joseph, D. 1960. *Am. J. Clin. Nutr.* 8:682.

Cohn, C. and Joseph, D. 1970. *J. Nutr.* 100:78.

Collins, J. M., Craig, M. C. and Nepekroeff, C. M. 1971. *Arch. Biochem. Biophys.* 143:343.

Conrad, E. A. and Bass, A. D. 1957. *J. Histochem. Cytochem.* 5:182.

Consolazio, C. E., Nelson, R. A., Johnson, H. L., Matoush, L. D., Krywicki, H. J. and Isaac, G. J. 1966. U.S. Army Med. Res. Lab. Rep. No. 289.

Conway, M. J., Goodner, C. J., Werrbach, J. H. and Gale, C. C. 1969. *J. Clin. Invest.* 48:1349.

Cooper, B., and Margolis, S. 1971. *J. Lipid Res.* 12:731.

Craig, M. C. and Porter, J. W. 1973. *Arch. Biochem. Biophys.* 159:606.

Craig, M. C., Dugan, R. E., Muesing, R. A., Slakey, L. L. and Porter, J. W. 1972a. *Arch. Biochem. Biophys.* 151:128.

Craig, M. C., Nepekroeff, C. M., Lakshmanan, M. R. and Porter, J. W. 1972b. *Arch. Biochem. Biophys.* 152:619.

Cuatrecasas, P. 1972. *J. Biol. Chem.* 247:1980.

Culp, C., Morrisey, J. and Hardesty, B. 1970. *Biochem. Biophys. Res. Commun.* 40:777.

D'Amour, M. D. and Keller, A. D. 1933. *Proc. Soc. Exp. Biol. Med.* 30:1175.

Dehlinger, P. J. and Schimke, R. T. 1970. *Biochem. Biophys. Res. Commun.* 40:1473.

De La Garza, S., Tepperman, H. M. and Tepperman, J. 1970. *J. Nutr.* 100:1027.

Desai, I. D. 1969. *Can. J. Biochem.* 47:785.

Desai, I. D. 1971. *Can. J. Biochem.* 49:170.

DeWulf, H. and Hers, H. G. 1968. *Eur. J. Biochem.* 6:558.

Dickson, R. C. and Abelson, J. 1975. *Science* 187:27.

Edwards, J. C. and Taylor, K. W. 1970. *Biochim. Biophys. Acta* 215:310.

Eggleston, L. V. and Krebs, H. A. 1969. *Biochem. J.* 114:877.

Eggleston, L. V. and Krebs, H. A. 1974. *Biochem. J.* 138:425.

Elias, H. and Kolb, L. 1913. *Biochem. Z. (Berlin)* 52:331.

Endo, Y., Seno, H., Tominage, H. and Natori, Y. 1973. *Biochim. Biophys. Acta* 299:114.

Enwonwu, C. O., Stambaugh, R., and Sreebny, L. 1971. *J. Nutr.* 101:337.

Exton, J. H. and Park, C. R. 1967. *J. Biol. Chem.* 242:2622.

Fábry, P. 1967. In *Handbook of physiology,* ed. C. Code and W. Heidel, vol. I, p. 31. Washington, D.C.: American Physiological Society.

Fábry, P. and Tepperman, J. 1970. *Am. J. Clin. Nutr.* 23:1059.

Fábry, P., Kleinfeld, R., Tepperman, H. M. and Tepperman, J. 1970. *Proc. Soc. Exp. Biol. Med.* 133:577.

Fajans, S. S., Floyd, J. C., Jr., Knopf, R. F., Guntsche, E. M., Rull, J. A., Thiffault, C. A. and Conn, J. W. 1967. *J. Clin. Endocrinol.* 27:1600.

Felig, P., Owen, O. E., Wahren, J. and Cahill, G. F., Jr. 1969. *J. Clin. Invest.* 48:584.

Felig, P., Marliss, E. B. and Cahill, G. F., Jr. 1971. *J. Clin. Invest.* 50:411.

Filkins, J. 1970. *Am. J. Physiol.* 219:923.

Flatt, J. P. and Blackburn, G. L. 1974. *Am. J. Clin. Nutr.* 27:175.

Florini, J. R. and Breuer, C. B. 1966. *Biochemistry* 5:1870.

Franková, S. and Barnes, R. H. 1968. *J. Nutr.* 96:447.

Freedland, R. A. 1967. *J. Nutr.* 91:489.

Freedland, R. A. and Szepesi, B. 1971. In *Enzyme synthesis and degradation in mammalian systems*, ed. M. Recheigl, Jr., p. 103. Switzerland: Karger Basel.

Freedland, R. A., Cunliffe, T. L. and Zinkl, J. B. 1966. *J. Biol. Chem.* 241:5448.

Frisch, R. 1970. *Am. J. Clin. Nutr.* 23:189.

Fröberg, S., Liljedahl, O. S. and Orö, L. 1964. *Acta Med. Scand.* 176:685.

Ganguly, J. 1960. *Biochim. Biophys. Acta* 40:110.

Garren, L. D., Howell, R. R., Tomkins, B. M. and Crocco, R. M. 1964. *Proc. Natl. Acad. Sci. U.S.A.* 52:1121.

Geisler, R. W. and Hansen, R. J. 1972. *Biochim. Biophys. Acta* 279:139.

Genuth, S. M. and Castro, J. 1974. *Metabolism* 23:375.

Gerschenson, L. E. and Andersson, M. 1971. *Biochim. Biophys. Acta* 43:1211.

Gibson, D. M. 1972. *Adv. Enzyme Regul.* 10:187.

Gibson, D. M., Hicks, S. E. and Allman, D. W. 1966. *Adv. Enzyme Regul.* 4:239.

Gilbert, C., Gillman, P. and Lutz, W. 1958. *Br. J. Cancer* 12:565.

Gilbertson, J. R. 1969. *Metabolism* 18:887.

Giorgio, N. A., Johnson, C. B. and Blecher, M. 1974. *J. Biol. Chem.* 249:428.

Glinsmann, W., Pank, G. and Hern, E. 1970. *Biochem. Biophys. Res. Commun.* 39:774.

Glock, B. E. and McLean, P. 1955. *Biochem. J.* 61:390.

Gold, A. J. and Costello, L. C. 1974. *Am. J. Physiol.* 227:1336.

Goodman, H. M. and Knobil, E. 1961. *Am. J. Physiol.* 201:1.

Goodridge, A. 1972. *J. Biol. Chem.* 247:6946.

Goodridge, A. 1973. *J. Biol. Chem.* 248:4318.

Goodridge, A. 1975. *Fed. Proc.* 34:117.

Gordon, C. W., Knowlton, S. D. and Martin, D. B. 1974. *J. Clin. Invest.* 54:1403.

Gozukara, E. M., Frolich, M. and Holten, D. 1972. *Biochim. Biophys. Acta* 286:155.

Graham, C. G. and Adrianzen, T. B. 1972. *Johns Hopkins Med. J.* 131:204.

Graham, G. G. and MacLean, W. C., Jr. 1975. *Fed. Proc.* 34(3):909.

Greene, H. L., Taunton, O. D., Stifel, F. B. and Herman, R. H. 1974. *J. Clin. Invest.* 53:44.

Grey, N. J., Goldring, S. and Kipnis, D. M. 1970. *J. Clin. Invest.* 49:881.

Griminger, P., Villamil, V. and Fisher, H. 1969. *J. Nutr.* 99:368.

Gross, M. 1974. *Biochim. Biophys. Acta* 366:275.

Gross, M. and Rabinovitz, M. 1972. *Proc. Natl. Acad. Sci. U.S.A.* 69:1565.

Gross, M. and Rabinovitz, M. 1973. *Biochem. Biophys. Res. Commun.* 50:832.

Gumaa, K. A. and McLean, P. 1971. *FEBS Lett.* 13:5.

Gunn, J. M. and Taylor, C. B. 1973. *Biochem. J.* 136:455.

Guynn, R. W., Veloso, D., Harris, R. L., Lawson, J. W. R. and Veech, R. L. 1973. *Biochem. J.* 136:639.

Habicht, J. P., Yarbrough, C., Lechtig, A. and Klein, R. E. 1973. *Nutr. Rep. Int.* 7:533.

Hahn, P. and Kirby, L. 1973. *J. Nutr.* 103:690.

Hahn, P. and Kirby, L. T. 1974. *Can. J. Biochem.* 52:739.

Hahn, P. and Koldovsky, O. 1966. In *Utilization of nutrients during postnatal development.* Oxford: Pergamon Press.

Haines, M. E., Carey, N. H. and Palmiter, R. D. 1974. *Eur. J. Biochem.* 43:549.

Halestrap, A. P. and Denton, R. M. 1973. *Biochem. J.* 132:509.

Halestrap, A. P. and Denton, R. M. 1974. *Biochem. J.* 142:365.

Halperin, M. L. 1970. *Can. J. Biochem.* 48:1228.

Hanson, R. W. 1974. *Nutr. Rev.* 32:1.

Hanson, R. W. and Ziporin, Z. Z. 1966. *J. Lipid Res.* 7:56.

Hanson, R. W., Garber, A. J., Reshef, L. and Ballard, R. J. 1973. *Am. J. Clin. Nutr.* 26:55.

Harrison, M. F. 1953. *Biochem. J.* 55:204.

Harrison, M. F. and Brown, L. M. 1951. *Biochem. J.* 48:151.

Hayes, L. W. and Larrabee, A. R. 1971. *Biochem. Biophys. Res. Commun.* 45:955.

Hayflick, L. 1975. *Fed. Proc.* 34:9.

Henshaw, E. C., Hirsch, C. A., Morton, B. E. and Hiatt, H. H. 1971. *J. Biol. Chem.* 246:436.

Hermbrough, F. B. and Link, R. P. 1968. *Proc. Soc. Exp. Biol. Med.* 128:1055.

Hermbrough, F. B. and Riedesel, D. H. 1970. *Am. J. Physiol.* 219:742.

Hers, H. G., DeWulf, H., Van den Berghe, G. and Stalmans, W. (1970). In *Metabolic interconversions of enzymes,* ed. E. H. Fischer, E. G. Krebs, H. Neurath, and E. R. Stadtman, p. 89. Berlin: Springer-Verlag.

Hicks, S. E., Allmann, D. W. and Gibson, D. M. 1965. *Biochim. Biophys. Acta* 106:441.

Higgins, M., Kawachi, T. and Rudney, H. 1971. *Biochem. Biophys. Res. Commun.* 45:138.

Hill, D. C. and Olsen, E. M. 1963. *J. Nutr.* 70:303.

Hill, R., Linazosoro, J. M., Chevallier, F. and Chaikoff, I. L. 1958. *J. Biol. Chem.* 233:305.

Hill, R., Webster, W. W., Linazasoro, J. M. and Chaikoff, I. L. 1960. *J. Lipid Res.* 1:150.

Hiroshi, Y. E., Tominga, H. and Natori, Y. 1971. *Biochim. Biophys. Acta* 240:215.

Hirsch, C. A. and Hiatt, H. H. 1966. *J. Biol. Chem.* 241:5936.

Hizi, A. and Yagil, G. 1974a. *Eur. J. Biochem.* 45:201.

Hizi, A. and Yagil, G. 1974b. *Eur. J. Biochem.* 45:211.

Hofmeister, F. 1890. *Arch. Exp. Pathol. Pharmakol. Leipzieg* 26:355.

Hogan, A. G. 1929. *Res. Bull. Mo. Agric. Exp. Stn.* 123:52.

Holliday, R. and Pugh, J. E. 1975. *Science* 187:226.

Holten, D. 1972. *Biochim. Biophys. Acta* 268:4.

Holzer, H. and Duntze, W. 1971. *Annu. Rev. Biochem.* 40:345.

Hopgood, M. F., Ballard, F. J., Reshef, L. and Hanson, R. W. 1973. *Biochem. J.* 134:445.

Hori, S. H. and Noda, S. 1971. *J. Histochem. Cytochem.* 19:299.

Hornbrook, K. R. and Lyon, J. B., Jr. 1970. *Biochim. Biophys. Acta* 215:29.

Hornichter, R. D. and Brown, J. 1969. *Diabetes* 18:257.
Howard, B. V., Howard, W. J. and Bailey, J. J. 1974. *J. Biol. Chem.* 249:7912.
Howarth, R. E. and Baldwin, R. L. 1971a. *J. Nutr.* 101:477.
Howarth, R. E. and Baldwin, R. L. 1971b. *J. Nutr.* 101:485.
Hsu, J. M. and Chow, B. F. 1973. *Nutr. Rep. Int.* 7:475.
Hsu, R. Y. and Lardy, H. A. 1967. *J. Biol. Chem.* 242:520.
Hsueh, A. M., Simonson, M. and Kellum, M. J. 1973. *Nutr. Rep. Int.* 7:437.
Hubbard, R. W. and Matthew, W. T. 1971. *J. Lipid Res.* 12:286.
Hue, L. and Hers, H. G. 1974a. *Biochem. Biophys. Res. Commun.* 58:540.
Hue, L. and Hers, H. G. 1974b. *Biochem. Biophys. Res. Commun.* 58:532.
Huggins, C. and Yao, F. 1959. *J. Exp. Med.* 110:899.
Hunter, W. R., Rigal, W. M. and Sukkar, M. Y. 1968. In *Growth hormone,* ed. A. Pecile and E. Müller. Milan: Excerpta Medica Foundation.
Inoue, H. and Lowenstein, J. M. 1972. *J. Biol. Chem.* 247:4825.
James, W. P. T. and Coore, H. G. 1970. *Am. J. Clin. Nutr.* 23:386.
Jansen, G. R., Hutchison, C. F. and Zanetti, M. E. 1966. *Biochem. J.* 99:323.
Jansen, G. R., Zanetti, M. E. and Hutchison, C. F. 1968. *Biochem. J.* 99:345.
Jervell, K. F., Christoffersen, T. and Morland, J. 1965. *Arch. Biochem. Biophys.* 111:15.
Johansson, J. E. 1909. *Skand. Arch. Physiol.* 21:1.
Johnson, B. C. and Sassoon, H. F. 1967. *Adv. Enzyme Regul.* 5:93.
Jomain, M., Loriette, C. and McCaire, I. 1970. *Nutr. Metab.* 12:245.
Jones, G. M. and Mayer, R. J. 1973. *Biochem. J.* 132:657.
Jourdan, M., Margen, S. and Bradfield, R. B. 1974. *Am. J. Clin. Nutr.* 27:850.
Jungas, R. L. 1971. *Metabolism* 20:43.
Kather, H., Rivera, M. and Brand, K. 1972. *Biochem. J.* 128:1089.
Kato, R. and Gilette, J. R. 1965. *J. Pharmacol. Exp. Ther.* 150:279.
Kazdová, B., Braun, T., Fábry, P. and Poledne, R. 1968. *Can. J. Physiol. Pharmacol.* 46:903.
Kelly, D., Watson, J., Mach, D. and Johnson, B. C. 1975. *Fed. Proc.* 34:881.
Kerwar, S. S., Spears, C. and Weissbach. H. 1970. *Biochem. Biophys. Res. Commun.* 41:78.
Keys, A., Brozek, J., Henschel, A., Michelsen, O., and Taylor, H. L. 1950. In *The biology of human starvation*. Minneapolis: University of Minnesota Press.
Khoo, J. C., Aquino, A. A. and Steinberg, D. 1974. *J. Clin. Invest.* 53:1124.
Knittle, J. 1972. *J. Nutr.* 102:427.
Koerker, D. J., Goodner, C. J., Toivola, P. T. K., Gale, C. C. and Ensinck, J. W. 1974. *Am. J. Physiol.* 227:520.
Korchack, H. M. and Masoro, E. J. 1964. *Biochim. Biophys. Acta* 84:750.
Korner, A. 1959. *Biochem. J.* 73:61.
Korner, A. 1968. *Ann. N.Y. Acad. Sci.* 148:408.
Kraegen, E. W., Chisholm, D. J., Young, J. D. and Lazarus, L. 1970. *J. Clin. Invest.* 49:524.
Kramer, J. W. and Freedland, R. A. 1971. *Fed. Proc.* 30:401.
Krebs, E. G. 1972. *Curr. Top. Cell. Regul.* 5:99.
Krebs, E. G., Gonzales, C., Posner, J. B., Love, D. S., Bratvold, G. E. and Fischer, E. H. 1964. *Ciba Found. Symp.* 200.
Krebs, H. A. 1966. *Adv. Enzyme Regul.* 4:339.
Kwan, S. W. and Webb, T. E. 1967. *J. Biol. Chem.* 242:5542.
Lakshmanan, M. R., Nepekroeff, C. M. and Porter, J. W. 1972. *Proc. Natl. Acad. Sci. U.S.A.* 69:3516.
Lambert, A. E., Kanazawa, Y., Orci, L., Burr, I. M., Christensen, H. N. and Renold, A. E. 1971. *Proc. Soc. Exp. Biol. Med.* 137:377.

Larner, J. and Villar-Palasi, C. 1971. *Curr. Top. Cell. Regul.* 3:195.

Latorre, J. and Perry, R. P. 1973. *Biochim. Biophys. Acta* 335:93.

Lebovitz, H. E. and Feldman, J. M. 1973. *Fed. Proc.* 32:1797.

Leclercq-Meyer, V., Brisson, G. R. and Malaisse, W. J. 1971. *Nature New Biol.* 231:248.

Lee, C. J. 1970. *J. Biol. Chem.* 245:1998.

Lee, K. L., Reel, J. R. and Kenney, F. T. 1970. *J. Biol. Chem.* 245:5806.

Lehmann, W. L. 1874. *Arch. Exp. Pathol. Pharmakol.* 2:463.

Leveille, G. 1966. *J. Nutr.* 90:449.

Leveille, G. 1972. *J. Nutr.* 102:549.

Leveille, G. A. 1967. *Proc. Soc. Exp. Biol. Med.* 125:85.

Leveille, G. A. and Chakrabarty, K. 1968. *J. Nutr.* 96:69.

Levitan, I. B. and Webb, T. E. 1969. *J. Biol. Chem.* 224:341.

Li, J. J., Ross, C. R., Tepperman, H. M. and Tepperman, J. 1975. *J. Biol. Chem.* 250:141.

Linn, T. C. 1967. *J. Biol. Chem.* 242:990.

Livingston, J. N., Cuatrecasas, P. and Lockwood, D. H. 1972. *Science* 177:626.

Lockard, R. E. and Lingrel, J. B. 1971. *Nature* 233:204.

Lockwood, D. H., Lipsky, J. J. and Meronk, F., Jr. 1971. *Biochem. Biophys. Res. Commun.* 44:600.

Lockwood, E. A., Bailey, E. and Taylor, C. B. 1970. *Biochem. J.* 118:155.

Luyckx, A. S. and Lefebvre, P. J. 1970. *Proc. Soc. Exp. Biol. Med.* 133:524.

Mahler, R. J. and Szabo, O. 1969. *Horm. Metab. Res.* 1:65.

Mahler, R. and Szabo, O. 1970. *Metabolism* 19:271.

Majerus, P. W. and Kilburn, E. 1969. *J. Biol. Chem.* 244:6254.

Malaisse, W. J., Malaisse-Lagae, F. and Wright, P. H. 1967. *Am. J. Physiol.* 213:843.

Manzoli, F. A. 1974. *Biochim. Biophys. Acta* 340:1.

Marliss, E. B., Aoki, T. T., Unger, R. H., Soeldner, J. C. and Cahill G. F., Jr. 1970. *J. Clin. Invest.* 49:2256.

Matschinsky, F. M. and Ellerman, J. 1973. *Biochem. Biophys. Res. Commun.* 50:193.

Matsuda, T. and Yugari, Y. 1967. *J. Biochem. (Tokyo)* 61:535.

McCay, C. M., Crowell, M. R. and Maynard, L. A. 1935. *J. Nutr.* 10:63.

McCay, C. M., Sperling, G. and Barnes, L. L. 1943. *Arch. Biochem.* 2:469.

McDonald, B. E. and Johnson, B. C. 1965. *J. Nutr.* 87:161.

McGarry, J. D. and Foster, D. W. 1974. *J. Biol. Chem.* 249:7984.

McGarry, J. D., Meier, J. M. and Foster, D. W. 1973. *J. Biol. Chem.* 248:270.

McManus, W. R., Reid, J. T. and Donaldson, N. E. 1972. *J. Agric. Sci. Camb.* 79:1.

McMeekan, C. P. 1941. *J. Agric. Sci.* 31:1.

Meikle, A. W. and Klain, G. J. 1972. *Am. J. Physiol.* 222:1246.

Menon, I. A. 1972. *Can. J. Biochem.* 50:807.

Meyer, J. H., Lueker, C. E. and Smith, J. D. 1956. *J. Nutr.* 60:121.

Meyer, J. H. and Clawson, W. J. 1964. *J. Anim. Sci.* 23:214.

Miller, T. B., Jr., and Larner, J. 1973. *J. Biol. Chem.* 248:3483.

Mirski, A. 1942. *Biochem. J.* 36:232.

Misbin, R. I., Edgar, P. J. and Lockwood, D. H. 1971. *Metabolism* 20:544.

Mortimore, G. E., Neely, A. N., Cox, J. R. and Guinivan, R. A. 1973. *Biochem. Biophys. Res. Commun.* 54:89.

Moser, P. B. and Berdanier, C. D. 1974. *J. Nutr.* 104:687.

Moulton, B. C. and Barker, K. L. 1974. *Proc. Soc. Exp. Biol. Med.* 146:742.

Müller, W. A., Faloona, G. R. and Unger, R. H. 1971. *J. Clin. Invest.* 50:1992.

Munro, H. N. 1964. In *Mammalian protein metabolism,* ed. H. N. Munro and J. B. Allison. New York: Academic Press.

Murai, T., Tokushige, M., Nugai, J. and Katsuki, H. 1971. *Biochem. Biophys. Res. Commun.* 43:875.

Murphy, G. and Walker, D. G. 1972. *Biochem. J.* 130:76P.

Murphy, G. and Walker, D. G. 1974. *Biochem. J.* 144:149.

Murphy, V. K. and Steiner, G. 1972. *Metabolism* 21:213.

Murphy, W. and Attardi, G. 1973. *Proc. Natl. Acad. Sci. U.S.A.* 70:115.

Musch, K., Ojakian, M. A. and Williams, M. A. 1974a. *Biochim. Biophys. Acta* 337:343.

Musch, K., Ojakian, M. A. and Williams, M. A. 1974b. *Biochim. Biophys. Acta* 337:348.

Muto, Y. and Gibson, D. M. 1970. *Biochem. Biophys. Res. Commun.* 38:9.

Nakanishi, S. and Numa, S. 1970. *Eur. J. Biochem.* 16:161.

Nakanishi, S., Adhya, S., Gottesman, M. E. and Pastan, I. 1973. *J. Biol. Chem.* 248:5937.

Nelson, N., Grayman, I. and Mirsky, A. 1941. *J. Biol. Chem.* 140:361.

Nepekroeff, C. M., Lakshmanan, M. R., Ness, G. S., Muesing, R. A., Kleinsek, D. A. and Porter, J. W. 1974. *Arch. Biochem. Biophys.* 162:340.

Nestel, P., Carroll, K. F. and Havenstein, N. 1970. *Metabolism* 19:1.

Newsholme, E. A. and Gevers, W. 1967. *Vit. Horm.* 25:1.

Niemeyer, H., Clark-Turri, L., Garcés, E. and Vergara, F. E. 1962. *Arch. Biochem. Biophys.* 98:77.

Nissley, S. P., Anderson, W. B., Gottesman, M. E., Perlman, R. L. and Pastan, I. 1971. *J. Biol. Chem.* 246:4671.

Norman, M., Gamulin, S. and Clark, K. 1973. *Biochem. J.* 134:387.

Novello, F., Guama, J. A. and McLean, P. 1969. *Biochem. J.* 111:713.

Numa, S., Ringelmann, E. and Lynen, F. 1965. *Biochem. Z.* 343:243.

Ochoa, S., Mehler, A. H. and Kornberg, A. 1948. *J. Biol. Chem.* 174:979.

O'Hea, E. K. and Leveille, G. A. 1969. *J. Nutr.* 99:345.

Ohneda, A., Parada, E., Eisentraut, A. M. and Unger, R. H. 1968. *J. Clin. Invest.* 47:2305.

Onishi, T. 1970. *Biochim. Biophys. Acta* 217:384.

Orci, L., Malaisse-Lagae, F., Ravazzola, M. and Amherdt, M. 1973. *Science* 181:562.

Oscai, L. B., Spirakis, C. N., Wolff, C. A. and Beck, R. J. 1972. *J. Lipid Res.* 13:588.

Owen, O. E., Morgan, A. P., Kemp, H. G., Sullivan, J. M., Herrera, M. G. and Cahill, G. F., Jr. 1967. *J. Clin. Invest.* 46:1589.

Owen, O. E., Felig, P., Morgan, A. P., Wahren, J. and Cahill, G. F., Jr. 1969. *J. Clin. Invest.* 48:574.

Owen, O. E., Reichard, G. A., Jr., Boden, G. and Shuman, C. 1974. *Metabolism* 23:7.

Ozols, R. F. and Hilf, R. 1973. *Proc. Soc. Exp. Biol. Med.* 144:73.

Pagliara, A. S., Stillings, S. N., Hover, B., Martin, D. M. and Matschinsky, F. M. 1974. *J. Clin. Invest.* 54:819.

Patel, M. S. and Mistry, S. P. 1969. *J. Nutr.* 98:235.

Patel, M. S., Jomain-Baum, M., Ballard, F. J. and Hanson, R. W. 1971. *J. Lipid Res.* 12:179.

Patzelt, G., Loffler, G., and Wieland, O. H. 1973. *Eur. J. Biochem.* 33:117.

Perley, M. J. and Kipnis, D. M. 1967. *J. Clin. Invest.* 46:1954.

Permutt, M. A. 1974. *J. Biol. Chem.* 248:2738.

Pfeifer, G. D. and Szepesi, B. 1974. *J. Nutr.* 104:1178.

Pfeifer, G. D., Michaelis, O. E., IV, and Szepesi, B. 1974. *Res. Commun. Chem. Pathol. Pharmacol.* 9:779.

Pilkis, S. J. 1970. *Biochim. Biophys. Acta* 215:461.

Pilkis, S. J. and Salaman, D. F. 1972. *Biochim. Biophys. Acta* 272:327.

Pitot, H. C., Inoue, H. and Kaplan, J. H. 1971. *Biochem. Pharmacol.* 20:1035.

Pontremoli, S., Melloni, E., Salamino, F., Franzi, A. T., De Flora, A. and Horecker, B. L. 1973. *Proc. Natl. Acad. Sci. U.S.A.* 70:3674.

Porte, D., Jr., Girardier, L., Seydous, J., Kanazawa, Y. and Posternak, J. 1973. *J. Clin. Invest.* 52:210.

Porte, D., Jr., and Robertson, R. P. 1973. *Fed. Proc.* 32:1792.

Porter, J. W. et al. 1975. *Fed Proc.* In press.

Potter, V. R. and Ono, T. 1961. *Cold Spring Harbor Symp. Quant. Biol.* 26:355.

Pozefsky, T., Felig, P., Tobin, J. D., Soeldner, J. S. and Cahill, G. F., Jr. 1969. *J. Clin. Invest.* 48:2273.

Quimby, F. H. 1948. *J. Nutr.* 36:177.

Quimby, R. H., Phillips, N. E. and White, I. U. 1948. *Am. J. Physiol.* 154:188.

Rathgeb, I., Steele, R., Winkler, B. and Altszuler, N. 1970. *Diabetes* 10:487.

Reichard, G. A., Jr. 1974. *J. Clin. Invest.* 53:508.

Reid, J. T. 1968. Publ. no. 1598, p. 19. Washington, D.C.: National Academy of Sciences.

Reiser, R., Williams, M. C., Sorrels, M. F. and Murty, N. L. 1963. *Arch. Biochem. Biophys.* 102:276.

Réthy, A., Tomasi, V. and Trevisani, A. 1971. *Arch. Biochem. Biophys.* 147:36.

Rider, A. A. and Simonson, M. 1973. *Nutr. Rep. Int.* 7:361.

Rizack, M. A. 1964. *J. Biol. Chem.* 239:392.

Robinson, D. S. and Wing, D. R. 1970. In *Adipose tissue*, ed. B. Jeanrenaud and D. Hepp, p. 41. New York: Academic Press.

Robinson, D. W. and Lambourne, L. J. 1970. *Growth* 34:235.

Rodbell, M., Krans, M. J., Pohl, S. L. and Biernbaumer, L. 1971. *J. Biol. Chem.* 246:1861.

Roeder, L. M. 1973. *Nutr. Rep. Int.* 7:271.

Rognstad, R. and Katz, J. 1973. *Biochem. J.* 132:349.

Rognstad, R., Clark, D. G. and Katz, J. 1973. *Biochem. Biophys. Res. Commun.* 54:1149.

Rolleston, F. S. 1972. *Curr. Top. Cell. Regul.* 5:47.

Rosenfeld, B. 1973. *J. Lipid Res.* 14:557.

Ross, M. H. and Bras, G. 1965. *J. Nutr.* 87:245.

Ross, M. H., Bras, G. and Ragbeer, M. S. 1970. *J. Nutr.* 100:177.

Roth, J. 1963. *Metabolism* 12:577.

Rudack, D. and Holten, D. 1972. *Fed. Proc.* 31:498.

Rudack, D., Davie, B. and Holten, D. 1971. *J. Biol. Chem.* 246:7823.

Ryan, N. T., George, B. C., Odessey, R. and Egdahl, R. H. 1974. *Metabolism* 23:901.

Saggerson, E. D. and Greenbaum, A. L. 1970. *Biochem. J.* 119:193.

Saito, T., Yoshimoto, A. and Tomita, K. 1971. *Jap. J. Biochem.* 69:127.

Sakurai, T., Miyazawa, S., Shindo, Y. and Hashimoto, T. 1974. *Biochim. Biophys. Acta* 360:275.

Salans, L. B. and Dougherty, J. W. 1971. *J. Clin. Invest.* 50:1399.

Sapag-Hagar, M., Lagunas, R. and Sols, A. 1973. *Biochem. Biophys. Res. Commun.* 50:179.

Sapir, D. G. 1974. *Clin. Res.* 22:42A.

Sapir, D. G. and Owen, O. E. 1975. *Metabolism* 24:23.

Sassoon, H. F., Dror, J., Watson, J. J. and Johnson, B. C. 1973. *J. Nutr.* 103:321.

Saxton, H. A., Sperling, G. A., Barnes, L. L. and McKay, C. M. 1948. *Acta Univ. Int. Contra Cancrum* 6:423.

Schiller, G. M., Taylor, W. M. and Halperin, M. L. 1974. *Can. J. Biochem.* 52:813.

Schimmel, R. J. and Knobil, E. 1969. *Am. J. Physiol.* 217:1803.

Schimmel, R. J. and Knobil, E. 1970. *Am. J. Physiol.* 218:1540.

Schirmer, M. D. and Harper, A. E. 1970. *J. Biol. Chem.* 245:1204.

Schmukler, M. 1970. *Biochim. Biophys. Acta* 214:309.

Schnakenberg, D. D., Krabil, L. F. and Weiser, P. C. 1971. *J. Nutr.* 101:787.

Scholz, R. W. and Rhodes, R. A. 1971. *Biochem. J.* 124:257.

Schwochau, M. E. and Hadwiger, L. A. 1969. *Arch. Biochem. Biophys.* 134:34.

Scrutton, M. L. 1971. *Metabolism* 20:168.

Scrutton, M. L. and Utter, M. F. 1968. *Annu. Rev. Biochem.* 37:249.

Segal, H. 1973. *Science* 180:25.

Selawary, H., Gutman, R., Fink, G. and Recant, L. 1973. *Biochem. Biophys. Res. Commun.* 51:198.

Sestoff, L. 1974. *Biochim. Biophys. Acta* 343:1.

Severson, A. R., Hubbard, D. D. and Gibson, D. M. 1973. *Anat. Rec.* 175:231.

Sharp, G. W. G., Wollheim, C., Muller, W. A., Gutzeit, A., Trueheart, P. A., Blondel, B., Orci, L. and Renold, A. E. 1975. *Fed. Proc.* 34:1537.

Sheppard, P., Hogan, K. and Roberts, K. B. 1970. *Biochim. Biophys. Acta* 217:159.

Shimazu, T. 1971. *Biochim. Biophys. Acta* 252:28.

Shimazu, T. and Fujimoto, T. 1971. *Biochim. Biophys. Acta* 252:18.

Shipley, G. G. 1974. *Science* 185:222.

Shlossberg, A. H. and Hollenberg, C. H. 1970. *Can. J. Biochem.* 48:113.

Sidransky, H., Sarma, D. S. R., Bongiorno, M. and Verney, E. 1968. *J. Biol. Chem.* 243:1123.

Sidransky, H. and Verney, E. 1971. *J. Nutr.* 101:1153.

Sidransky, H., Verney, E. and Sarma, D. S. R. 1971. *Am. J. Clin. Nutr.* 24:779.

Silpananta, P. and Goodridge, A. G. 1971. *J. Biol. Chem.* 246:5754.

Simonson, M., Hanson, H. M., Roeder, L. M. and Chow, B. F. 1973. *Nutr. Rep. Int.* 7:321.

Sladek, C. D. and Snarr, J. F. 1974. *Proc. Soc. Exp. Biol. Med.* 148:194.

Slakey, L. L., Craig, M. C., Beytia, E., Briedis, A., Feldbruegge, D. H., Dugan, R. E., Qureshi, A. A., Subbarayan, C. and Porter, J. W. 1972. *J. Biol. Chem.* 247:3014.

Slayton, C. A. and Szepesi, B. 1973. *Proc. Soc. Exp. Biol. Med.* 144:876.

Slayton, C. A. and Szepesi, B. 1974. *Fed. Proc.* 33:663.

Smith, G. S. 1964. *J. Nutr.* 82:173.

Snook, J. T. 1971. *Am. J. Physiol.* 221:1383.

Söling, H. D., Willms, B., Friedrichs, D. and Kleineke, J. 1968. *Eur. J. Biochem.* 4:364.

Söling, H. D., Willms, B. and Janson, G. 1970. *FEBS Lett.* 11:324.

Soskin, S., Allweiss, M. D., and Cohen, D. J. 1934. *Am. J. Physiol.* 109:155.
Soskin, S., Levine, R., and Lehmann, W. 1939. *Am. J. Physiol.* 127:463.
Spergel, G., Levy, L. J. and Goldner, M. G. 1971. *Metabolism* 20:401.
Srivastava, L. M., Shakespeare, P. and Hübscher, G. 1968. *Biochem. J.* 109:35.
Staehelin, T., Verney, E. and Sidransky, H. 1967. *Biochim. Biophys. Acta* 145:105.
Stearns, G. and Moore, D. L. R. 1931. *Am. J. Dis. Child.* 42:774.
Steggles, A. W., Spelsberg, T. C. and O'Malley, B. W. 1971. *Biochem. Biophys. Res. Commun.* 43:20.
Stephan, J. K., Chow, B., Frohman, L. A. and Chow, B. F. 1971. *J. Nutr.* 101:1453.
Stern, J. S. and Johnson, P. R. 1975. *Fed. Proc.* 34 (3):909.
Stevenson, J. A. F. 1969. *Ann. N.Y. Acad. Sci.* 157:1069.
Stewart, A. M. 1974. *Proc. Nutr. Soc.* 33:54A.
Stewart, R. J. C. 1973. *Nutr. Rep. Int.* 7:487.
Struck, E., Ashmore, J. and Wieland, O. 1965. *Biochem. Z.* 343:107.
Stubbs, D. W. and Griffin, J. F. 1973. *Proc. Soc. Exp. Biol. Med.* 144:195.
Sudilovský, O. and Pitot, H. N. 1973. *Proc. Soc. Exp. Biol. Med.* 144:113.
Sullivan, A. C., Miller, O. N., Wittman, J. S., III, and Hamilton J. S. 1971. *J. Nutr.* 101:265.
Szepesi, B. 1973. *Nutr. Rep. Int.* 7:133.
Szepesi, B. 1974a. *Nutr. Rep. Int.* 9:15
Szepesi, B. 1974b. *Nutr. Rep. Int.* 10:189.
Szepesi, B. and Berdanier, C. D. 1971. *J. Nutr.* 101:1563.
Szepesi, B. and Freedland, R. A. 1969. *J. Nutr.* 99:449.
Szepesi, B. and Freedland, R. A. 1970. *Proc. Soc. Exp. Biol. Med.* 135:709.
Szepesi, B. and Moser, P. 1971. *Proc. Soc. Exp. Biol. Med.* 136:200.
Szepesi, B. and Vojnik, C. 1975. *Nutr. Rep. Int.* 11:4.
Szepesi, B., Vegors, R., and Demouy, J. M. 1972. *Nutr. Rep. Int.* 5:281.
Szepesi, B., Vegors, R. M. and DeMouy, J. M. 1973. *Proc. Soc. Exp. Biol. Med.* 142:1036.
Szepesi, B., Slayton, C. A. and Michaelis, O. E., IV. 1974a. *Proc. Soc. Exp. Biol. Med.* 145:729.
Szepesi, B., Michaelis, O. E., IV, and Slayton, C. A. 1974b. *Nutr. Rep. Int.* 9:91.
Taketa, K. and Watanabe, A. 1971. *Biochim. Biophys. Acta* 235:19.
Taketa, K., Kaneshige, Y. and Kosaka, K. 1972. *Enzyme* 14:105.
Tannenbaum, A. 1947. *Ann. N.Y. Acad. Sci.* 49:5.
Tanner, J. M. 1963. *Child Dev.* 34:817.
Taunton, O. D., Stifel, F. B., Greene, H. L. and Herman, R. H. 1972. *Biochem. Biophys. Res. Commun.* 48:1633.
Taylor, H. L. 1945. *Am. J. Physiol.* 143:148.
Taylor, K. W. 1972. *Clin. Endocrinol. Metab.* 1:601.
Tepperman, H. M. and Tepperman, J. 1958a. *Diabetes* 7:478.
Tepperman, H. M. and Tepperman, J. 1962. *Am. J. Physiol.* 202:401.
Tepperman, H. M. and Tepperman, J. 1963. *Adv. Enzyme Regul.* 1:121.
Tepperman, H. M. and Tepperman, J. 1965. *Am. J. Physiol.* 209:773.
Tepperman, H. M., De La Garza, S. A. and Tepperman, J. 1968. *Am. J. Physiol.* 214:1126.
Tepperman, H. M., Fábry, P. and Tepperman, J. 1970. *J. Nutr.* 100:837.
Tepperman, J. and Tepperman, H. M. 1958b. *Am. J. Physiol.* 193:55.
Tepperman, J. and Tepperman, H. M. 1961. *Am. J. Physiol.* 200:1069.
Tepperman, J. and Tepperman, H. M. 1970. *Fed. Proc.* 29:1284.

Tepperman, J., Brobeck, J. R. and Long, C. N. H. 1943a. *Yale J. Biol. Med.* 15:855.
Tepperman, J., Brobeck, J. R. and Long, C. N. H. 1943b. *Yale J. Biol. Med.* 15:875.
Teufel, H., Menahan, L. A., Shipp, J. C., Böning, S. and Wieland, O. 1967. *Eur. J. Biochem.* 2:182.
Thaler, M. 1972. *Nature. New Biol.* 236:140.
Thomson, R. Y., Heagy, F. C., Hutchison, W. C. and Davidson, J. N. 1953. *Biochem. J.* 53:460.
Tomi, M. 1961. *Jikei Med.* 8:25.
Tomkins, G. M. 1972. *Nature. New Biol.* 239:9.
Tomkins, G. M. and Chaikoff, I. L. 1952. *J. Biol. Chem.* 196:569.
Tomkins, G. M., Gelehrter, T. D., Granner, D. K., Martin, D. W., Jr., Samuels, H. H. and Thompson, E. B. 1969. *Science* 166:1474.
Trenkle, A. 1970. *J. Nutr.* 100:1323.
Tuerkisher, E. and Wertheimer, D. 1942. *J. Physiol.* 100:385.
Turkington, R. W. 1970. *Biochem. Biophys. Res. Commun.* 41:1362.
Turkington, R. W. and Riddle, M. 1969. *J. Biol. Chem.* 244:6040.
Tzagournis, M. and Skillman, T. G. 1970. *Metabolism* 19:170.
Umaña, C. R. 1970. *Proc. Soc. Exp. Biol. Med.* 135:925.
Umaña, C. R. 1971a. *Proc. Soc. Exp. Biol. Med.* 137:385.
Umaña, C. R. 1971b. *Proc. Soc. Exp. Biol. Med.* 138:31.
Umaña, C. R. and Feldman, G. 1971. *Proc. Soc. Exp. Biol. Med.* 138:28.
Unger, R. H., Eisentrout, A. M., McCall, M. S. and Madison, L. L. 1962. *J. Clin. Invest.* 41:682.
Unger, R. H., Eisentrout, A. M. and Madison, L. L. 1963. *J. Clin. Invest.* 42:1031.
Varandani, P. T. 1973. *Biochim. Biophys. Acta* 304:642.
Vaughan, D. A., Drury, H. F., Hannon, J. P., Vaughan, L. N. and Larson, A. M. 1959. *J. Nutr.* 67:99.
Vaughan, D. A. and Winders, R. L. 1964. *J. Physiol.* 206:1081.
Venkatesan, N., Arcos, J. C. and Argus, M. F. 1970. *Cancer Res.* 30:2563.
Villar-Palasi, C. and Larner, J. 1968. *Vit. Horm.* 26:65.
Wagle, S. R. 1974. *Biochem. Biophys. Res. Commun.* 59:1366.
Wagle, S. R., Ingebretsen, W. R. and Sampson, L. 1973. *Biochem. Biophys. Res. Commun.* 53:937.
Walsh, D. A., Perkins, J. P. and Krebs, E. G. 1968. *J. Biol. Chem.* 243:3763.
Wardlaw, J. M., Henney, D. J. and Clarke, R. H. 1969. *Can. J. Physiol. Pharmacol.* 47:47.
Watanabe, A. and Taketa, K. 1973. *Arch. Biochem. Biophys.* 158:43.
Webb, T. E., Blobel, G. and Potter, V. R. 1966. *Cancer Res.* 26:253.
Weber, G., Lea, M. A. and Stamm, N. B. 1968. *Adv. Enzyme Regul.* 6:101.
Weinsier, R. L. 1971. *Am. J. Med.* 50:233.
Weiser, M. M., Quill, H. and Isselbacher, K. J. 1971. *Am. J. Physiol.* 221:844.
Weller, L. A., Margen, S. and Calloway, D. 1969. *Am. J. Clin. Nutr.* 22:1577.
Wettenhall, R. E. H., Leader, D. P., and Wool, I. G. 1971. *Biochem. Biophys. Res. Commun.* 43:994.
Wick, A. N. and Drury, D. R. 1941. *J. Biol. Chem.* 138:129.
Widdowson, E. M. and Kennedy, G. C. 1962. *Proc. Roy. Soc. B.* 156:96.
Widdowson, E. M. and McCance, R. A. 1963. *Proc. Roy. Soc. B.* 158:329.
Wiley, J. and Leveille, G. A. 1970. *J. Nutr.* 100:85.
Wilhelmj, C. M., Waldman, E. B. and McGuire, T. F. 1951. *Am. J. Physiol.* 166:296.

B. Szepesi

Wilhelmj, C. M., Shutput-Meyers, D. and McCarthy, H. H. 1956. *Exp. Med. Surg.* 14:286.

Wilhelmj, C. M., Carnazzo, A. J. and McCarthy, H. H. 1957. *Am. J. Physiol.* 191:103.

Willmer, J. S. and Foster, T. S. 1965. *Can. J. Biochem.* 43:1375.

Wilmurst, J. M. and Manchester, K. L. 1973. *Biochem. J.* 134:143.

Wilson, P. N. 1960. *J. Agric. Sci.* 54:105.

Wilson, P. N. and Osbourn, D. F. 1960. *Biol. Rev.* 35:324.

Wittman, J. S., III, Lee, K. L. and Miller, O. N. 1969. *Biochim. Biophys. Acta* 174:536.

Wolpert, L. and Lewis, J. H. 1975. *Fed. Proc.* 34:14.

Wool, I. G. 1960. *Am. J. Physiol.* 198:54.

Wool, I. G. 1972. *Proc. Nutr. Soc.* 31:185.

Wool, I. G. and Cavicchi, P. 1967. *Biochemistry* 6:1231.

Wool, I. G. Stirewalt, W. S., Kurihara, K., Low, R. B., Bailey, P. and Oyer, D. 1968. *Recent Progr. Horm. Res.* 24:139.

Yagil, G., Shimron, F., and Hizi, A. 1974. *Eur. J. Biochem.* 45:189.

Yatvin, M. B. 1971. *Proc. Soc. Exp. Biol. Med.* 136:1010.

Yeh, Y. Y. and Leveille, G. A. 1970. *J. Nutr.* 100:1389.

Yeh, Y. Y. and Leveille, G. A. 1971. *J. Nutr.* 101:803.

Yu, H. L. and Burton, D. N. 1974. *Biochem. Biophys. Res. Commun.* 61:483.

Yuwiler, A., Geller, E. and Schapiro, S. 1969. *Can. J. Physiol. Pharmacol.* 47:317.

Zakim, D., Pardini, R. S., Herman, R. H. and Sauberlich, H. E. 1967. *Biochim. Biophys. Acta* 114:242.

Zamenhof, S., Van Marthens, E. and Grauel, L. 1973. *Nutr. Rep. Int.* 7:371.

Zimmerman, E. F. and Greenberg, S. A. 1965. *Mol. Pharmacol.* 1:113.

Zinder, O. Eisenberg, E. and Shapiro, B. 1973. *J. Biol. Chem.* 248:7673.

Zunz, E. and LaBarre, J. 1928. *Soc. Biol. (Paris)* 98:1435.

Chapter 8

SEX DIFFERENCES IN THE METABOLIC RESPONSE TO DIETARY CARBOHYDRATES

Ian Macdonald
Physiology Department
Guy's Hospital Medical School
London, England

INTRODUCTION

In any account of differences in metabolism due to the sex of the individual, it is necessary to distinguish those quantitative differences associated with variations in body size, occupation, etc., from those metabolic differences that are more directly under the influence of the sex hormones. The awareness that the sex hormones may have effects on the metabolism of tissues, other than the sexual appendages, has been reinforced recently by the knowledge that, in age-matched groups, cardiovascular disease is more common in young males than females. It has been reported (Diet and coronary heart disease, 1974) that osteoporosis is more common in older women than in older men (Albright et al., 1941), that vitamin C requirements are less for women than for men (Brook and Grimshaw, 1968), and that females are more resistant to malnutrition than are men (Widdowson, 1968). A sex difference in the metabolism of carbohydrates was mentioned as long ago as 1931 when it was pointed out that male rats had a higher liver glycogen and a lower liver fat content than did female animals on similar diets (Greisheimer, 1931). More recently, the advent of the oral contraceptive with its widespread effects on metabolism and the suggestion that dietary carbohydrates may be atherogenic in some people (Fredrickson et al., 1961), coupled with the lesser incidence of atherosclerotic complications in women, has promoted a closer look at the influence of sex hormones on dietary carbohydrate metabolism, especially in its relation to endogenous lipid formation. Though it might be tempting to ascribe sex differences in the frequency of certain diseases to altered metabolism due to sex hormones, this would, at this stage, be unwise; such evidence as there is on the sex differences in the metabolic response to dietary carbohydrate needs much more substantiation.

EVIDENCE THAT A DIFFERENCE EXISTS BETWEEN
THE SEXES IN THE RESPONSE TO
DIETARY CARBOHYDRATE

The most likely fate of dietary carbohydrate is either to be metabolized to carbon dioxide and water with the release of energy or to be converted to lipid in the liver, adipose tissue, or plasma. It is in the measurements of the latter parameters that differences in response between the sexes have been uncovered.

When fructose is given intravenously, it is cleared from the blood more rapidly by male than by mature female baboons (Jourdan, 1969a). No such differences between the sexes could be detected in the fall in serum glucose concentration after the rapid intravenous injection of glucose (Jourdan, 1969b). Following the intravenous administration of glucose the plasma triglyceride concentration falls more markedly in men than in women (Perry and Corbett, 1964). These findings suggest a metabolic rather than absorptive mechanism that responds in a different quantitative manner between males and females. As the response to the intravenous injection of carbohydrate can show a sex difference, it is not, therefore, surprising to find that the carbohydrates in the diet can also be found to exhibit a response that depends on the sex of the consumer. When a fat-free diet is given to men and women students, the level of triglyceride in the fasting serum increases in the men but remains unchanged in the women (Beveridge et al., 1964). It was not until a closer look was taken at the metabolic effects of dietary fructose that the sex difference became more apparent. It appears that fructose in the diet—taken either as such or in combination with glucose as sucrose—is the only carbohydrate at present known to elicit different metabolic responses attributable to sex.

EVIDENCE THAT THE DIFFERENCE IN RESPONSE
DOES NOT APPLY TO ALL DIETARY
CARBOHYDRATES

The evidence that it is the fructose component of the dietary carbohydrate that is processed differently by the body comes from a series of experiments in which a fat-free diet was given to free-living men and women. When sucrose as the sole source of carbohydrate in a fat-free diet is given to men, the fasting level of serum triglyceride rises at least for 25 days; no such rise is seen when raw corn starch replaces the sucrose (Macdonald and Braithwaite, 1964). When the experiment was repeated, using young women instead of men as subjects, the fasting serum triglyceride concentration did not rise when the subjects were fed the high-sucrose diet, but fell; the results using raw corn starch were similar to those found in the men (Macdonald, 1965b). In a similar study using postmenopausal women, the fasting triglyceride levels in subjects on the sucrose regimen were similar to those seen in the men and the opposite to those found in the young women (Macdonald, 1966a).

In an attempt to determine which aspect of sucrose was responsible for the rise in fasting serum triglyceride levels in men, various dietary carbohydrates were given, including the disaccharide maltose. It was found that neither starch, an incomplete hydrolysate of starch, nor maltose, nor glucose caused an elevation of the fasting serum triglycerides; only sucrose seemed capable of evoking this response (Macdonald, 1965a). As it is not possible to take fructose in large quantities, because it produces an osmotic diarrhea, it was decided to construct a fat-free diet in which the carbohydrate component was a mixture of two of the three carbohydrates: raw corn starch, glucose, and fructose.

It was found in young men that only those carbohydrate mixtures containing fructose raised the fasting serum triglyceride level. Very similar findings were seen in postmenopausal women. In the premenopausal women consuming these carbohydrate mixtures, however, the diets that contained fructose did not cause any rise in the level of triglyceride in fasting serum (Macdonald, 1966b). These findings have received support in the report that young women have a similar endogenous triglyceride response to wheat starch and to sucrose (Klugh and Irwin, 1966); in a diet that contained a high proportion of "simple sugars" the serum phospholipid increased more in men than in premenopausal women (Antar and Ohlson, 1965). Further reports that would be compatible with a difference between the sexes in their response to fructose include the finding that in men the level of triglyceride in the fasting serum is directly related to the extent to which the serum fructose rises after an acute load of sucrose. In young women no such relationship exists (Crossley, 1967). In an attempt to learn where the different response to fructose might originate in its metabolic pathway, glycerol (which is not only chemically a carbohydrate but as α-glycerophosphate is an intermediate in fructose metabolism) was given to young men and young women and the serum triglyceride levels after "acute" and "chronic" ingestion studied. In the men the triglyceride levels rose more markedly than in the young women where no significant rise occurred (Macdonald, 1970). It has been suggested that the difference in response to sucrose lies not in the equal increases in lipogenesis seen in men and women but in the fact that women clear serum triglycerides more rapidly than men (Kekki and Nikkila, 1971; Olefsky et al., 1974).

ROLE OF VARIOUS SEX HORMONES

The fluctuations in the output of the female hormones during a normal menstrual cycle enable the investigator to study the physiologic response to any variables that may be introduced. For example, the glucose tolerance test varies with the phase of the menstrual cycle such that the blood glucose levels are highest at the time of ovulation (Jarrett and Graver, 1968; Macdonald and Crossley, 1970; Okey and Robb, 1925). Administering estrogens (Buchler and Warren, 1960) but not progestogens (Larsson-Cohn et al., 1969) impairs the oral glucose tolerance. At first sight it therefore seems, that the production of estrogen is responsible for these changes, but the effect is probably mediated via changes in gastrointestinal motility because when the glucose is given intravenously there is no cyclic variation (Larsson-Cohn et al., 1969; Spellacy et al., 1967).

If the triglycerides in fasting serum are endogenous and susceptible to the level of dietary carbohydrate intake (Fredrickson et al., 1961), then variations in the level of this serum lipid fraction in association with the physiologic fluctuations of female hormones would provide pointers to the more detailed understanding of the effect of these hormones of carbohydrate metabolism. During the menstrual cycle, for example, the plasma triglyceride level was lower at the 23rd day compared with the 8th day of a 28-day cycle (Svanborg and Vikrot, 1967). In pregnancy there is a marked increase in the level of triglyceride in the fasting serum; it is highest in the third trimester, despite the hypervolemia (Aurell and Cramer, 1966; Svanborg and Vikrot, 1965; Taylor, 1972). After menopause not only is the serum triglyceride raised, but so is the level of cholesterol and phospholipid in the blood (Hallberg et al., 1966). Earlier, the effects of age and weight gain, as well as ovarian functions on circulating triglyceride concentration, have been described (Feldman et al., 1963). Thus, there is ample evidence to expect that that part of carbohydrate metabolism concerned with the production of triglyceride would be influenced by the sex hormones. The limited fluctuations in androgen output in the male make comparable studies more difficult; nevertheless, the androgens affect lipid metabolism and thereby indirectly carbohydrate metabolism. Thus, it seems that although all dietary carbohydrates can be influenced by the sex hormones to some extent, it is only dietary fructose that shows a markedly different response between the sexes.

Little is known of the effect of sex hormones on either the metabolism of carbohydrate when it is being utilized directly or on the storage compound glycogen. However, more information is available on the end product triglyceride and the effect of sex hormones on the level of this lipid. If the level of triglyceride is affected by hormones, it appears likely that any role that carbohydrate might play in triglyceride metabolism could also be affected by sex hormones.

Effect of Estrogens on Triglyceride Metabolism

Most of the evidence suggests that the administration of estrogens raises the concentration of triglyceride in the serum (Hagopian and Robinson, 1965; Robinson and Lebeau, 1965; Steiner et al., 1955). In fact, iatrogenic disorders of triglyceride metabolism resulting from estrogen administration have been reported (Glueck et al., 1972; Molitch et al., 1974).

Effects of Progestogens on Triglyceride Metabolism

The progestogens have little effect on normal levels of serum triglyceride but produce decrements in those persons whose triglyceride concentration is raised (Beck, 1970, 1973; Glueck et al., 1971a).

As far as is known no studies have been conducted on the carbohydrate-lipid interrelationships during the physiologic fluctuations in female hormonal levels. However, it would not be improper to presume that as estrogens raise serum triglyceride levels and as carbohydrate, especially fructose, in the diet has a tendency to produce a similar response, then the combination of raised estrogen levels and increased carbohydrate in the diet would be synergistic. It would be of interest to study the effect of a high-carbohydrate diet in the presence of an increase in the level of progestogens. The triglyceride response to the dietary carbohydrate may then fail to appear.

Effects of Androgens on Triglyceride Metabolism

Little is known about the effect of androgens on triglyceride metabolism, but it seems that in patients with raised triglyceride levels oxandrolone, a synthetic anabolic–androgenic steroid reduces the triglyceride level (Glueck et al., 1971b). Androgens, by injection, can reduce the serum triglyceride level (Dufault et al., 1961; Furman and Howard, 1962; Hellman et al., 1959), and striking falls in a patient with hypertriglyceridemia have been reported when androgens were administered (Stone, 1963).

More direct, but unphysiologic studies, in nonhuman primates have, to some extent, been consistent with the conclusions that might be expected from the effects noted above. In these studies a high-sucrose diet raised the level of fasting serum triglyceride in the male but not in the female animals. When the female animals were given androgen, together with a high-sucrose diet, no increase in serum triglyceride concentration occurred (Coltart and Macdonald, 1971).

POSSIBLE SYNERGISTIC EFFECTS OF SEX HORMONES ON CARBOHYDRATE METABOLISM

While it is simpler in experimental practice to alter only one variable at a time, it would be unwise to draw conclusions from this type of experiment as to the behavior of that variable in the intact organism. In the first half of the menstrual cycle estrogen is the predominating hormone, in the second half progesterone is added to the hormonal pool, and in early pregnancy a third hormone appears (namely, chorionic gonadotropin). Each of these hormones may influence carbohydrate metabolism in a manner that is quite different from that when two or more of the hormones are administered together.

The danger of assuming the action of a hormone when given alone, as compared with its administration when combined with another hormone, was well illustrated in some experiments on rats given high-sucrose-containing diets (Jeffreys and White, 1973). Male rats on this diet had an increase in the amount of liver triglyceride. When estradiol was given to rats consuming this high-sucrose diet, the liver triglyceride was not raised as markedly. When progesterone was given, no difference in the amount of liver triglyceride was observed. However, when the animals on the high-sucrose diet were given both the estrogen and progesterone together, then the amount of triglyceride in the liver was greater than any value found in the previous three groups. In further experiments these authors found that the nature of the carbohydrate in the diet affects the nutritional status of the male but not of the female (Jeffreys and White, 1974).

Thus, the precise role of a sex hormone may be difficult to determine since in the physiologic state its actions may be modified by the presence of other variables, including other sex hormones. In the male, where fluctuations of sex hormonal output are less evident, it is easier to define more precisely the role of the hormone in the whole organism.

INFLUENCE OF ORAL CONTRACEPTIVES ON THE METABOLIC RESPONSE TO DIETARY CARBOHYDRATES

Prior to 1963 studies on the effect of ovarian steroids on carbohydrate metabolism were confined to pancreatomized or alloxan-treated rats. These experiments led to the conclusion that progesterone was without effect, whereas estrogen impaired and later improved carbohydrate tolerance (Carrasco and Vargas, 1949; Houssay et al., 1954; Lewis et al., 1950). Although oral contraceptives were introduced initially in 1956, it was not until 1963 (Waine et al., 1963) that the first report of an alteration in carbohydrate metabolism associated with this method of contraception was published.

The level of glucose in the fasting blood in women taking oral contraceptives has been found by some to increase (Besch et al., 1965; Di-Paola et al., 1968; Javier and Gershberg, 1964); others have reported no change in this level (Spellacy and Carlson, 1966; Wynn and Doar, 1966). The glucose tolerance is impaired by the oral contraceptive whether the glucose is given by mouth or intravenously. Plasma insulin levels and serum triglyceride concentrations have been reported to be raised by oral contraceptives (Wynn and Doar, 1969a, b). It is considered that the impaired glucose tolerance is due to the estrogenic component (Goldman et al., 1968; Jabor et al., 1972), while progesterone seems to have no effect or even to improve glucose metabolism (Adams and Wynn, 1972; Beck, 1969; Benjamin and Casper, 1966; Goldman et al., 1968). Very-low-dose oral contraceptives have also been found to improve the glucose tolerance (Clinch et al., 1969).

In view of the impaired glucose tolerance and, especially, the raised serum triglyceride levels in women taking an estrogen-containing oral contraceptive (Wynn et al., 1966), it is obviously of interest to learn whether there is some synergism between effect of the oral contraceptive and the metabolic response to dietary sucrose or fructose. Little work, however, has been reported on this aspect. It has been found, in a small series, that women on an oral contraceptive have higher than normal serum glucose values after the ingestion of fructose and that these values were similar to those seen in men (A. R. Macrae, personal communication).

In a study of nonhuman primates in which the animals were given diets high in sucrose or glucose, it was found that the level of triglyceride in the serum was significantly raised when animals were given oral contraceptives, compared with when no contraceptive was given (Stovin and Macdonald, 1975). If a synergism exists between the estrogen given with oral contraceptives and the fructose in the diet, then it might be expected that the result of this could be an increase in the incidence of that disorders, such as atherosclerosis, associated with "carbohydrate sensitivity." A recent report has shown that the risk of a fatal myocardial infarct is greater in women using an oral contraceptive, particularly in the older age groups (Mann and Inman, 1975) but does not provide evidence that the risk is associated with hypertriglyceridemia.

FACTORS MODIFYING THE SEX DIFFERENCE IN RESPONSE TO DIETARY CARBOHYDRATES

Nature of Dietary Fat Accompanying the Carbohydrate

Many of the investigations into the role of dietary carbohydrate in metabolism that have been reported have been carried out with an abnormally high intake of carbohydrate. The rationale for this is that if large quantities do not affect the aspect of metabolism under study, then smaller or more usual quantities are unlikely to have any effect. The criticism that can be leveled, justifiably, is that the body reacts in an abnormal fashion to abnormal quantities; therefore, results are of little physiologic consequence. As the replacement of high levels of carbohydrate in the diet is usually with fat, it would be sensible to study the effect that the nature of dietary fat has on the metabolic fate of dietary carbohydrate.

In men the replacement of some of the dietary sucrose with a saturated fat, such as cream, has no effect on the raised serum triglyceride levels associated with a high-sucrose intake. Conversely, if sunflower seed oil, a polyunsaturated fat, is given instead of the cream, the rise in serum triglyceride concentration does not occur (Macdonald, 1968). In further experiments studying the effect of the type of fat on dietary carbohydrate metabolism it was again found that, irrespective of the type of dietary carbohydrate consumed, sunflower seed oil always reduced the level of serum triglycerides both in young men and young women, whereas with cream the reverse tended to occur in the men but not in the women (Macdonald, 1972).

The effect that the nature of the dietary fat has on the serum cholesterol level is very well documented, and there is also evidence that the serum triglycerides can be altered in a comparable way (Ahrens, et al., 1957). Moreover, the chain length of the saturated fat determines its effect on the serum triglyceride concentration (see Macdonald, 1973a). Also, in patients with hypertriglyceridemia a synergistic effect has been found between dietary sucrose and animal fat, whereas dietary starch instead of sucrose is not a hypertriglyceridemic mixture (Antar et al., 1970).

Thus, the sex difference in response to dietary sucrose disappears or lessens when men consuming sucrose use polyunsaturated fat to accompany the sucrose. Although the precise mechanism for this effect is not known, in rats it has been shown that polyunsaturated fats increase the activity of lipoprotein lipase (Pawar and Tidwell, 1968).

Individual Differences

The response of an individual to dietary carbohydrates depends not only on the sex of the individual but also on whether that individual is "sensitive" to dietary carbohydrate. About 13–15% of men have abnormally raised triglycerides in response to the carbohydrate in their diet. This proportion is less for women, and of those women who are "sensitive" most are postmenopausal (Stone and Dick, 1973; Wood et al., 1972). Thus, though there is a difference between sexes in some of the metabolic responses to fructose, there is wide interindividual variation within the sexes.

Adaptation

In the raised serum triglyceride response to carbohydrate, especially sucrose, seen in men, adaptation takes place such that after several weeks the triglyceride levels in the serum have returned to values that are, at most, only slightly higher than the control level (Antonis and Bersohn, 1960; Bierman and Hamlin, 1961) Also, there are many people in the world who subsist on a high-carbohydrate diet and do not develop hypertriglyceridemia (Schwartz et al., 1963). One possible explanation is that adaptation (implying enzyme induction) has taken place in these people. However, other variables, such as the nature of the dietary fat and the genetic makeup of these people, could supply an equally valid explanation for this fact.

Other Factors

In men it has been found that in short-term experiments when the dietary nitrogen is in the form of amino acids instead of protein, the hypertriglyceridemia in response to sucrose is much more marked (Coles and Macdonald, 1972). Again in men, the frequency of consuming sucrose affects the levels of lipid in the fasting serum (Macdonald et al., 1970). Though there is as yet no evidence that similar responses occur in young women, it seems not unreasonable to expect that they may also vary in their response to sucrose, depending on the nature of the dietary protein and the meal pattern.

CLINICAL CONSEQUENCES OF THE SEX DIFFERENCE
IN RESPONSE TO DIETARY CARBOHYDRATE

Atherosclerosis

Atherosclerosis of the coronary arteries is 10–40 times more common in young men than in women of comparable age (Taylor et al., 1947), a difference lost in women who have had bilateral oophorectomy before menopause (Parrish et al., 1967; Wuest et al., 1953). On the other hand, the administration of estrogens to castrated women did not reduce the manifestations of coronary disease (Higano et al., 1963); in fact, estrogen could lead to a metabolic situation where atherosclerosis and its consequences would be more likely to occur (Glueck and Fallat, 1974).

In view of the findings that the glucose tolerance test is impaired with estrogen administration and that fasting serum triglycerides [which are not only a risk factor for myocardial infarction (Carlson and Bottiger, 1972) but may reflect abnormal carbohydrate metabolism] are raised with estrogen administration, it is tempting to relate the female sex hormones (plainly not estrogen per se) to the capacity to prevent the more harmful effects of dietary carbohydrates, at least in certain individuals. As estrogen has been reported many times to disimprove the body's ability to handle dietary carbohydrate, then any protection that the premenopausal woman is afforded by her hormones is not due to estrogen. This leaves progesterone. Unfortunately, there is little evidence to support this seemingly logical conclusion. It may well be it is the combination of the two hormones with their special dose and time relationship that is responsible for the seemingly beneficial effects of womanhood.

Skin

The skin has long been known to reflect the adequacy of the dietary intake, and the dermatologist has recognized that the amount of dietary carbohydrate can influence the course of certain skin lesions (Barber, 1930). Some laboratory evidence to support this clinical observation was found when the fatty acid pattern of the skin surface lipid in man changed on an experimental high-carbohydrate diet; furthermore, the change was not the same for starch as for sucrose in the diet (Macdonald, 1964). Later work showed that in men the amount of triglyceride on the surface of the skin decreased when corn starch was a major component of an experimental diet and increased when sucrose replaced the starch (Llewellyn, 1967). Men on a diet where the composition of both the type of carbohydrate and type of fat in the diet was altered showed that the amount of triglyceride and cholesterol content of skin surface lipid was altered by the changes in diet, but no changes were seen in these two skin surface lipids in young women on comparable diets (Macdonald, 1973b). The female hormones can offset lipid metabolism in the skin as is seen in the variation in sebum excretion rate (Burton et al., 1972) and in skin surface lipid changes (Macdonald and Clarke, 1970) that occur during the menstrual cycle. A sex difference in the handling of carbohydrate by the skin has been found in rats where skin from female rats incorporated more $[^{14}C]$ glucose into lipid than did skin from male rats (T. Rebello, personal communication).

The effect of dietary carbohydrates on the metabolism of the skin is an area relatively unexplored—one of great potential. There are hints that there is a sex difference in the lipid response, and it seems possible that some long-known clinical observations may receive support from modern biochemical findings.

SUMMARY

There is evidence that the premenopausal woman shows a different metabolic response to dietary carbohydrate from a man or a postmenopausal woman. This difference is especially marked with dietary fructose when the role of dietary carbohydrate in lipid metabolism is considered. As estrogen appears to raise the fasting serum triglyceride level and as fructose in the male and postmenopausal woman exhibits a similar effect, it is postulated that estrogen therapy, together with dietary fructose (as such or in sucrose), would combine to produce high levels of endogenous triglyceride in the serum. There is some evidence to support this.

Factors such as the nature of the dietary fat accompanying the dietary carbohydrate, the "sensitivity" of the individual to carbohydrate, etc., can modify the metabolic response to dietary carbohydrate in both men and women. These factors need to be assessed before any clinical implications can be ascribed to the sex difference in the response to dietary carbohydrate.

REFERENCES

Adams, P. W. and Wynn, V. 1972. *J. Obstet. Gynaecol. Br. Commonw.* 79:744.

Ahrens, E. H., Hirsch, J., Insull, W., Tsaltas, T. T., Blomstrand, R. and Peterson, M. L. 1957. *Lancet* 1:943.

Albright, F., Smith, P. H. and Richardson, A. M. 1941. *J. Am. Med. Assoc.* 116:2465.

Antar, M. A. and Ohlson, M. A. 1965. *J. Nutr.* 85:329.

Antar, M. A., Little, J. A., Lucas, P., Buckley, G. C. and Csima, A. 1970. *Atherosclerosis* 11:191.

Antonis, A. and Bersohn, I. 1960. *Lancet* 1:998.

Aurell, N. and Cramer, K. 1966. *Clin. Chem. Acta* 13:278.

Barber, H. W. 1930. In *Taylor's practice of medicine,* p. 937. London: Churchill.

Beck, P. 1969. *Diabetes* 18:146.

Beck, P. 1970. *J. Clin. Endocrinol. Metab.* 30:785.

Beck, P. 1973. *Metab. Clin. Exp.* 22:841.

Benjamin, F. and Casper, D. J. 1966. *Am. J. Obstet. Gynecol.* 94:991.

Besch, P. K., Vorys, N., Ullery, J. C., Stevens, V. and Barry, R. D. 1965. *Metab. Clin. Exp.* 14:387.

Beveridge, J. M. R., Jagannathan, S. N. and Connell, W. F. 1964. *Can. J. Biochem.* 42:999.

Bierman, E. L. and Hamlin, J. T. 1961. *Diabetes* 10:432.

Brook, M. and Grimshaw, J. J. 1968. *Am. J. Clin. Nutr.* 21:1254.

Buchler, D. and Warren, J. C. 1960. *Am. J. Obstet. Gynecol.* 95:479.

Burton, J. L., Cartidge, M. and Shuster, S. 1972. *Acta Dermato-Venereol.* 53:81.

Carlson, L. A. and Bottiger, L. E. 1972. *Lancet* 1:865.

Carrasco, R. and Vargas, L. 1949. *Bol. Soc. Biol. Santiago (Chile)* 6:61.

Clinch, J., Turnbull, A. C. and Khosla, T. 1969. *Lancet* 1:857.

Coles, B. L. and Macdonald, I. 1972. *Nutr. Metab.* 14:238.

Coltart, T. M. and Macdonald, I. 1971. *Br. J. Nutr.* 25:323.

Crossley, J. N. 1967. *Proc. Nutr. Soc.* 26:iii.

Diet and coronary heart disease. 1974. In *Report on health and social subjects*, vol. 7, p. 4. London: H.M.S.O.

Di-Paola, G., Puchulu, F., Robin, M., Nicholson, R. and Mart, M. 1968. *Am. J. Obstet. Gynecol.* 101:206.

Dufault, C., Tremblay, G., Nowaczynski, W. and Genest, J. 1961. *Can. Med. Assoc. J.* 85:1025.

Feldman, E. B., Benkel, P. and Nayak, R. U. 1963. *J. Lab. Clin. Med.* 62:437.

Fredrickson, D. S., Levy, R. I. and Lees, R. S. 1961. *New Engl. J. Med.* 276:34, 94, 148, 215, 273.

Furman, R. H. and Howard, R. P. 1962. *Metab. Clin. Exp.* 11:76.

Glueck, C. J. and Fallat, R. 1974. *Proc. R. Soc. Med.* 67:23.

Glueck, C. J., Levy, R. I. and Fredrickson, D. S. 1971a. *Ann. Intern. Med.* 75:345.

Glueck, C. J., Swanson, F. and Fishback, J. 1971b. *Metab. Clin. Exp.* 20:691.

Glueck, C. J., Sheel, D., Fishback, J. and Steiner, P. 1972. *Metab. Clin. Exp.* 21:657.

Goldman, J. A., Ouadia, J. L. and Eckerling, B. 1968. *Isr. J. Med. Sci.* 4:878.

Greisheimer, E. M. 1931. *J. Nutr.* 4:411.

Hagopian, M. and Robinson, R. W. 1965. *Circulation Suppl.* II 32:16.

Hallberg, L., Hogdahl, A. M., Svanborg, A. and Vikrot, O. 1966. *Acta Med. Scand.* 180:697.

Hellman, L., Bradlow, H. L., Zumoff, G., Fukushima, D. K. and Gallagher, T. F. 1959. *J. Clin. Endocrinol.* 19:936.

Higano, N., Robinson, R. W. and Cohen, W. D. 1963. *New Engl. J. Med.* 268:1123.

Houssay, B. A., Foglia, V. G., Rodriquez, R. R. 1954. *Acta Endocrinol. (Copenhagen)* 17:146.

Jabor, L. N. A., Tsai, C. C., Vela, P. and Yen, S. S. C. 1972. *Am. J. Obstet Gynecol.* 113:383.

Jarrett, R. J. and Graver, H. J. 1968. *Br. Med. J.* 2:528.

Javier, Z. and Gershberg, H. 1964. *Clin. Res. Proc.* 12:458.

Jeffreys, D. B. and White, I. R. 1973. *Nutr. Rep. Int.* 8:201.

Jeffreys, D. B. and White, I. R. 1974. *Proc. Nutr. Soc.* 33:25A.

Jourdan, M. H. 1969a. *Proc. Nutr. Soc.* 28:10A.

Jourdan, M. H. 1969b. *J. Physiol. (London)* 201:27P.

Kekki, M. and Nikkila, E. A. 1971. *Metab. Clin. Exp.* 20:878.

Klugh, C. A. and Irwin, M. I. 1966. *Fed. Proc.* 25:672.

Larsson-Cohn, U., Tengstrom, B. and Wide, L. 1969. *Acta Endocrinol. (Copenhagen)* 62:242.

Lewis, J. T., Foglia, V. G. and Rodriguez, R. R. 1950. *Endocrinology* 46:111.

Llewellyn, A. F. 1967. *Proc. Nutr. Soc.* 26:ii.

Macdonald, I. 1964. *Nature (London)* 203:1067.

Macdonald, I. 1965a. *Clin. Sci.* 29:193.

Macdonald, I. 1965b. *Am. J. Clin. Nutr.* 16:458.

Macdonald, I. 1966a. *Am. J. Clin. Nutr.* 18:86.

Macdonald, I. 1966b. *Am. J. Clin. Nutr.* 18:369.

Macdonald, I. 1968. *Am. J. Clin. Nutr.* 20:345.

Macdonald, I. 1970. *Br. J. Nutr.* 24:537.

Macdonald, I. 1972. *Clin. Sci.* 43:265.

Macdonald, I. 1973a. *Progr. Biochem. Pharmacol.* 8:216.

Macdonald, I. 1973b. *Br. J. Dermatol.* 88:267.

Macdonald, I. and Braithwaite, D. M. 1964. *Clin. Sci.* 27:23.

Macdonald, I. and Clarke, G. 1970. *Br. J. Dermatol.* 83:473.

Macdonald, I., Coles, B. L., Brice, J. and Jourdan, M. H. 1970. *Br. J. Nutr.* 24:413.

Macdonald, I. and Crossley, J. N. 1970. *Diabetes* 19:450.

Mann, J. I. and Inman, W. H. W. 1975. *Br. Med. J.* 2:245.

Molitch, M. E., Oill, P. and Odell, W. D. 1974. *J. Am. Med. Assoc.* 227:522.

Okey, R. and Robb, E. I. 1925. *J. Biol. Chem.* 65:165.

Olefsky, J. Farquhar, J. W. and Reaven, G. M. 1974. *Eur. J. Clin. Invest.* 4:121.

Parrish, H. M., Carr, C. A., Hall, D. G. and King, T. M. 1967. *Am. J. Obstet. Gynecol.* 99:155.

Pawar, S. S. and Tidwell, H. C. 1968. *J. Lipid. Res.* 9:334.

Perry, W. F. and Corbett, B. N. 1964. *Can. J. Physiol. Pharmacol.* 42:353.

Robinson, R. W. and Lebeau, R. 1965. *J. Atheroscler. Res.* 5:120.

Schwartz, M. J., Rosenweig, B., Toor, M. and Lewitus, Z. 1963. *Am. J. Cardiol.* 12:157.

Spellacy, W. N. and Carlson, K. L. 1966. *Am. J. Obstet. Gynecol.* 95:474.

Spellacy, W. N., Carlson, K. L. and Schade, S. L. 1967. *Am. J. Obstet. Gynecol.* 99:382.

Steiner, A., Payson, H. and Kendall, F. E. 1955. *Circulation* 5:605.

Stone, M. C. 1963. *Lancet* 1:477.

Stone, M. C. and Dick, T. B. S. 1973. *Br. Heart. J.* 35:954.

Stovin, V. and Macdonald, I. 1975. *Proc. Nutr. Soc.* 34:55A.

Svanborg, A. and Vikrot, O. 1965. *Acta Med. Scand.* 178:615.

Svanborg, A. and Vikrot, O. 1967. *Acta Med. Scand.* 181:93.

Taylor, G. O. 1972. *J. Obstet. Gynaecol. Br. Commonw.* 79:68.

Taylor, R. D., Corcoran, A. C. and Page, I. H. 1947. *Am. J. Med. Sci.* 213:475.

Waine, H., Frieden, E. H., Caplan, H. I. and Cole, R. 1963. *Arthritis Rheum.* 6:796.

Widdowson, E. M. 1968. In *Calorie deficiency and protein deficiency,* ed. R. A. McCance and E. M. Widdowson, p. 225. London: Churchill.

Wood, P. D. S., Stern, M. P., Silvers, A., Reaven, G. M. and Groenen, J. 1972. *Circulation* 45:114.

Wuest, J. H., Dry, T. J. and Edwards, J. E. 1953. *Circulation* 7:801.

Wynn, V. and Doar, J. W. H. 1966. *Lancet* 1:715.

Wynn, V. and Doar, J. W. H. 1969a. *Lancet* 2:756.

Wynn, V. and Doar, J. W. H. 1969b. *Lancet* 2:761.

Wynn, V., Doar, J. W. H. and Mills, G. L. 1966. *Lancet* 2:720.

Chapter 9

GENETIC-DIET INTERACTION IN CARBOHYDRATE NUTRITION

A. M. Cohen and Shlomo Eisenberg
*Diabetic Unit and Isotope Laboratory for Endocrine Research
and Department of Medicine B
Hadassah University Hospital and
The Hebrew University–Hadassah Medical School
Jerusalem, Israel*

INTRODUCTION

Until recently it was generally accepted that all carbohydrates are equally broken down in the body to glucose and are metabolized as such. This is now known not to be so. Furthermore, it has been established that the metabolism of carbohydrates differs among species and that they do not provoke a uniform metabolic, enzymic, and hormonal response. Recent studies have, moreover, demonstrated a genetic difference among individuals of the same species in the metabolism of the same carbohydrate molecule, especially refined sugars: sucrose, glucose, and fructose. Thus, the metabolic consequences of ingested carbohydrates are dependent on the nature of the carbohydrate molecule and the genetic makeup of the recipient. Depending on these two factors, the ensuing metabolic and hormonal response will determine whether individuals of the species will remain "normal" or will develop a specific metabolic disorder. Studying the individual response to a specific carbohydrate may therefore serve as a tool to discover whether an individual is susceptible to this carbohydrate and enable the prevention of the development of disease by a proper dietary regime.

In this chapter we shall not deal with the intermediary metabolic pathways resulting from the ingestion of carbohydrates but will concentrate on the results of the interaction between the "genetic" background of the individual and the ingested carbohydrate.

LIPID METABOLISM EFFECTS IN EXPERIMENTAL ANIMALS

Numerous experiments have been performed to determine the influence of dietary carbohydrates on serum lipid levels. These studies have shown that

A. M. Cohen and S. Eisenberg

dietary carbohydrates not only cause a rise in the blood glucose level but also are readily converted in the body to fat, resulting in carbohydrate-induced elevation of serum lipids in both humans and experimental animals. In most studies, variable responses to different carbohydrates were observed between species and among individuals of the same species.

Serum Cholesterol Levels

Rat. Portman et al. (1956) observed that in rats fed cholesterol- and cholic acid-enriched diets serum cholesterol levels were lower when starch replaced sucrose, fructose, or glucose in the diet. However, Anderson (1969) reported lower serum and liver cholesterol levels in rats fed sucrose, compared with rats fed various forms of modified food starches.

Rabbits. Rabbits fed diets with added cholesterol were reported to have higher serum cholesterol levels when the diet contained sucrose than when it contained glucose (Grant and Fahrenbach, 1959). Rabbits fed diets containing 29% lactose and 0.35% cholesterol have higher serum cholesterol levels than rabbits fed a similar diet containing sucrose (Wells and Anderson, 1959).

Dogs. No significant change in serum cholesterol levels was observed in dogs either before or after removal of the thyroid gland when the diet contained starch or sucrose (48% of the total caloric intake) (Schultz and Grande, 1968).

Chickens. Diets containing cholesterol and sucrose caused higher serum cholesterol levels than those containing glucose (Grant and Fahrenbach, 1959). Germfree chickens fed a high-sucrose diet had higher serum cholesterol than chickens fed a high-glucose diet (Kritchevsky et al., 1959).

Acomys cahirinus. A marked rise (from 222 to 364 mg%) in blood cholesterol levels was observed in these animals following sucrose feeding (Shafrir et al., 1972).

Serum Triglyceride Levels

Rats. Serum triglyceride concentration was shown to be higher when rats were fed diets containing different sugars, compared with rats fed diets containing equivalent amounts of starch (Bar-On and Stein, 1968; Kritchevsky and Tepper, 1969; Naismith and Kahn, 1970a, b; Nath et al., 1959). However, different strains of rats differ in the magnitude of their blood level response to dietary sucrose (Berdanier, 1974a; Marshall and Hildebrand, 1963; Taylor et al., 1967). Nikkila and Ojala (1965) reported that fructose-rich diets produced higher levels of serum triglycerides than diets containing glucose. Macdonald and Roberts (1965), however, reported that diets containing sucrose produced higher levels of total serum lipids in male rats than diets containing either glucose or fructose after a 12-wk feeding period. The elevation of serum triglycerides produced by diets containing sugars in rats is influenced by the age of the animal. Chevalier et al. (1972) have reported that diets containing either fructose or sucrose produced elevation of serum triglycerides in mature rats but not in weanling rats.

Dogs. No significant difference in the serum of triglyceride levels of dogs was observed following diets containing starch and sucrose, respectively (48% of total caloric intake) (Schultz and Grande, 1968). However, when the experiment was repeated with the same dogs after removal of the thyroid gland, the serum triglyceride levels were higher in dogs fed sucrose diet.

Acomys cahirinus. This animal shows a very marked increase of the serum lipids when fed a sucrose diet; the triglyceride levels rose from 653 to 1479 mg%. The hepatic triglyceride content also rose from 13.7 to 40 mg/g in animals fed the starch and sucrose diets, respectively (Shafrir et al., 1974).

Guinea pigs. In these animals, fructose and glucose feeding evoke a similar response with respect to plasma triglyceride levels (Bar-On and Stein, 1968).

Some of the species difference with regard to the hypertriglyceridemic effect of fructose seems to be related to the form in which this sugar is absorbed. Because of the low activity of glucose-6-phosphatase in the intestine of rats, fructose is absorbed without being converted to glucose. In guinea pigs, where the intestine is very efficient in converting fructose to glucose, the absorption of fructose occurs predominantly as glucose (Ginsburg and Hers, 1960; Kiyasu and Chaikoff, 1957).

Synthesis of Lipids in the Liver

The synthesis and content of lipids in the liver is affected to a different degree by the nature of the dietary carbohydrates, starch, sucrose, fructose, or glucose (Cohen and Teitelbaum, 1964, 1968; Kritchevsky et al., 1959; Macdonald, 1962; Moser and Berdanier, 1974). Different responses of body weight, size of liver, and content of fat and cholesterol in the liver by dietary carbohydrates were described (Marshall and Hildebrand, 1963). Bender et al. (1970) have shown that the effects of dietary sucrose as against starch (60% of calories) on glucose utilization, and glucose-6-phosphatase activity in the liver differs among five strains of rats. Sucrose ingestion significantly depressed fat synthesis from glucose in liver slices of three strains of rats (Sprague-Dawley, Wistar and Lister), while it did not affect hepatic lipogenesis in the two Hooded strains. In the Lister, Wistar, and one Hooded strain, a depressed rate of hepatic glucose oxidation and an increased activity of glucose-6-phosphatase were found. These and other observations, while indicating differences between the dietary carbohydrates with respect to their effect on the level of blood lipids and hepatic fat content and fat synthesis, cannot be duplicated in all animal species or even in the same species under different experimental conditions. The following effects of carbohydrates on plasma lipid levels and hepatic fat content and fat synthesis seem to be reasonably well established at the present:

1. Different species (rat, dog, rabbit, *Acomys cahirinus,* and chicken) and different strains of the same species respond differently to the same dietary manipulations (Berdanier, 1974a; Portman et al., 1956; Schultz and Grande, 1968; Taylor et al., 1967; Wells and Anderson, 1959).

2. Several reports indicate that the elevation of serum cholesterol observed when feeding different carbohydrates are not manifested when the diets do not contain exogenous cholesterol (Bedö and Szigeti, 1967; Fillios et al., 1958; Grant and Fahrenbach, 1959). On the other hand, other authors have found higher serum cholesterol levels with diets containing sucrose than with diets containing starch, in the absence of added cholesterol (Allen and Leahy, 1966).

3. Modification of other constituents of the diet, for instance, the protein, may change the effect of dietary carbohydrate on serum lipid levels in man (Keys and Anderson, 1957; Olson et al., 1958) and in experimental animals (Farnell and Burns, 1962).

This summary illustrates the complexity of the problem and demonstrates that there is no single pattern of response of plasma lipid levels common to all species studied.

LIPID METABOLISM EFFECTS IN HUMANS

Diets, in which carbohydrates account for more than 50% of calories, cause elevation of plasma triglyceride levels and the levels of very-low-density lipoproteins. Of the different carbohydrates, sucrose and fructose seem to have a more pronounced effect than starch or glucose. Since cholesterol accounts for 10–15% of the very-low-density lipoprotein mass (Eisenberg et al., 1973), carbohydrate-rich diets that cause elevation of this lipoprotein are expected to increase the serum cholesterol levels. However, most studies report a decrease in plasma cholesterol during periods of feeding carbohydrate-rich diets. This observation may be explained by the fact that in most instances carbohydrate-rich diets are necessarily carbohydrate rich and fat poor. Since low-fat diets accelerate the catabolism of low-density lipoprotein (the major transport vehicle of cholesterol in circulation) (Langer et al., 1972), the overall effect of the diet on plasma cholesterol levels is variable.

Serum Lipids in Normal Humans

Studies of the effects of carbohydrate-rich diets on plasma lipid levels have demonstrated a remarkably variable response in the percent increment of plasma triglyceride levels among individuals. During the 1950s, several investigators (Ahrens et al., 1957; Hatch et al., 1955; Nichols et al., 1957) have shown that carbohydrate-rich diets (70–80% of calories from complex carbohydrates, disaccharides, and monosaccharides) caused an average rise in plasma triglyceride ("neutral fat") levels of about 100%, individual variation ranging from 0 to 500%; in addition, the increased plasma triglyceride levels were found to be associated with an increase of the very-low-density lipoprotein fraction, and plasma cholesterol levels generally either were not affected or were reduced during periods of high-carbohydrate feeding. These basic observations have been verified many times in both short- and long-term experiments. In a long-term study carried out among white and Bantu prisoners in South Africa, Antonis and Bersohn (1961) were able to distinguish groups of hyperresponders and hyporesponders in the two races. The groups differed in both the magnitude of the triglyceridemia and its duration. An important consequence of the study was the recognition that the triglyceride response was determined by the genetic background of the subject and his metabolic status. In a more recent report, Glueck et al. (1969) extended the earlier observations of Lees and Fredrickson (1965) and determined the peak triglyceride response during 7 days of carbohydrate-rich (80% of calories) diets among 23 "young" (18–23 yr) and "middle-age" (40–58 yr) normal humans. The mean percent increase of plasma triglyceride level was 99 and 139%, respectively; individual response varied between 30 and 326%. Twelve of the 23 subjects demonstrated increments of plasma triglycerides greater than 100%. These studies, and many more, strengthened the hypothesis that "carbohydrate induction" is a highly individual property, one that varies remarkably among normal humans.

The effects of different carbohydrates (starch, sucrose, glucose, and fructose) on plasma lipid levels was studied in the 1960s (Cohen et al., 1966b; Kaufmann et al., 1966a, b; Macdonald, 1965, 1966a, b, 1967; Macdonald and Braithwaite, 1964). The studies demonstrated that carbohydrate induction is more pronounced with sucrose than with starch and that this property is possibly ascribed to the fructose moiety of the sucrose molecule. Subsequently, Macdonald (1968) reported an increased incorporation of radioactivity into triglycerides from fructose, compared with glucose.

In most studies, the changes in serum cholesterol with the feeding of carbohydrate-rich diets were also recorded. Generally, it was found that the serum cholesterol level decreased. Groen et al. (1966) have reported an average decrease of 12% of plasma cholesterol when 16 normal adults were fed a "bread" diet (62% of calories from carbohydrates and 19.3% fat) as against a "western" diet (48.2% and 35.4%, respectively). However, a different response was recorded when sucrose was substituted for the bread isocalorically. Under these conditions, plasma cholesterol levels were only minimally reduced from those recorded when the western diet was fed, and were significantly elevated over those recorded when the bread diet was fed.

Serum Lipids in Hyperlipemic Patients

A group of hyperlipemic patients who achieve extremely high levels of triglycerides when challenged with diets rich in carbohydrates, especially sucrose or fructose, has been established since the original report of Ahrens et al. (1961) on carbohydrate-induced lipemia (Antar et al., 1970; Cohen et al., 1966b; Farquhar et al., 1966; Kaufmann et al., 1966a, b; Kuo and Bassett, 1965; Nestel et al., 1970). In most patients, plasma triglyceride levels actually decreased on starch-rich diets to levels below those measured during periods on a self-selected diet. In these patients, control of hypertriglyceridemia is dependent on a "rational" diet—one poor in carbohydrates and especially low in sucrose.

The largest study of the effects of a carbohydrate-rich diet on the response of plasma triglycerides in patients with defined hyperlipoproteinemia was published by Glueck et al. Fifty-two patients with types II, III, and IV familial hyperlipoproteinemia, defined according to the "typing" system of Fredrickson et al. (1967), were included in the study. In this study the individual response among patients was also extremely variable and ranged in the three groups from 25-129%, 36-338%, to 35-213%. Mean percent increase of plasma triglycerides among patients with types II, III, and IV hyperlipoproteinemia was 87, 147, and 105%, respectively. The study has thus demonstrated two basic phenomena in the response of hyperlipemic patients to carbohydrate-rich diets: (1) No consistent pattern of carbohydrate induction was recorded among the groups. When the 23 normals (see above) are included, plasma triglyceride levels more than doubled during the period of carbohydrate-rich diet in about half the individuals in each group. (2) The absolute increment of plasma triglycerides during the diet was as much as 1,900 mg% and was commonly more than 500 mg% (11 of the 52 patients). In some individuals, therefore, a very pronounced increase of plasma triglycerides is attained by dietary manipulation.

The data presented above leave no doubt as to the important role of the dietary carbohydrates in determining the levels of plasma lipids and lipoproteins in humans. The most prominent effect of feeding carbohydrate-rich diets is the increased level of triglycerides, associated with very-low-density lipoproteins. A decrease in plasma low-density lipoprotein is often observed and is presumably due to the low-fat content of these experimental diets. An even more important consequence of these studies is the heterogenous and even divergent effects of carbohydrates on an individual basis among both normal and hyperlipemic humans, irrespective of their primary lipoprotein pattern.

EFFECT OF CARBOHYDRATES ON CARBOHYDRATE METABOLISM

Sugars, sugar derivatives, and polyols can cause insulin secretion from mammalian islets, or can function as powerful potentiators of insulin release. Among the sugars, D-glucose is the most thoroughly investigated compound (Table 1).

Glucose ingestion causes an immediate rise in blood glucose levels; together with the simultaneous rise in gastrointestinal hormones, this sugar leads to rapid insulin release. Other hormones affected are glucagon and growth hormone, both of which decline. Conversely, small to insignificant increases in circulating insulin levels have been observed after oral or intravenous administration of fructose in man (Aitken and Dunnigan, 1969; Modigliani et al., 1970; Steinke, 1972). Ingestion of fat in man results in a very slight and transient rise of insulin (Pi-Sunyer et al., 1969).

Considerable evidence has accumulated to indicate that the amount of ingested carbohydrate profoundly modifies the ensuing glucose and insulin

TABLE 1 Insulin Response to Different Carbohydrates
in Different Animals

Carbohydrate	Animal	Reference
Glucose	Rabbit	Coore and Randle (1964)
	Rat	Grodsky et al. (1963)
		Lambert et al. (1969)
Fructose	Dogs	Kuzuya et al. (1969)
	Rat	Lambert et al. (1969)
Sucrose	Rat	Berdanier (1974a)
		Cohen et al. (1974b)
Mannose	Rabbit	Coore and Randle (1964)
Galactose	Rat	Landgraf (1971)

response. High-carbohydrate diets were shown by Brunzell et al. (1971) to cause a concomitant decrease in the fasting blood glucose and insulin levels in normal and mild diabetic subjects. However, Grey and Kipnis (1971) did not find in obese subjects a change in basal insulin levels when comparing diets with either 62 or 45% of calories from carbohydrates. Reaven and Olefsky (1974) found that in 20 nondiabetic adult men feeding isocaloric diets containing 42% fat/43% carbohydrate and 30% fat/55% carbohydrate affected the blood insulin levels differently: the low-fat–high-carbohydrate diet led to an approximate 40% increase in plasma insulin levels. As mentioned above, Grey and Kipnis (1971) noted that in obese patients serum insulin levels increased, regardless of the amount of carbohydrate in the diet. They suggested that islet hypertrophy and hyperinsulinemia result from the usual high intake of carbohydrate in the obese and that antagonism to insulin develops as a mechanism of protection against the hyperinsulinemia.

Sims et al. (1974) have studied the metabolic responses of high-carbohydrate (300 g/m²) and low-carbohydrate (100 g/m²) diets in five subjects. An increased plasma insulin, decreased glucose tolerance, and resistance to insulin were demonstrated in subjects fed the carbohydrate-rich diet. These effects were more pronounced when body weight gain was achieved by an increase of the total caloric intake from 1,800 to 2,700 per day.

Cohen and Teitelbaum (1964) have described increased insulin-like activity in albino rats fed a high-sucrose diet, compared with their siblings fed a high-starch diet. However, individual and species variations do occur. Berdanier (1974a) found a difference between the Wistar and the BHE rats as to their insulin response to a high-sucrose diet. The BHE rats exhibited a lower degree of insulinemia when not fasting than do Wistar rats.

Abnormalities of insulin secretion, both in the basal state and in response to acute glucose load, do occur in all rodent species or strains developing hyperglycemia or obesity [Chinese hamster (Carpenter et al., 1967), Ob Ob mice (Coleman and Hummel, 1968), New Zealand obese mice (NZO) (Sneyd, 1964), yellow A$_y$ (Weitze, 1963)]. The obese *Acomys cahirinus* bred in Geneva showed impaired immunoreactive insulin response (Stauffacher et al., 1971).

Starch, sucrose, glucose, and fructose affect the fasting blood glucose levels and the glucose tolerance differently. Himmsworth (1953) has shown that previous consumption of a high-carbohydrate diet may improve glucose tolerance, but the possible effect of different carbohydrates was not studied. Cohen et al. (1966a) have shown that in normal humans fed isocaloric low-fat–high-carbohydrate diets the average glucose tolerance curve was significantly lower during periods on bread-rich diet as compared with periods on sucrose-rich diet. Individual variations were noted and emphasized.

Uram et al. (1958) found that sucrose-fed rats have higher blood glucose values during a glucose tolerance test than starch-fed rats and suggested the presence of a hypoglycemic substance in the starch-fed group. Cohen and Teitelbaum (1964) have shown that in albino rats of the Hebrew University strain, substituting dietary sucrose for starch (other ingredients of the diet being constant) resulted in impaired oral or intravenous glucose tolerance. The period required to develop the impaired glucose tolerance varied with the concentration (percentage) of the sucrose in the diet. In animals fed a diet containing 67% sucrose this period was 21–40 days, whereas about 100 days of feeding a diet with 33–40% of the calories from sucrose were needed to develop the impairment of the glucose tolerance. The sucrose-fed animals had a greater percentage of fat in the liver and the serum insulin-like activity was reduced. Berdanier (1974b) did not observe a difference in fasting or nonfasting blood glucose levels in young rats of the Wistar or the BHE strain fed a 65% sucrose diet until 50 or 100 days of age. In the *Acomys cahirinus* domesticated from the native habitat in the Negev part of Israel, a high-sucrose diet (55%) resulted in an impaired glucose tolerance (Shafrir et al., 1972).

The data presented above demonstrate conclusively that a different metabolic response to carbohydrate-rich diets exists between species and among individuals within the species. They indicate, therefore, a genetic predisposition of the individual to specific carbohydrates, particularly sucrose, and suggest the possibility of selection of susceptible subpopulations.

INTERACTIONS BETWEEN GENETIC FACTOR(S) AND INGESTED CARBOHYDRATES

A dietary survey among Yemenite Jews in Israel has shown that while their diet in Yemen had contained no sucrose, the quantities consumed in Israel equalled those consumed by the western Jew (Cohen et al., 1961). It was suggested that this dietary difference might be one reason for the rarity of diabetes among newly arrived Yemenite immigrants, compared with its greater prevalence in old-established Yemenite settlers and the population in general (Cohen, 1961). Indeed, as cited above, sucrose-rich diets given to man and rats

TABLE 2   Mean Blood Glucose (mg/100 ml) at 60 min
Following Glucose Load (350 mg/100 g) of Rats
after 60 Days on Diet

Group	Diet	No. of animals	Mean blood glucose ($\pm$ SEM)
Parent generation	Starch	40	108 ± 3.8
Parent generation	Sucrose	47	135 ± 4.9
Upward line			
S_1	Sucrose	21	176 ± 7.9
S_2	Sucrose	46	159 ± 7.8
S_3	Sucrose	20	167 ± 6.5
S_4	Sucrose	11	269 ± 12
S_5	Sucrose	20	270 ± 9
Downward line			
S_1	Sucrose	25	122 ± 4.3
S_2	Sucrose	41	137 ± 1.9
S_3	Sucrose	38	130 ± 1.7
S_4	Sucrose	27	153 ± 7.0
S_5	Sucrose	15	135 ± 8

may cause an impaired glucose tolerance (Cohen and Teitelbaum, 1964; Cohen et al., 1966a).

To determine whether there is a genetic predisposition to develop impaired glucose tolerance on feeding high concentrations of sucrose, the interaction between glucose intolerance and sucrose feeding was studied in rats (Cohen et al., 1972b) by brother–sister matings using the method of two-way selection (Falconer, 1953). To this end, 28 male and 19 female (parent generation, P) albino rats of the Sabra Hebrew University strain, weighing 60–70 g, were fed a high-sucrose synthetic diet *ad libitum* (18% casein, 5% butter, 72% sucrose, and 5% salts and vitamins) for 2 months. At the end of this period an oral glucose tolerance test (gtt) was performed (350 mg/100 g body weight) (Table 2). The male and two females with the highest blood glucose values at 1 hr after the glucose load were selected and mated (upward selection). In addition, the male and female with the lowest blood glucose values were selected and mated (downward selection). After mating and during breeding, the rats were fed the regular animal house rations.

The offspring of each line were separated at age 21 days and the litters were kept apart. The animals continued to be fed the animal house rations until they weighed 60 g. They were then fed the high sucrose diet for 2 months, after which time a gtt was taken. The same upward and downward selection procedure, using brother–sister mating as outlined above, was applied, respectively, to subsequent generations (S_2, S_3, S_4, and S_5).

Table 2 shows the blood glucose values 60 min after an intragastric glucose load in the upward and downward selected lines. Note that in the succeeding generations of the upward selected line (fed sucrose) the level of blood glucose rose to significant levels and that a considerable number of animals developed a diabetic syndrome with spontaneous hyperglycemia and glucosuria (Table 2). In a separate experiment the litters of the S_5 generation were divided into two groups. One group was fed the sucrose diet for 2 months; their siblings, used as controls, were fed the starch diet. Both groups were tested for their spontaneous blood glucose at 9, 13, and 21 hr (Table 3). While the animals of the upward line developed high blood-glucose values, the siblings fed starch, did not show such a rise. On the other hand, in the offspring of the downward selected line, blood glucose did not rise, whether fed the sucrose or the starch diet. This finding points to the need for interaction between the genetic factor(s) and the dietary factor for expression of the diabetic syndrome. There was no significant difference in body weight between the hyperglycemic sucrose-fed rats of the upward selected line and the sucrose-fed normoglycemic rats of the downward selected line. Starch-fed siblings of either line weighed more than the sucrose-fed rats. Thus, obesity, which usually accompanies genetically transmitted diabetes in rodents (except for the Chinese hamster), is not present in our model.

The appearance of diabetic features in the animals of the upward selected line was studied with the aid of the following parameters: hyperglycemia, glucosuria, activities of liver enzymes (glycolysis, lipogenesis, and gluconeo-genesis), serum insulin on fasting and after a glucose stimulus, and retinal and renal angiopathy (vascular complications).

Biochemical features. As mentioned above, the sucrose-fed rats of the upward selected line developed hyperglycemia and glucosuria. The activities of the hepatic enzymes of the pathways of glycolysis, gluconeogenesis, and lipogenesis in the upward selected line are shown in Table 4. The activity of these enzymes is expressed as a ratio of values in rats fed sucrose vs. those fed starch, both in the parent generation and in the siblings of the selected generations, after 5 and 10 months on the respective diets. Since the enzyme activity changes with age, a separate comparison was made for each group of sucrose-fed animals

TABLE 3 Spontaneous Blood Glucose (Mean ± SEM)
at 9, 13, and 21 hr of the Upward and Downward
Selected Animals Fed Starch or Sucrose

Line	Diet	No. of animals	Hours		
			9	13	21
Upward	Starch	15	118 ± 2.9	128 ± 1.9	134 ± 4.2
	Sucrose	12	134 ± 11	165 ± 2.1	230 ± 4.2
Downward	Starch	12	98 ± 1.6	106 ± 1.2	115 ± 3.6
	Sucrose	12	110 ± 2.5	121 ± 1.6	128 ± 2.5

TABLE 4   Liver Enzyme Activity Expressed as Ratio Sucrose/Starch[a] of Parents and Upward Selected Generations

		Glycolysis	Lipogenesis			Gluconeogenesis	
Group	Time on diet (months)	Pyruvate kinase	G6PDH	Malate enzyme	Acetyl CoA carboxyl- ase	Phos- phoenol pyruvate carboxy- kinase	Alanine amino- (GPT) trans- ferase
Parents (9)[b]	10	150	255	170	180	95	0
Selected generations							
(9)	5	460	315	320	130	70	115
(6)	10	98	150	115	80	150	155

[a]Activities in starch-fed animals taken as 100%.
[b]Numbers in parentheses are numbers of animals.

with respect to their starch-fed siblings, which were taken as 100%. In the parent generation, the activity of glycolysis and lipogenesis enzymes increased more in the sucrose-fed animals than in the starch-fed controls. There was no significant change in the activity ratio of the enzymes involved in gluconeogenesis. In the upward selected generations, 5 months of sucrose feeding produced a much larger increase in the ratio of the activity of enzymes involved in lipogenesis and glycolysis. Continuation of sucrose feeding for 9 months in the upward selected line markedly decreased the activity ratio in the case of glycolysis and lipogenesis enzymes; in contrast, the activity ratio of enzymes associated with gluconeogenesis increased, indicating a shift of enzyme activities into a diabetic pattern (Cohen et al., 1974a).

The fasting plasma insulin levels of the upward selected line of the sucrose-fed (hyperglycemic) animals were not significantly greater than those of their starch-fed siblings, nor of the sucrose-fed animals of the downward selected line. The dynamics of insulin release at 30 and 60 min following a glucose load are shown in Table 5. With glucose stimulation, the sucrose-fed animals of the downward selected line exhibit a smaller insulin response than the sucrose- and starch-fed animals of the upward selected line. There is no direct relationship between the plasma glucose level and the insulin response, and different animals with high glucose values may have high-, normal-, or low-insulin responses. This finding is similar to that of adult-onset diabetes in man.

Vascular complications. Renal vascular lesions (intercapillary glomerulo- sclerosis), microaneurysms in the retina, and progressive thickening of the capillary basement membrane in different organs are considered specific for diabetes mellitus.

TABLE 5 Plasma Insulin Response to Oral Glucose Load
(350 mg/100 g body wt) in the Upward and Downward
Selected Line Fed Sucrose or Starch Diet

Line	Diet	No. of animals	Plasma insulin (μU/ml)		
				min after glucose load	
			Fasting	30	60
Upward	Sucrose	16	68.2 ± 8.6	122 ± 14.6	118 ± 11.2
	Starch	12	70.8 ± 13.4	108.3 ± 8.8	92.3 ± 9.5
Downward	Sucrose	15	51 ± 5.6	76 ± 5.5	64 ± 8.7

Specimens from the kidney, examined by light and electron microscopy, showed that the renal alterations in the sucrose-fed rats consisted of diffuse intercapillary glomerulosclerosis. In several instances, exudative or lipohyaline glomerular lesions were conspicuous. Arterial and arteriolar sclerosis was prominent in a few cases (Cohen and Rosenmann, 1971). The electron microscopic examination corroborated and extended the findings observed by the light microscope. Such changes were not observed in any of the starch-fed siblings (Rosenmann et al., 1971). These renal changes are similar to those found in experimental diabetic animals, induced by surgical removal of the pancreas or its chemical destruction or in spontaneous diabetic animals and humans (Beaser et al., 1964; Bloodworth, 1965; Dachs and Churg, 1964; Farquhar et al., 1959; Foglia et al., 1950; Lawe, 1962; Lundback et al., 1967; Mann et al., 1951; Orskov et al., 1965; Patz et al., 1965). However, the specific renal lesions of human diabetes (nodular glomerulosclerosis) were not observed.

The retinal changes observed in human diabetics were also observed in our experimental animals. The retinal changes (Cohen et al., 1972a) consisted of a loss (mural and endothelial), narrowing and closure (strand formation), and sacculation (microaneurysms) of the capillaries. These changes have been observed only rarely in other experimental diabetic models.

Relation of microangiopathy to metabolic or genetic factor(s). When considering the development of microvascular complications, especially retinopathy and nephropathy, and its relation to effective control of the metabolic disturbances in diabetes, there are two main viewpoints. According to Siperstein (1970), muscular capillary basement membrane thickening results from the genetic defect responsible for diabetes mellitus and is found independently of the metabolic changes. This, however, was not confirmed in a similar study (Williamson et al., 1971).

To answer the question of whether angiopathy results from metabolic changes accompanying the state of diabetes, or is independent and solely related to a genetic factor, sucrose- and starch-fed siblings of the upward selected line were studied. Table 6 shows the incidence of renal vascular disease (diffuse glomerulosclerosis) and the vascular retinopathy in sucrose-fed animals and their starch-fed siblings. In 138 sucrose-fed animals of the upward selected line (those with hyperglycemia and other metabolic changes), the incidence of nephropathy varied from 8 to 14% in all age groups, whereas no renal disease was found in the 65 starch-fed siblings who had no metabolic derangements. The incidence of the vascular retinopathy in the 53 animals of the upward selected line of sucrose-fed rats was as high as 32%, while no vascular changes were observed in their 22 starch-fed siblings. In animals of the downward selected line (47 sucrose-fed and 45 starch-fed siblings) kept for 12 months on their respective diets, no renal or retinal vascular changes were detected.

These findings clearly demonstrate that the sucrose-fed animals of the upward selected line that developed hyperglycemia also developed retinal and renal angiopathy. Their starch-fed siblings with the same genetic pattern remained normoglycemic and did not develop angiopathy, nor did the downward selected animals, whether fed sucrose or starch. This indicates that there are individual responses to the feeding of the same carbohydrate and to different carbohydrates. Animals susceptible to sucrose feeding will develop abnormal metabolic changes which will be followed by pathologic–structural changes. On the other hand, the downward selected animals which are *not* susceptible to sucrose feeding will not develop metabolic changes nor vascular complications. Furthermore, these findings indicate that the genetic factor(s) alone is not sufficient to induce the pathologic angiopathy, unless the animal develops "diabetes," i.e., hyperglycemia with its accompanying metabolic changes. This experiment supports the view that the development of diabetic angiopathy is not independent of the metabolic changes and that it is not related solely to the genetic factors(s). By preventing the metabolic changes in an individual with the genetic tendency to develop vascular angiopathy, it may be possible to prevent or delay the appearance of vascular changes.

TABLE 6   Incidence of Glomerulosclerosis and
Diabetic Retinopathy in the Upward and
Downward Selected Lines Fed
Starch or Sucrose

Age (months)	Retinopathy (%)		Glomerulosclerosis (%)	
	Sucrose	Starch	Sucrose	Starch
3–5	9	0	14	0
6–8	0	0	8	0
9–11	31	0	9	0
12–14	50	0	13	0

SUMMARY

The data presented conclusively demonstrate that different metabolic responses to the different dietary carbohydrates are found among the species and among individuals in the same species. These metabolic responses are expressed in the metabolism of lipids, carbohydrates, and in the hormonal status of these animals. The ultimate metabolic behavior is thus determined by the interaction between the genetic makeup of the individual and the ingested carbohydrate. In susceptible individuals the ingestion of the specific carbohydrate moiety may result in the development of a metabolic disorder.

The genetic studies have demonstrated that in a selected population with a genetic predisposition, high-sucrose intakes lead to the appearance of diabetes, while the same population fed a starch diet remains normal. Furthermore, the unsusceptible selected population exposed to the same carbohydrate (sucrose) also remains normal. The diabetes appearing in these experimental animals exhibits parameters similar to human adult-onset diabetes (namely, hyperglycemia, glucosuria, a diabetic–enzymic pattern, changes in serum insulin levels, and retinal and renal vascular complications). The experiments with animals duplicate the observations in the Yemenites, in whom an increased prevalence of diabetes on transition from a limited caloric and sucrose intake to the high-caloric, sucrose-rich diet adopted by these immigrants in the so-called developed countries was observed. Therefore, individuals or groups with different genetic sensitivities to a high intake of a specific carbohydrate may develop high glucose and/or high lipid levels, whereas other individuals will retain normal values on consuming the same amounts of the carbohydrate. This explains why, in the same community, only a certain percentage of the population will develop diabetes or carbohydrate-induced lipemia while others will not.

REFERENCES

Ahrens, E. H., Insull, W., Blomstrand, R., Hirsch, J., Tsaltas, T. T. and Peterson, M. L. 1957. *Lancet* 1:943.
Ahrens, E. H., Hirsch, J., Oette, K., Farquhar, J. W. and Stein, Y. 1961. *Trans. Assoc. Am. Physicians* 74:134–146.
Aitken, J. N. and Dunnigan, M. G. 1969. *Br. Med. J.* 3:276.
Allen, R. J. L. and Leahy, J. S. 1966. *Br. J. Nutr.* 20:339–347.
Anderson, T. A. 1969. *Proc. Soc. Exp. Biol. Med.* 130:884–887.
Antar, M. A., Little, J. A., Lucas, C., Buckley, G. C. and Csima, A. 1970. *Atherosclerosis* 11:191.
Antonis, A. and Bersohn, I. 1961. *Lancet* 1:3–9.
Bar-On, H. and Stein, Y. 1968. *J. Nutr.* 94:95–105.
Beaser, S. B., Matthew, F. S., Donaldson, G. W., McLaughlin, R. J. and Sommers, S. C. 1964. *Diabetes* 13:49–53.
Bedö, M. and Szigeti, A. 1967. *Nahrung* 11:305–310.
Bender, A. E., Damji, K. B. and Yapa, C. G. R. 1970. *Biochem. J.* 119:351–352.

Berdanier, C. D. 1974a. *J. Nutr.* 104:1246–1256.

Berdanier, C. D. 1974b. *Diabetologia* 10:691–695.

Bloodworth, J. M. B., Jr. 1965. *Arch. Pathol. (Chicago)* 79:113–125.

Brunzell, J. D., Lerner, R. L., Hazzard, W. R. and Porte, D. 1971. *New Engl. J. Med.* 284:521.

Carpenter, A. M., Gerritsen, G. C., Dulin, W. E. and Lazarow, A. 1967. *Diabetologia* 3:92–96.

Chevalier, M., Wiley, J. H. and Leveille, G. A. 1972. *Proc. Soc. Exp. Biol. Med.* 139:220–222.

Cohen, A. M. 1961. *Metab. Clin. Exp.* 10:50–58.

Cohen, A. M. and Rosenmann, E. 1971. *Diabetologia* 7:25–28.

Cohen, A. M. and Teitelbaum, A. 1964. *Am. J. Physiol.* 206:105–108.

Cohen, A. M. and Teitelbaum, A. 1968. *Life Sci.* 7:23–29.

Cohen, A. M., Bavly, S. and Poznanski, R. 1961. *Lancet* 1:399–401.

Cohen, A. M., Teitelbaum, A., Balogh, M. and Groen, J. J. 1966a. *Am. J. Clin. Nutr.* 19:59–62.

Cohen, A. M., Kaufmann, N. A., Poznanski, R., Blondheim, S. H. and Stein, Y. 1966b. *Br. Med. J.* I:339.

Cohen, A. M., Michaelson, I. C. and Yanko, L. 1972a. *Am. J. Ophthal.* 73:863–868.

Cohen, A. M., Teitelbaum, A. and Saliternik, R. 1972b. *Metabolism* 21:235.

Cohen, A. M., Teitelbaum, A., Briller, S., Rosenmann, E., Yanko, L. and Shafrir, E. 1974a. *Horm. Metab. Res.* Suppl. no. 4:117–123.

Cohen, A. M., Teitelbaum, A., Briller, S., Yanko, L., Rosenmann, E. and Shafrir, E. 1974b. *Experimental models of diabetes. Sugars in nutrition,* ed. H. L. Sipple and K. W. McNutt, pp. 484–511. New York: Academic Press.

Coleman, D. L. and Hummel, K. D. 1968. In *Jornees annuelles de diabetologie Hotel-Dieu,* ed. M. Deorot, pp. 19–30. Paris: Editions Medicales, Flammarion.

Coore, H. G. and Randle, P. J. 1964. *Biochem. J.* 93:66–78.

Dachs, S. and Churg, J. 1964. *Am. J. Pathol.* 44:155–168.

Eisenberg, S., Bilheimer, D. W., Levy, R. I. and Lindgren, F. T. 1973. *Biochim. Biophys. Acta* 326:361–377.

Falconer, D. S. 1953. *J. Genet.* 51:470.

Farnell, D. R. and Burns, J. J. 1962. *Metab. Clin. Exp.* 11:566–571.

Farquhar, M. G., Hopper, J. and Moon, H. D. 1959. *Am. J. Pathol.* 35:721–753.

Farquhar, J. W., Frank, A., Gross, R. C. and Reaven, G. N. 1966. *J. Clin. Invest.* 45:1648–1656.

Fillios, L. C., Naito, C., Andrus, S. B., Portman, O. W. and Martin, R. S. 1958. *Am. J. Physiol.* 194:275–279.

Foglia, V. G., Mancini, R. E. and Cardeza, A. F. 1950. *Am. Med. Assoc. Pathol.* 50:75–83.

Fredrickson, D. S., Levy, R. I. and Lees, R. S. 1967. *New Engl. J. Med.* 276:34–44, 94–103, 148–156, 215–226, 273–281.

Ginsburg, V. and Hers, H. G. 1960. *Biochim. Biophys. Acta* 38:427–434.

Glueck, C. J., Levy, R. I. and Fredrickson, D. S. 1969. *Diabetes* 18:739–747.

Grant, W. C. and Fahrenbach, M. J. 1959. *Proc. Soc. Exp. Biol. Med.* 100:250–252.

Grey, N. and Kipnis, D. M. 1971. *New Engl. J. Med.* 285:827.

Grodsky, G. M., Batts, A. A., Bennett, L. L., Vcella, C., McWilliams, N. B. and Smith, D. F. 1963. *Am. J. Physiol.* 205:638–644.

238

A. M. Cohen and S. Eisenberg

Groen, J. J., Balogh, M., Yaron, E. and Cohen, A. M. 1966. *Am. J. Clin. Nutr.* 19:46–62.

Hatch, F. T., Abell, L. L. and Kendall, F. E. 1955. *Am. J. Med.* 19:48.

Himmsworth, H. P. 1953. *Clin. Sci.* 1:1.

Kaufmann, N. A., Poznanski, R., Blondheim, S. H. and Stein, Y. 1966a. *Am. J. Clin. Nutr.* 18:261.

Kaufmann, N. A., Poznanski, R., Blondheim, S. H. and Stein, Y. 1966b. *Isr. J. Med. Sci.* 2:715–726.

Keys, A. and Anderson, J. J. 1957. *Am. J. Clin. Nutr.* 5:29.

Kiyasu, J. Y. and Chaikoff, I. L. 1957. *J. Biol. Chem.* 224:935–939.

Kritchevsky, D. and Tepper, S. A. 1969. *Med. Exp.* 19:329–341.

Kritchevsky, D., Kolman, R. R., Guttmacher, R. M. and Forbes, M. 1959. *Arch. Biochem. Biophys.* 85:444–451.

Kuo, P. T. and Bassett, D. R. 1965. *Ann. Int. Med.* 62:1199.

Kuzuya, T., Kanazawa, Y. and Kosaka, K. 1969. *Endocrinology* 84:200–207.

Lambert, A. E., Junod, A., Stauffacher, W., Jean Remeaud, B. and Renold, A. E. 1969. *Biochim. Biophys. Acta* 184:529–539.

Landgraf, R., Kotler-Brajtburg, J. and Matschinsky, F. M. 1971. *Proc. Natl. Acad. Sci. U.S.A.* 68:536.

Langer, T., Strober, W., and Levy, R. I. 1972. *J. Clin. Invest.* 51:1528–1536.

Lawe, J. E. 1962. *Arch. Pathol.* 73:88–96.

Lees, R. S. and Fredrickson, D. S. 1965. *J. Clin. Invest.* 44:1968–1977.

Lundback, K., Steen-Olsen, T., Orskov, H. and Osterby-Hansen, R. 1967. *Acta Med. Scand. Suppl.* 476:160–173.

Macdonald, I. 1962. *J. Physiol. (London)* 160:306.

Macdonald, I. 1965. *Clin. Sci.* 29:193.

Macdonald, I. 1966a. *Am. J. Clin. Nutr.* 18:86.

Macdonald, I. 1966b. *Am. J. Clin. Nutr.* 18:369.

Macdonald, I. 1967. *Am. J. Clin. Nutr.* 20:345.

Macdonald, I. 1968. *Am. J. Clin. Nutr.* 21:1366.

Macdonald, I. and Braithwaite, D. M. 1964. *Clin. Sci.* 27:123–130.

Macdonald, I. and Roberts, J. B. 1965. *Metab. Clin. Exp.* 14:991–999.

Mann, G. V., Goddard, J. W. and Adams, L. 1951. *Am. J. Pathol.* 27:857–864.

Marshall, M. W. and Hildebrand, H. E. 1963. *J. Nutr.* 79:227–238.

Modigliani, E., Strauch, G. and Odievre, M. 1970. *Rev. Eur. Etud. Clin. Biol.* 15:882.

Moser, P. B. and Berdanier, C. D. 1974. *J. Nutr.* 104:687–694.

Naismith, D. J. and Khan, N. A. 1970a. *Proc. Nutr. Soc.* 29:63A–64A. (Abstr.)

Naismith, D. J. and Khan, N. A. 1970b. *Proc. Nutr. Soc.* 29:64A–65A. (Abstr.)

Nath, N., Harper, A. E. and Elvehjem, C. A. 1959. *Proc. Soc. Exp. Biol. Med.* 102:571–574.

Nestel, P. J., Carrol, K. F. and Halenster, N. 1970. *Metabolism* 19:1–18.

Nichols, A. V., Dobbin, V. and Gofman, J. W. 1957. *Geriatrics* 12:7–17.

Nikkila, E. A. and Ojala, K. 1965. *Life Sci.* 4:937–943.

Olson, R. E., Vester, J. W., Gursey, D. and Longman, D. 1958. *Am. J. Clin. Nutr.* 310:6.

Orskov, H., Olsen, T. S., Nielson, K., Rafaelson, O. and Lundbaek, K. 1965. *Diabetologia* 1:172–179.

Patz, A., Berkow, J. W., Maumenee, A. E. and Cox, J. 1965. *Diabetes* 14:700–708.

Pi-Sunyer, F. X., Hashim, S. A. and Van Itallie, T. B. 1969. *Diabetes* 18:96–100.
Portman, O. W., Lawry, E. Y. and Bruno, D. 1956. *Proc. Soc. Exp. Biol. Med.* 91:321–323.
Reaven, G. M. and Olefsky, J. M. 1974. *J. Clin. Endocrinol. Metab.* 38:151–154.
Rosenmann, E., Teitelbaum, A. and Cohen, A. M. 1971. *Diabetes* 20:803–810.
Schultz, A. L. and Grande, F. 1968. *J. Nutr.* 94:71–73.
Shafrir, E., Teitelbaum, A. and Cohen, A. M. 1972. *Isr. J. Med. Sci.* 8:990–992.
Shafrir, E., Gutman, A. and Cohen, A. M. 1974. In *Lipid metabolism, obesity, and diabetes mellitus: Impact upon atherosclerosis*, International Symposium, April 1972. *Horm. Metab. Res.* Suppl. no. 4:102–110.
Sims, E. A. H., Bray, G. A., Danforth, E., Glennon, J. A., Jr., Horton, E. S., Salans, L. B. and Connel, M. 1974. *Horm. Metab. Res.* Suppl. no. 4:70–77.
Siperstein, M. D. 1970. In *13th Nobel symposium: Pathogenesis of diabetes mellitus*, ed. E. Cerasi and R. Luft, pp. 81–96. Uppsala: Almqvist and Wiksell.
Sneyd, J. G. T. 1964. *J. Endocrinol.* 28:163–172.
Stauffacher, W., Orci, L., Cameron, D. P., Burr, I. M. and Renold, A. E. 1971. *Recent Progr. Horm. Res.* 27:41–91.
Steinke, J. 1972. In *Nutrition and diabetes*, ed. E. Froesh and J. Yudkin, p. 297. Milano: VI Capri Conference, "Il Ponte."
Taylor, D. D., Conway, E. S., Schuster, E. M. and Adams, M. 1967. *J. Nutr.* 91:275–282.
Uram, J. A., Friedman, L. and Kline, O. L. 1958. *Am. J. Physiol.* 192:521.
Weitze, M. 1963. *Metab. Clin. Exp.* 12:527.
Wells, W. W. and Anderson, S. C. 1959. *J. Nutr.* 68:541–549.
Williamson, J. R., Vogler, N. J. and Kilo, C. 1971. *Med. Clin. N. Am.* 55:847–860.

Chapter 10

GENETIC ERRORS IN CARBOHYDRATE METABOLISM

Carolyn D. Berdanier

Departments of Biochemistry and Medicine
University of Nebraska College of Medicine
and Veterans Administration Hospital
Omaha, Nebraska

I. INTRODUCTION

Heredity has been recognized for many years as playing an important role in the etiology of a number of diseases affecting man. Diabetes, the "classical" disorder in carbohydrate metabolism, has long been known to have a strong genetic component. Other genetically determined disorders of carbohydrate metabolism have been described as interest in inborn errors in metabolism (i.e., errors due to missing or deficient enzymes) has increased. More than 24 such disorders relating to carbohydrate nutrition and metabolism have been identified and described (Table 1).

Genetic aberrations that result in missing enzymes are usually the result of a single-gene mutation. These mutations can result in mild, moderate, or severe alterations in metabolism and produce mildly, moderately, or severely impaired individuals. The severity of the impairment depends largely on the relative importance of the enzyme itself in the metabolism of carbohydrate, whether alternate pathways are available for the metabolism of the accumulated substrate(s), and whether the substrate(s) or one of its metabolites accumulates and becomes toxic. In addition, it is possible for a metabolic defect to occur with no evidence of its existence until the individual is subjected to unusual physiologic stress or to particular medications. Inborn errors may also be multifactorial diseases involving more than one gene and perhaps environmental factors as well.

Simple gene mutations have been shown to affect all areas of carbohydrate metabolism from digestion, absorption, storage, and utilization. Multifactorial genetic errors in carbohydrate metabolism, having more than one identifiable defect site and affecting more than one enzyme and perhaps several hormones as

TABLE 1 Inherited Disorders of Carbohydrate Metabolism

Process affected	Disease	Cellular error or enzyme affected	Symptoms
Digestion	Lactose intolerance	Lactase	Chronic or intermittent diarrhea, flatulence, nausea, vomiting, growth failure in young children
	Sucrose intolerance	Sucrase	Diarrhea, flatulence, nausea, poor growth in infants
Intestinal transport	Glucose–galactose intolerance	Glucose–galactose carrier	Diarrhea, growth failure in infants, stools contain large quantities of glucose and lactic acid
Interconversion of sugars	Galactosemia	Galactose-1-P-uridyl transferase	Increased cellular content of galactose 1-phosphate, eye cataracts, mental retardation, increased cellular levels of galactitol
		Galactokinase	Cataracts, cellular accumulation of galactose and galactitol
		Galactoepimerase	No severe symptoms
	Fructosemia	Fructokinase	Fructosuria, fructosemia
		Fructose-1-P-aldolase	Hypoglycemia, vomiting after fructose load, fructosemia, fructosuria; in children: poor growth, jaundice, hyperbilirubinemia, albuminuria, amino-aciduria
		Fructose-1,6-diphosphatase	Hypoglycemia, hepatomegaly, poor muscle tone, increased blood lactate levels
	Pentosuria	NADP-linked xylitol dehydrogenase	Elevated levels of xylose in urine
Glucose catabolism	Hemolytic anemia	Glucose-6-phosphate dehydrogenase	Low erythrocyte levels of NADPH, hemolysis of the erythrocyte
		Pyruvate kinase	Nonspherocytic anemia, accumulation of phosphorylated glucose metabolites in the cell, jaundice in newborn
	Type VII glycogenosis	Phosphofructokinase	Intolerance to exercise, elevated muscle glycogen levels, accumulation of hexose monophosphates in muscle
Gluconeogenesis	Von Gierke's disease (Type I glycogenosis)	Glucose-6-phosphatase	Hypoglycemia, hyperlipemia, brain damage in some patients, excess liver glycogen levels, shortened lifespan, increased glycerol utilization

Pathway	Disease	Enzyme Defect	Characteristics
Glycogen synthesis	Amylopectinosis (Type IV glycogenosis)	Branching enzyme [Liver amylo(1,4→1,6)-transglucosidase]	Tissue accumulation of long-chain glycogen that is poorly branched, intolerance to exercise
Glycogenolysis	Pompe's disease (Type II glycogenosis)	Lysosomal α-1,4-glucosidase (acid maltase)	Generalized glycogen excess in viscera, muscles, and nervous system, extreme muscular weakness, hepatomegaly, enlarged heart
	Forbe's disease (Type III glycogenosis)	Amylo-1,6-glucosidase (debranching enzyme)	Tissue accumulation of highly branched, short-chain glycogen, hypoglycemia, acidosis, muscular weakness, enlarged heart
	McArdle's disease (Type V glycogenosis)	Muscle phosphorylase	Intolerance to exercise
	Her's disease (Type VI glycogenosis)	Liver phosphorylase	Hepatomegaly, increased liver glycogen content, elevated serum lipids, growth retardation
	Type IX glycogenosis	Phosphorylase kinase	Hepatomegaly, increased liver glycogen levels, decreased phosphorylase activity in hepatocytes and leukocytes, elevated blood lipids, hypoglycemia after prolonged fasting, increased gluconeogenesis
Lipogenesis	Type I lipoproteinemia	Lipoprotein lipase	Elevated chylomicrons in serum, eruptive xanthomas, abdominal discomfort, hepatomegaly, splenomegaly
	Type II lipoproteinemia	β-lipoprotein receptors	Lipid deposits in skin, eyes, tendons, and vascular tissue, elevated β-lipoprotein levels, elevated serum cholesterol levels, shortened lifespan, elevated serum triglyceride levels (in Type IIb)
	Type III lipoproteinemia	Primary defect unknown	Elevated levels of serum cholesterol, phospholipids, and triglycerides, elevated β- and pre-β-lipoprotein levels, tuberous, planar and tendon xanthomas, vascular atheromas, ischemic heart disease, glucose intolerance
	Type IV lipoproteinema	Primary defect unknown	Elevated serum triglyceride levels, elevated pre-β-lipoprotein levels, premature atherosclerosis, ischemic heart disease, obesity, impaired glucose tolerance
	Type V lipoproteinemia	Primary defect unknown	Elevated chylomicrons and triglycerides in the serum, reduced fat tolerance
Cellular glucose utilization	Diabetes mellitus	Primary defect unknown; all enzymes of glucose metabolism and lipogenesis affected	Glucose intolerance, glucosuria, glucosemia, polyuria, excessive rapid weight loss, acidosis, coma, shortened lifespan

well, have also been described. It is entirely possible that these multifactorial diseases also have a single genetic defect as yet unidentified. It is the purpose of this chapter to summarize and describe those disorders of carbohydrate metabolism that have a strong genetic component.

II. ERRORS AFFECTING DIGESTION AND ABSORPTION

The diet of man contains a number of mono-, di-, and polysaccharides that must be degraded to their simple absorbable components in order to be of nutritional value. In turn, these components must be converted to the metabolic fuel of choice: glucose. The process of degradation prior to or during absorption (see Chapter 3) requires the presence of the appropriate enzymes that, if absent, lead to a disease state chiefly characterized by diarrhea. The diarrhea is the result of the osmotic effect of the undigested and/or unabsorbed carbohydrates present in the gut (Weijers et al., 1960, 1961). Congenital enzyme defects in the digestion of lactose (Dahlqvist, 1974; Holzel et al., 1959, 1962), maltose (Auricchio et al., 1963; Semenza et al., 1965), and sucrose (Prader et al., 1961; Weijers et al., 1960, 1961) have been described as have several secondary or acquired disaccharidase disorders (Bayless and Christopher, 1969). The latter disorders appear to result from gastrointestinal mucosal damage as in celiac disease or tropical sprue or secondary to decreases in protein synthesis as in kwashiorkor (Bowie et al., 1967), or neomycin administration (Paes et al., 1967), or associated with diseases that in themselves shorten gut transit time, such as small bowel resection or ulcerative colitis (Cady et al., 1967; Gaviser, 1948; Kern et al., 1963; Newcomer and McGill, 1967).

A. Lactase Deficiency

Lactose, the primary carbohydrate in milk, constitutes approximately 40% of the energy consumed by the newborn infant. The utilization of lactose for energy or to provide galactose for the synthesis of glycoproteins and lipids in nervous tissue involves the hydrolysis of this disaccharide to its component monosaccharides—glucose and galactose. The hydrolysis is accomplished through the activity of the enzyme lactase. Most of the activity of this enzyme is localized in the brush border fraction of the mucosal cells of the small intestine (Miller and Crane, 1961). Lactase activity appears to be more sensitive to digestive disturbances that affect mucosal cell integrity than the other disaccharidases (Littman and Hammond, 1965; Plotkin and Isselbacher, 1964). With lactase deficiency, lactose accumulates in the intestine followed by an increase in fluid volume, increased gut motility, and the subject may complain of bloating, intestinal cramps, malaise, and diarrhea (Dahlqvist, 1974; Gudmand-Hoyer et al., 1970; Holzel et al., 1959; McMichael et al., 1965).

Whether lactase deficiency is congenital or induced is subject to question. In populations that traditionally consume large quantities of dairy products, the incidence of lactase deficiency is relatively low; in populations whose postweaning diets contain little milk, lactase deficiency is prevalent. Lactase deficiency has been assessed by a lactose tolerance test or by jejunal biopsies or by both techniques. Lactose intolerance when assessed by the lactose tolerance test alone may also include individuals with genetic errors in galactose metabolism (see section on Glucose–Galactose Malabsorption).

Lactase deficiency has been reported in 55% of Mexican-American males (Dill et al., 1972); 73.8% of adult Mexicans from rural Mexico (Lisker et al., 1974); 44.7% of Greeks, 56% of Cretans, and 66% of Greek Cypriots (Kanaghinis et al., 1974); 68.8% of North American Jews (Leichter, 1971); 50% of Indian adults and 20% of Indian children (Reddy and Pershad, 1972); 45% of Negro children in the United States (Paige et al., 1971); 80% of Alaskan Eskimos (Duncan and Scott, 1972); and greater in Oriental adults compared with Caucasian adults (Davis and Bolin, 1967; Huang and Bayless, 1968; Nandi and Parham, 1972). Current evidence indicates that lactose intolerance is more common than lactose tolerance. Notable exceptions to these observations are Caucasians of Scandinavian or Northern European background. These populations have less than 5% with lactose intolerance and traditionally consume diets containing large amounts of milk and milk products.

Lactose intolerance appears to be age related. Prevalence of lactose intolerance is greater in adult populations than in populations of children, suggesting that if there is a genetic tendency toward lactase deficiency, this tendency may be modified by such environmental factors as milk availability, sanitation, adequacy of diet with respect to essential nutrients, and the presence of parasites (Bayless et al., 1971; Kretchmer et al., 1971; Paige and Graham, 1971). That lactose intolerance does not appear until after weaning and is related to milk drinking or avoidance suggests that high milk consumption may be a stimulus for prolonging lactase activity in the mucosal brush border during the postweaning period. (Lebenthal et al., 1975). Genetic studies of lactose intolerant families suggest that true lactase deficiency is an autosomal recessive trait (Flatz et al., 1969; Gudmand-Høyer et al., 1970; Sahi et al., 1973; Sowers and Winterfeld, 1975; Welsh, 1970; Welsh et al., 1968).

Therapy for lactose intolerant individuals consists simply of restricting lactose intakes. Some individuals tolerate fermented products such as yogurt and cheese fairly well, while varying amounts of milk or ice cream induce the typical symptoms of diarrhea and flatulence.

B. Sucrase–Isomaltase Deficiency

Sucrose, the most common disaccharide in the diet of modern man, provides up to 50% of the carbohydrate calories consumed. The hydrolysis of sucrose through the activity of sucrase yields glucose and fructose. In the absence of this enzyme, sucrose accumulates, and diarrhea, flatulence, nausea, and poor growth in infants result. The degree of severity of the symptoms varies with the amount of sucrose consumed. Sucrose intolerance has been described by Weijers et al. (1960, 1961) and Prader et al. (1961). In addition to sucrase deficiency, isomaltase deficiency is also present (Auricchio et al., 1963; Dahlqvist, 1962; Dahlqvist et al., 1963). These two enzymes are closely related and appear to be bound together in a complex in the mucosal brush border (Koluiska and Semenza, 1967).

Sucrase-isomaltase deficiency is quite rare with less than 100 cases reported (Bayless and Christopher, 1969; Prader and Auricchio, 1965). The disease appears to be a recessive trait; heterozygotes exhibit less than normal enzyme activity and may be mildly intolerant of sucrose (Burgess et al., 1964; Kerry and Townley, 1965). Infant homozygotes are more severely affected than adults. With age there is an apparent increase in sucrose tolerance indicating a possible diet induced increase in sucrase and isomaltase activity (Rosensweig and Herman, 1967).

Therapy consists of limiting sucrose intake so as to prevent the occurrence of diarrhea. Isomaltose, present in small quantities in starch, does not need to be restricted.

C. Maltase, Amylase Deficiencies

Maltose, a disaccharide composed of two molecules of glucose, is hydrolyzed through the activity of the enzyme maltase. Maltase intolerance cannot occur unless four or five enzymes (maltases) are missing simultaneously (Dahlqvist, 1966). Maltase deficiency is extremely rare having been described in only one patient (Weijers et al., 1961). Dahlqvist (1974) suggests in his review that this patient probably had a secondary disaccharidase deficiency rather than an inborn error in metabolism.

Amylase deficiency is similarly thought to be secondary to pancreatic dysfunction rather than to genetic error.

III. ERRORS AFFECTING INTESTINAL TRANSPORT

A. Glucose-Galactose Malabsorption

A syndrome characterized by growth failure in infants and diarrhea, described by Lindquist and Meeuwisse (1962, 1963) and by Laplane et al. (1962), has been shown to result from glucose-galactose malabsorption. The syndrome appears to be rare with 20 cases reported as of 1974 (Dahlqvist, 1974). Severe diarrhea with the stools containing large quantities of glucose and lactic acid is characteristic of the condition that, if untreated, results in death. Slight glucosuria and a lowered renal threshold for glucose has also been reported (Dubois et al., 1966). In patients with glucose-galactose intolerance, the association of impaired sugar transport by the intestine, slight glucosuria, and lowered renal threshold for glucose suggests the existence of two renal sugar carriers, such as has been demonstrated for lysine, only one of which is related to the intestinal sugar carrier (Scriver, 1967).

Malabsorption of glucose and galactose in the presence of normal absorption of fructose and passively absorbed sugars indicates that the genetic error resides within the sodium-dependent, glucose–galactose carrier in the small intestine brush border (Holzel, 1968). Further evidence that the error resides within the carrier can be seen in the determination of the transport of 3-*O*-methylglucose. If the subject has the syndrome, 3-*O*-methylglucose will be recovered in the feces; if not, this synthetic sugar will be recovered in the urine (Holzel, 1968). Linneweh et al. (1966) found that affected individuals could accumulate less than 10% of the administered sugars in the mucosal cells, whereas nonaffected individuals could accumulate up to nine times that amount. Intravenously administered glucose and galactose appear to be well tolerated (Holzel, 1968).

Family studies permit the conclusion that the disease is inherited by an autosomal recessive mode (Lindquist et al., 1963). Infants with the disorder have apparently healthy parents. Although both sexes are affected, of the cases reported, 75% were female. The few studies of siblings of affected infants showed that two out of eight also have the disorder (Anderson et al., 1965; Laplane et al., 1962; Linneweh et al., 1966). Studies of the pedigrees of six Swedish patients showed a high frequency of consanguineous marriage among ancesters, thus documenting the recessive mode of inheritance (Lindquist, 1967; Melin and Meeuwisse, 1969).

Treatment of patients with glucose–galactose malabsorption consists of feeding a glucose–galactose free diet. Prompt recovery is observed.

IV. ERRORS IN THE INTERCONVERSION OF SUGARS

While the metabolic fuel of choice is glucose, all tissues can use carbohydrates other than glucose as a significant source of energy and metabolic intermediates. The variety of compounds that can be utilized varies with the tissues from the highly versatile liver to the highly selective nervous system. A number of mechanisms exist for the interconversion and metabolism of the various sugars. Conversion or utilization of these sugars requires a number of different enzymes; the absence of any one of these enzymes could be detrimental to the individual. Genetic errors in the metabolism of galactose (galactosemia), fructose (fructosemia), and xylulose (pentosuria) have been observed.

A. Galactosemia

Galactose utilization by mammals depends largely on the Leloir (1951) pathway in the liver and red blood cells. Galactose is phosphorylated in the presence of magnesium and ATP to galactose 1-phosphate through the activity of galactokinase (Ballard, 1966). Galactose 1-phosphate is converted by galactose UDP by the enzyme galactose 1-phosphate uridyl transferase (Kalckar, 1965). This reaction can also be catalyzed by hepatic UDP-galactose pyrophosphatase, an enzyme with a higher K_m for galactose 1-phosphate than the transferase. Galactose UDP is necessary for the synthesis of galactose derivatives (lactose, galactolipids, chondroitin sulfate, etc.). Galactose UDP can be converted to glucose UDP through the activity of UDP galactose epimerase.

In galactosemia, the enzyme galactose-1-P transferase may be missing or deficient, resulting in an accumulation of galactose 1-phosphate. When galactose accumulates, the presence of aldose reductase and reduced pyridine nucleotide promotes the formation of galactitol, a nonmetabolizable sugar alcohol. Intracellular accumulation of galactitol leads to osmotic swelling of the peripheral nerves of rats (Gabbay and Snider, 1972), and motor nerve dysfunction results. The withdrawal of galactose from the diet reverses this effect. Galactitol accumulates in the brain and the lens causing the formation of cataracts (Gitzelmann et al., 1967; Wells et al., 1964). As galactose 1-phosphate accumulates, galactose, galactitol, and galactonic acid are excreted in the urine (Bergren et al., 1972).

Symptoms of galactosemia usually manifest themselves shortly after birth and are causally related to the ingestion of milk. The main clinical features include cataract formation, mental retardation, hepatosplenomegaly, and nutritional failure. Reduced blood glucose levels and reduced mutase, dehydrogenase, and pyrophosphorylase enzyme activities have also been reported (Sidbury, 1957; Sidbury et al., 1962). Reduced mutase activity would be expected to affect glycogen synthesis, whereas reduced dehydrogenase and pyrophosphorylase activities would affect glucose metabolism.

Defects in galactose metabolism other than a deficiency in transferase activity have also been reported (Gitzelmann, 1967). Galactokinase has been shown to be deficient in a number of families with galactose and galactitol but not galactose 1-phosphate accumulating in the tissues (Dahlqvist et al., 1963; Gitzelmann, 1967; Olambiwonnee et al., 1974; Pickering and Howell, 1972). The other toxic features of galactosemia were not noted with the exception of cataract formation in the lens. Thus, it appears that galactitol is the causative agent for the lens defect.

A deficiency of the erythrocyte epimerase has also been reported (Gitzelmann, 1972) as has a variant of the transferase enzyme (the Duarte variant) that has half the activity of the normal transferase enzyme (Beutler et al., 1965). Individuals with these errors appear to be able to tolerate larger quantities of dietary lactose than individuals with a true transferase or kinase deficiency. As patients grow older it appears that they can tolerate larger quantities of galactose in their diets (Komrower et al., 1956); however, restriction of galactose intake is essential in the infant and child to prevent the formation of cataracts and the development of mental retardation.

All evidence to date indicates that all forms of galactosemia are genetic disorders involving a single autosomal recessive gene. Heterozygotes can be identified on the basis of lower than normal enzyme activity (transferase, kinase or epimerase) (Brettauer et al., 1959; Dahlqvist et al., 1963; Hugh-Jones et al., 1960; Kirkman, 1959; Pickering and Howell, 1972).

B. Fructosemia

Fructose, the ketohexose in fruits and sucrose, is metabolized primarily by the liver, kidney, and intestinal mucosa (Bollman and Mann, 1931; Levine and Huddleston, 1947; Mendeloff and Weichselbaum, 1953; Reinecke, 1944). While fructose can theoretically be phosphorylated and metabolized in all tissues, the hexokinase responsible for this phosphorylation in the peripheral tissues has a greater affinity for glucose than for fructose (Mackler and Guest, 1953; Nakada, 1956). Likewise, hepatic hexokinase has a greater affinity for glucose and, therefore, phosphorylates glucose in preference to fructose or mannose (Sols and Crane, 1954). Fructose is phosphorylated through the action of fructokinase to fructose 1-phosphate (Cori et al., 1951). The reaction requires Mg, ATP, and K^+ (Hers, 1952a, b; Sanchez et al., 1971). Fructokinase also catalyzes the phosphorylation of other ketosugars, depending on the concentration of potassium (Adelman et al., 1967; Sanchez et al., 1971). Fructose 1-phosphate is then split to yield D-glyceraldehyde and dihydroxyacetone phosphate. Two moles of the latter triose phosphate can be recombined to form fructose 1,6-diphosphate through the action of phosphofructoaldolase (Hers and Kusaka, 1953; Leuthardt et al., 1953). Fructose 1,6-diphosphate then is hydrolyzed to yield glyceraldehyde 3-phosphate and dihydroxyacetone phosphate; these triose phosphates are then metabolized via the glycolytic pathway.

Three errors in fructose metabolism have been identified. One relatively harmless error called essential fructosuria is characterized by the absence of fructokinase in the liver (Schapira et al., 1961), elevations in serum fructose levels, and excretion of fructose in the urine. The second disorder, called hereditary fructose intolerance, is characterized by a severe hypoglycemic response to a fructose load, hypophosphotemia, vomiting, and a decreased activity of hepatic fructose-1-phosphate aldolase (Hers and Joassin, 1961). The decreased activity has been shown to be due to a structural alteration of the enzyme protein that results in a reduced affinity for fructose 1-phosphate (Koster et al., 1975). The hypoglycemic response to fructose appears to be unresponsive to glucagon (Hers, 1974) and is thought to be the result of an inhibition of glycogenolysis by the accumulated fructose 1-phosphate (Froesch, 1966; Hers and Joassin, 1961; Morris et al., 1967; Nisell and Linden, 1968). High hepatic glycogen levels have been reported causing some patients to be misdiagnosed initially as having glycogen storage disease (Cain and Ryman, 1971). In patients consuming large quantities of fructose, damage to the renal proximal convoluted tubules has been observed (Kranhold et al., 1969).

A third disorder in fructose metabolism has been described. This disorder is characterized by a striking deficiency of hepatic fructose-1,6-diphosphatase activity (Baker and Winegrad, 1970; Corbeel et al., 1970; Pagliara et al., 1972). Oral glucose and galactose tolerance is normal, but hypoglycemia and metabolic acidosis is observed in the fasted patient. While hepatic fructose-1,6-diphosphatase is deficient, muscle fructose-1,6-diphosphatase is normal, suggesting that these two enzymes are as genetically distinct in the human as they are in the rabbit (Euser et al., 1969). More properly, this disorder is an error in gluconeogenesis rather than in fructose metabolism.

All three disorders are apparently inherited as an autosomal recessive trait (Froesch, 1966; Landau et al., 1971). These conclusions are based on the reports that siblings of both sexes but not parents or offspring had the disorder. Three families have been reported with hereditary fructose intolerance that do not fit into the usual pattern of autosomal recessive inheritance (Froesch, 1966; Wolf et al., 1959). In these families, both parents and offspring had the trait, suggesting a dominant inheritance. However, since heterozygotes cannot be readily identified, recessive inheritance cannot be ruled out in these families. The offspring could have had an affected homozygous parent and a normal heterozygous parent.

C. Pentosuria

While glucose, fructose, and sucrose are the main sugars in the human diet, small amounts of the five-carbon sugars are also consumed. Xylose or xylulose (the keto sugar) is present in plums, cherries, grapes, and certain fruit juices (Johnstone, 1906). D-xylulose is a normal constituent of the hexosemono-phosphate shunt; however, the naturally occurring compound is the L-isomer. If this isomer is to be utilized, it must be converted to the D-form. This is done by converting L-xylulose to xylitol through the action of NADP-linked xylitol dehydrogenase (Wang and van Eys, 1970). The xylitol is then oxidized in an NAD-dependent reaction to D-xylulose. D-xylulose, after conversion to D-xylu-lose 5-phosphate with ATP as the phosphate donor, is further metabolized via the hexose monophosphate shunt.

In pentosuria, the NADP-linked xylitol dehydrogenase is either missing or deficient (Wang and van Eys, 1970). This rather minor defect results in an increased (1–4 g/day) excretion of L-xylulose in the urine (Garrod, 1908; Touster, 1959) and is related to the activity of the glucuronic pathway (Hiatt, 1965). Increased levels of ribose in the urine (up to 0.03 g/day) have been reported for patients with muscular dystrophy; however, it is thought that this ribose arises from excessive muscle coenzyme breakdown (Hiatt, 1965). Increased levels of xylulose in the urine have been observed when large quantities of xylose-containing fruits are consumed or when large doses of glucuronic acid are administered (Hiatt, 1965). Knox (1958) has suggested that renal tubule reabsorption of xylulose may also be defective. This suggestion, however, has been disputed (Hiatt, 1965). The increased levels of xylulose in the urine can lead to a misdiagnosis of diabetes mellitus since the pentose is a reducing sugar giving a false positive reaction when the urine is not specifically tested for glucose. Sometimes, the misdiagnosis is corrected when the patient suffers an episode of insulin-induced hypoglycemia. There appears to be no relationship between diabetes and pentosuria.

Estimates of the incidence of pentosuria vary. Since the defect produces no impairment of health, it is likely that many persons with the defect go undetected. From life insurance statistics, it is estimated that 1 in 50,000 persons are affected. All of the reported cases were Jews primarily of Eastern European origin (Larson et al., 1941; Wright, 1961). The defect appears to be an autosomal recessive characteristic with the homozygous state required for the expression of the defect. Heterozygotes can be identified on the basis of their reduced ability to metabolize a load dose of glucuronolactone (Freedberg et al., 1959).

V. ERRORS IN GLUCOSE CATABOLISM

Glucose, once it has entered the cell, is phosphorylated through the action of gluco- or hexokinase. Glucose 6-phosphate then may be used for the synthesis of glycogen or metabolized to pyruvate via the glycolytic pathway or the hexosemonophosphate shunt; glucose 6-phosphate may also be dephosphorylated to yield glucose through the activity of glucose-6-phosphatase. Several errors (and their variations) in glucose catabolism have been studied and reported extensively. Errors that occur in the erythrocyte may result in hemolytic anemia.

A. Glucose-6-Phosphate Dehydrogenase Deficiency

In the red blood cells, the activity of glucokinase is low relative to the activities of the enzymes involved in later reactions of glucose catabolism. Once the glucose is phosphorylated, most of it is metabolized via the glycolytic pathway to lactate and pyruvate. A small percentage of the glucose is metabolized via the hexose monophosphate shunt. The degree to which glycolysis predominates over the shunt in the catabolism of glucose depends on the pH of the fluid surrounding the erythrocyte, the activity of glucose-6-phosphate dehydrogenase (G6PD), and the rate of oxidation of NADPH (Kellermeyer et al., 1961; Murphy, 1960).

G6PD catalyzes the initial reaction in the hexose monophosphate shunt. It is a NADP-linked enzyme, generating reducing equivalents for hydroxylation reactions. The most important of these reactions in the red blood cell is the reduction of oxidized glutathione via the NADPH-requiring glutathione reductase (Gaetini et al., 1974). Erythrocytes from G6PD-deficient individuals appear to be unable to provide NADPH at a rate sufficient to maintain the glutathione in a reduced form during exposure to drugs whose metabolism is also NADPH dependent (Gaetani et al., 1974; Welt et al., 1971). Drugs such as acetanilid and related analgesics, sulfonamides, primaquine and related antimalarials, non-sulfonamide antibacterial agents, and several miscellaneous compounds have been identified as precipitating agents (Beutler, 1965).

More than 80 variants of G6PD, distinguishable by their various physical and chemical characteristics, have been reported (Yoshida et al., 1971). Half of these 80 variants have normal enzyme activity and are not associated with any clinical abnormalities. About half of the remaining variants result in chronic enzyme deficiency but require exogenous agents such as antimalarial drugs, naphthalene, or methylene blue for hemolysis to occur. The remaining variants result in chronic nonspherocytic hemolytic anemia, even in the absence of precipitating agents. Some of the enzyme variants have a low affinity for glucose 6-phosphate; however, this is not the case for other variants.

The severity of the enzyme deficiency does not correlate well with the clinical severity of the anemia. While the kinetic characteristics of the enzyme itself cannot totally explain this discrepancy, studies of the variant enzymes have shown that these enzymes are strongly inhibited by physiologic concentrations of NADPH and are sensitive to inhibition by ATP (Yoshida, 1973). Thus, the variant enzymes cannot generate enough NADPH to maintain an adequate concentration of reduced glutathione that, in turn, appears to be necessary for the maintenance of sulfhydryl groups within the red cell and the red cell membrane. When the levels of oxidized glutathione exceed tolerable limits, hemolysis of the cell results.

G6PD deficiency, one of the most common genetic errors in metabolism, probably affects more than 100 million persons (Marks, 1966; Yoshida, 1973). The gene determining G6PD structure (and hence G6PD activity) is located on the X chromosome (Kirkman and Henderson, 1963) and almost twice as many females as males carry the genetic code for G6PD deficiency. Because the code is sex-linked, more males than females are affected. The defect is of intermediate dominance, with homozygous males and females having full expression of the trait. Heterozygous females may not show the trait on screening and may be free of any clinical symptoms.

The incidence of G6PD deficiency varies markedly in different populations (Motulsky et al., 1971). An incidence of 60% among Kurdish Jews, 5-7% among Asian Indians, 0.4% among Ashkanazee Jews, and 2% among Chinese has been reported (Jolly et al., 1972; Marks, 1966). G6PD deficiency has been found to be prevalent in populations subject to malaria (Luzzatto, 1973; Motulsky and Stamatoyannopoulos, 1966; Piomelli and Siniscalco, 1969) and carrying the sickle cell anemia trait (Beutler et al., 1974). It seems debatable whether the G6PD trait has survival value to populations residing in endemic malarial regions.

B. Pyruvate Kinase Deficiency

When glucose is metabolized via the glycolytic pathway, it is hydrolyzed to two three-carbon fragments that are then converted to phosphoenolpyruvate (PEP). PEP is converted to pyruvate through the activity of pyruvate kinase. For each mole of glucose two moles of ATP are produced from ADP. In the subsequent reaction, pyruvate is converted to lactate through the action of lactate dehydrogenase with the simultaneous oxidation of NADH to NAD. In patients with nonspherocytic anemia there is a deficiency in pyruvate kinase activity with a consequent 70-75% reduction in glucose oxidation by the erythrocyte (Robinson et al., 1961; Selwyn and Dacie, 1954). The disease is characterized by an accumulation of phosphorylated glucose metabolites in the red blood cells and by jaundice and anemia, particularly in the newborn. Some patients have little or no jaundice and no anemia until adulthood, while others are severely handicapped as children. An enlarged spleen and liver are sometimes observed, and there is a severe shortening of the red cell lifespan.

Since pyruvate kinase catalyzes a reaction that provides for the regeneration of ATP from ADP, it is to be expected that defective cells would have lowered ATP (Robinson, 1963), as well as lowered NAD, levels (Oski and Diamond, 1963). The lowered ATP level is related to the hemolysis of the red cell by an as yet unknown mechanism.

Pyruvate kinase deficiency of the red cell is transmitted as an autosomal recessive trait (Oski et al., 1964). Homozygotes have hemolytic anemia and deficient pyruvate kinase activity. Heterozygotes have no anemia but have lower than normal enzyme activity. There is considerable variation in enzyme activity among heterozygotes. The frequency of defect is unknown but has been reported to occur in populations from Northern Europe, Mexico, and Syria. Both sexes are affected equally (Tanaka et al., 1962).

C. Muscle Phosphofructokinase Deficiency (Type VII Glycogenosis)

A rare defect in the phosphorylation of fructose 6-phosphate has been described in three siblings (Nishikawa et al., 1965; Tarui et al., 1965, 1969) who were easily fatigued by exercise. In these patients, it has been shown that there was a deficiency in the activity of muscle phosphofructokinase. This enzyme catalyzes the conversion of fructose 6-phosphate to fructose 1,6-diphosphate, one of the rate-limiting steps in the glycolytic pathway. This step is also an essential step in glycogenolysis. Patients with this defect accumulate glucose and fructose phosphates in their muscles because they are unable to metabolize these sugars further to lactic acid during or immediately after exercise. Since this metabolic block occurs prior to the formation of ATP, energy is not available to the muscles for work from either glucose or glycogen. Apparently normal levels of phosphofructokinase activity are found in the leukocytes or hepatocytes. A slightly lower enzyme activity is found in erythrocytes (Layzer et al., 1967). While only a few patients and their families have been studied, it appears likely that this disorder is inherited as an autosomal recessive trait.

VI. ERRORS IN GLUCONEOGENESIS

Gluconeogenesis, or the synthesis of glucose from nonglucose precursors, takes place primarily in the liver and kidney. Gluconeogenesis provides glucose during starvation or during periods of high-fat feeding, allows the free utilization of lactate (via the Cori cycle) and the utilization of glycerol. The main enzymes of gluconeogenesis are those involved in the conversion of pyruvate to oxalacetate and phosphoenolpyruvate, hexose diphosphatase and glucose-6-phosphatase (G6Pase). Genetic errors responsible for deficiencies in the last two enzymes have been reported. Fructose-1,6-diphosphatase deficiency has been described under errors in fructose metabolism (see section on Fructosemia above).

A. Glucose-6-Phosphatase Deficiency
(Von Gierke's Disease:
Type I Glycogenosis)

In 1929, Von Gierke described two patients having enlarged livers, elevated liver glycogen levels, and hypoglycemia upon fasting. It was assumed that this disease was caused by a defect in the breakdown of glycogen to glucose. This defect was identified by Cori and Cori (1952) as a deficiency in G6Pase activity. This enzyme is required not only for glycogenolysis but also for gluconeogenesis. The enzyme is found primarily in the liver and kidney, where it is bound to the endoplasmic reticulum of the cell and catalyzes the release of free glucose from glucose 6-phosphate. Microsomal G6Pase and pyrophosphatase activity appear to reside within the same enzyme complex and both activities are deficient in patients with type I glycogenolysis (Illingworth and Cori, 1965). Both liver and kidney are involved in this type of glycogenosis; muscle, however, is normal. G6Pase deficiency is accompanied by a diminished triglyceride clearance and a decreased postheparin lipoprotein lipase activity (Forget et al., 1974). Hyperlipemia is a common finding (Fernandes and Pikaar, 1969; Howell et al., 1971; Jacovic et al., 1966). Liver biopsies from patients with this disease have been found to have high *de novo* fatty acid synthesizing activity from citrate (Hulsmann et al., 1970). Acidosis, ketosis, retarded growth and development, and shortened lifespan have also been observed (Fine et al., 1969; Hers, 1974).

The deficiency in G6Pase can adequately explain the fasting hypoglycemia, the lack of hyperglycemic response to glucagon and epinephrine, and the failure of administered galactose or fructose to be converted to glucose (Hug, 1962; Mason and Anderson, 1955; Schwartz et al., 1957). G6Pase activity is essential for rapid glucose recycling time (Hers et al., 1974).

The lack of a hyperglycemic response to glucagon cannot be interpreted as an unresponsiveness to glucagon per se, but as a difference in the end result of glucagon action. In G6Pase-deficient patients, glucagon administration results in an increase in blood lactate levels (Sarcione et al., 1970). This observation suggests that the excess glycogen in the liver in G6Pase-deficient individuals is not a consequence of the enzyme deficiency but is secondary to factors that enhance glycogen synthesis and inhibit its breakdown. Among such factors might be insulin. Initially, G6Pase-deficient patients tend to be hyperinsulinemic but with age their peripheral tissues become more resistant to insulin (Lockwood et al., 1969). The decreased sensitivity and normalization of glucose tolerance with age may thus explain the normalization of blood glucose levels as the patients grow older.

There appears to be some variation in the severity of the disease due in part to the ability of the individual to circumvent the enzyme deficiency. Severely affected children die early in childhood, while less severely affected individuals adapt in some manner to the defect. This adaptation may involve hyposensitivity to insulin, as well as to other mechanisms developed for the stabilization of blood glucose levels during fasting. Studies of glycerol disappearance in G6Pase-deficient subjects showed that glycerol disappeared more rapidly in the deficient subjects than in the normal subjects (Senior and Loridan, 1968). It has been suggested that glycerol is utilized to form a highly branched glycogen that when subject to glycogenolysis yields free glucose rather than phosphorylated glucose from each branch (1,6-linkage) point (Sadeghi-Nejad et al., 1970). This suggestion is based on the findings of greater amylo-α-1,6-glucosidase and fructose-1,6-diphosphatase activities in G6Pase-deficient subjects than in normal subjects (Sadeghi-Nejad et al., 1970). It is also possible that glucose released by the livers of G6Pase-deficient patients may be due to an increase in the activities of nonspecific phosphatases and/or an increase in the activity of a lysosomal acid maltase acting on the α-1,4-linkages of glycogen (Hers, 1964).

G6Pase deficiency is rare and usually fatal. It is inherited as an autosomal recessive trait (Sokal et al., 1962). Of all the patients with glycogenesis, 25% are G6Pase deficient (Ockerman, 1972). G6Pase deficiency has been detected more frequently in Israel than in the United States or Northern Europe. Both sexes are equally affected.

VII. ERRORS IN GLYCOGEN SYNTHESIS

Some of the glucose consumed in excess of immediate energy needs is stored in the liver, muscles, and other tissues as a complex polysaccharide, glycogen. Glycogen synthesis begins with the phosphorylation of glucose to form glucose 6-phosphate. Glucose 6-phosphate is isomerized through the action of phosphoglucomutase to glucose 1-phosphate. Glucose 1-phosphate can also be synthesized directly from glucose, in the presence of ATP, through the action of L-glucose-1-phosphate kinase and d-glucose-1-phosphate dismutase (Smith et al., 1968). Glucose 1-phosphate is then converted to uridine diphosphate glucose (UDP-glucose) through the action of UDPG pyrophosphorylase. UDP-glucose is added to a "primer" glucosyl 1,4-unit increasing its length by one glucose unit; this reaction is catalyzed by the enzyme UDPG-glycogen transglucosylase. Finally, the complex, branched-chain polysaccharide, glycogen, is formed by transferring a glucosyl 1,4-unit to another glucosyl unit in a 1,6-linkage instead of a 1,4-linkage. This is done through the action of amylo(1,4 → 1,6)transglucosidase (the branching enzyme). This enzyme becomes active when a peripheral chain of growing glycogens reaches between 7 and 21 glycosyl units by means of successive transfers from UDPG; the transglucosidase transfers a string of 1,4-linked glucosyl units from their proximal 1,4-attachment on the main chain to a 1,6-attachment to the same or another growing chain of glycosyl units (Larner, 1953).

A. Amylopectinosis (Type IV Glycogenesis)

One of the rarest of the glycogen storage diseases is one in which the enzyme amylo(1,4 → 1,6)transglucosidase is deficient (Brown and Brown, 1966). The disease is characterized by the accumulation of glycogen with very long, nonbranched chains (Anderson, 1956) and of low molecular weight (Krivit et al., 1973). This low-molecular-weight glycogen cannot serve as a "primer" for glycogen synthesis (Shen et al., 1972). Infants with this disorder appear normal at birth but soon fail to thrive. Enlarged livers, poor weight gains, hypotonia, and enlarged spleens have been observed in these infants (Howell et al., 1971). The branching enzyme has been found to be deficient in liver, leukocytes, and skin fibroblasts (Brown and Brown, 1966; Fernandes and Huijing, 1968; Howell et al., 1971). Patients with this disease have not survived beyond childhood.

Family studies suggest that this disorder is genetically transmitted as an autosomal recessive trait. Heterozygotes can be identified on the basis of decreased branching enzyme activity in their leukocytes (Howell et al., 1971; Legum and Nitowsky, 1969).

VIII. ERRORS IN GLYCOGEN UTILIZATION

In times of glucose need, glycogen serves as a ready source of glucose units. Glycogen breakdown is rapid and is stimulated or enhanced by glucagon and epinephrine; glycogenolysis is inhibited by insulin. Glycogenolysis proceeds by a pathway similar to glycogenesis but separate from it (Leloir and Cardini, 1957). Glycogenolysis is initiated through the activation of phosphorylase. Phosphorylases from several different tissues have been studied, and it has become apparent that they are not identical. The differences in structure and cofactor requirements possibly reflect the differences in metabolism in the different tissues. In general, however, glycogen is degraded through the action of phosphorylase, in the presence of PO_4^{3-}, producing glucose 1-phosphate.

The outer chains of glycogen constitute approximately 60% of the total glucose residues; therefore, a relatively large proportion of the glucose liberated from glycogen is liberated through the action of phosphorylase alone (Smith et al., 1968). The very rapid rate of glycogen degradation in mammalian cells is probably due to the high affinity of the phosphorylase enzyme for the branched chain glycogen and to the high concentration of the enzyme in the cell. However, in order for the phosphorylase to act on the glycogen it must be activated. Part of the activation consists of the attachment of the prosthetic group pyridoxal phosphate (Cori and Illingworth, 1957; Hedrick et al., 1966). In muscle the inactive phosphorylase *b* in the presence of AMP and phosphorylase *b* kinase becomes the active phosphorylase *a* (Krebs et al., 1958). The activation of the phosphorylase in other tissues is similar to that occurring in muscle. The phosphorylase enzyme cannot attack the α-1,6-linkage in the glycogen structure. As a result, the next step in glycogenolysis is accomplished through the activity of amylo-1,6-glucosidase (the debranching enzyme). This reaction can result in free or phosphorylated glucose.

The α-1,4-linkage of glycogen can also be attacked by a group of enzymes known as α-amylases. These enzymes contain at least one calcium atom per molecule; the calcium appears to stabilize the tertiary structure and the catalytic activity of the enzyme (Fischer and Stein, 1960; Vallee et al., 1959; Whelan, 1960). The products of α-amylase action are maltose, maltotriose, and limit dextrin containing α-1,6-linkages (Whelan, 1960). Maltotriose is gradually hydrolyzed to maltose and glucose (Walker and Whelan, 1960).

Glycogen can be hydrolyzed from the nonreducing end by a group of enzymes called α-glucosidases. In muscle and liver several forms of the α-glucosidases exist (Smith et al., 1968). None is present in large amounts. The enzymes can be distinguished by the pH at which they are optimally active. "Acid" α-glucosidases occur chiefly in the microsomal and supernatant fractions of cell homogenates (Lejeune et al., 1963). Although the significance of the glucosidases is as yet unclear, one inherited disorder of glycogen utilization has been described in which the lysosomal α-glucosidase is absent (Pompe's disease). Other errors in glycogenolysis have also been identified and described (Hers, 1963, 1964).

A. Pompe's Disease (Type II Glycogenosis)

Generalized glycogen storage in the viscera, skeletal, and cardiac muscle and muscle weakness was described almost simultaneously by Pompe and Putschar in 1932. As excessive glycogen accumulates in the affected organs, their functionality is affected. Although glycogen accumulates in all tissues, the usual cause of death in infants with this disorder is due to cardiac failure. Individuals with Pompe's disease rarely survive childhood; however, several cases in their second decade have been reported (Courtecuisse et al., 1965; Engel, 1970; Illingworth-Brown and Zellweger, 1966; Roth and Williams 1967; Swaiman et al., 1968). A deficiency in lysosomal α-1,4-glucosidase (acid maltase) has been identified as the defect leading to tissue glycogen accumulation (Hers, 1963). In addition to the glycogen, other nonglycogenic carbohydrates have been reported to accumulate (Wolfe and Cohen, 1968). This material is present in the form of granular to globular intracytoplasmic deposits. The amount deposited varies from site to site, and the degree of storage does not always parallel the degree of glycogen storage. An increased excretion of a glucose-containing tetrasaccharide in urine has been reported (Hallgren et al., 1974). It has been suggested that this compound is an end product of α-amylase action on glycogen.

In addition to acid maltase deficiency, Pompe's disease may involve the relative deficiency of other enzymes as well. Garancis (1968) suggested that differences in glycogen deposition patterns indicate that another enzyme not bound to the lysosomes might be deficient as well. This suggestion has not been followed in subsequent work, although Koster et al. (1975) have reported that patients with a variant of Pompe's disease had some acid maltase in their leukocytes while having none at all in muscle.

Pompe's disease is a genetic disease inherited in an autosomal recessive manner. There is a 40–50% incidence in affected families, which is, however, twice the predicted 25% of the Mendelian ratio for recessives (Spach et al., 1966). The reason for this increase in incidence is unknown.

B. Forbe's Disease (Type III Glycogenosis)

Forbe's disease is characterized by a partial or complete deficiency of the glycogen-debranching enzyme system. The glycogen debranching system catalyzes the debranching of glycogen in two steps: uncovering the branching point by oligo(1,4 → 1,4)glucantransferase followed by the hydrolysis of the 1,6-glucosidic linkage by amylo-1,6-glucosidase (Brown and Illingworth, 1964). The two enzymes appear to be closely associated perhaps within a single protein or enzyme complex (Nelson et al., 1969; Taylor and Whelan, 1968). The symptoms of Forbe's disease are similar to those of Von Gierke's disease and Hers' disease (liver phosphorylase deficiency). The main symptoms are enlarged liver, hypoglycemia, acidosis, muscular weakness, and enlarged heart. Absence of the debranching enzyme has been shown in the leukocytes, erythrocytes, muscle, and liver (Moses et al., 1968; Steinitz, 1962; Van Creveld and Huijing, 1964). The polysaccharide that accumulates in the tissues has the structure of a phosphorylase limit dextrin in which the outer chains are much shorter than in normal glycogen. There are several variants of type III glycogenosis; for example, in type IIIa the debranching enzyme is missing in all tissues. In other variants the enzyme is missing or inactive in some tissues but not in others. These variants probably result from allelic mutations of the same gene (Hers, 1974; Van Hoof and Hers, 1968). In all variants the glycogen-rich cells have a more rapid utilization of glucose as evaluated by [^{14}C]glucose utilization studies (Moses et al., 1968). This increase in glucose utilization is not reflected by a higher lactate production (Moses et al., 1968), and it is possible that the increased utilization was due to an incorporation of the radioactive glucose into newly formed or extended glycogen.

Family studies by Williams and Field (1968) and by Esmann et al. (1969) indicate that amylo-1,6-glucosidase deficiency is inherited as an autosomal recessive trait. Homozygotes can be identified on the basis of their leukocyte enzyme activity. Heterozygotes cannot be clearly identified, and both sexes are affected.

C. McArdle's Disease (Type V Glycogenosis)

The disease caused by muscle phosphorylase deficiency consists of painful muscle cramps with exercise followed occasionally by muscle necrosis and myoglobinuria. The disease was originally described by McArdle in 1951 and later by Schmid and Mahler (1959). Excessive levels of glycogen in the muscles have been noted in some patients but not in others (Mellick et al., 1962).

A characteristic feature of the disorder is the lack of lactate formation during muscular activity (Porte et al., 1966). Patients with this disease have a reduced (50%) oxygen uptake, reduced (15–20% of normal) oxygen debt (Anderson et al., 1969), and an increased alanine metabolism during exercise (Wahren et al., 1973). Only muscle phosphorylase is deficient; fibroblast, erythrocyte, and hepatic phosphorylase activity is normal (Pearson et al., 1961; Schmid and Mahler, 1959).

The disease appears to be essentially benign. While most patients appear to be intolerant of exercise from childhood, two instances of late-onset disease have been recorded (Engel, 1970). Of these two patients, muscle wasting was apparent in one but not in the other. Acute renal failure, accompanied by rhabdomyolysis and transient hypercalcemia, has been reported in two patients (Grunfeld et al., 1972). Nonetheless, involvement of the kidneys does not appear to be a common feature.

Family studies of patients with McArdle's disease indicate that the disease is transmitted by an autosomal recessive mode of inheritance (Dawson et al., 1968; Tobin and Coleman, 1965). Patients of both sexes have been studied and reported.

D. Hers' Disease (Type VI Glycogenosis)

Excess glycogen stores in the liver due to a deficiency in liver phosphorylase was described by Hers in 1959. In these patients, the low residual phosphorylase activity is not stimulated by 5'-AMP (Koster et al., 1975) or by the addition of phosphorylase kinase (Hug and Schubert, 1970). Only a few cases of true liver phosphorylase deficiency have been reported; other cases thought to be phosphorylase deficient have now been found to be deficient in the phosphorylase activating system. (The latter deficiency has been classed as type IX glycogenosis and will be discussed below.) Type VI glycogenosis is characterized by hepatomegaly, growth retardation, and an elevated serum lipid level (Hug et al., 1974). The muscular and cardiovascular systems are normal. Aside from the enlarged liver and the growth retardation, the disease is relatively mild. From the few cases shown to be truly deficient in phosphorylase activity, it appears that this inherited defect is transmitted in an autosomal recessive manner (Hug et al., 1974).

E. Type IX Glycogenosis

While type IX glycogenosis is characterized by low phosphorylase activity in the liver and leukocytes, the disease is not due to a deficiency in the enzyme per se but to a deficient activating system (Hug et al., 1966, 1969; Huijing, 1967, 1968, 1970). The phosphorylase enzyme exists in an active form (phosphophosphorylase) and an inactive form (dephosphophosphorylase). Phosphophosphorylase phosphatase catalyzes the conversion of the active to the inactive form; dephosphophosphorylase kinase catalyzes the inactive to the active form. The latter reaction requires ATP, bivalent ions, and the presence of cAMP. Evidence that the reduced phosphorylase activity was due to a deficiency in the activating system was provided by the studies of Huijing (1967, 1968), which showed that phosphorylase activity could be restored in tissues from type IX glycogenosis patients by the addition of cAMP or dephosphophosphorylase kinase. Hug et al. (1969) showed that treatment of such patients with long-lasting glucagon activated the kinase enzyme. This led Huijing (1970) to suggest that the deficient activation was due to a low affinity of the enzyme (kinase) for its substrate (phosphorylase). Muscle phosphorylase kinase and cAMP kinase have also been shown to be deficient in one subject with type IX glycogenosis (Hug et al., 1970).

Type IX glycogenosis manifests itself only in childhood, mainly as hepatomegaly (Huijing, 1970). Although enlarged, the liver maintains normal or nearly normal function. There may be some muscle weakness, but both the enlarged liver and muscle weakness disappear by puberty. Blood lipids are frequently elevated (Fernandes and Pikaar, 1969) and hypoglycemia can be observed after prolonged fasting (Fernandes et al., 1969). Patients can be identified on the basis of low leukocyte phosphorylase activity; true hepatic phosphorylase deficient (type VI) patients have normal leukocyte phosphorylase activity (Hulsmann et al., 1961; Schwartz et al., 1970; Williams and Field, 1961). Gluconeogenesis is greater in patients with type IX glycogenosis than in normal subjects (Huijing, 1970). This increase is probably compensatory to the decreased availability of glucose from glycogen in times of need. The increase in gluconeogenesis places an added burden on the protein requirement for these patients, since protein is needed not only for tissue protein synthesis but also to supply glucose via gluconeogenesis during those periods when the patients are without food.

The disease is relatively mild with no clear-cut reduction in lifespan or fertility (Huijing and Fernandes, 1969). The patients studied have been males (homozygotes) and heterozygote carrier females indicating a sex-linked recessive mode of inheritance (Esman et al., 1969; Huijing, 1970; Huijing and Fernandes, 1969).

IX. ERRORS LEADING TO ABNORMAL CARBOHYDRATE CONVERSION TO LIPID

The idea that genetic factors contribute to the development of hyperlipemia, heart disease, and abnormal glucose tolerance is not new. However, the mechanism of this genetic involvement or indeed the locus of the genetic error has not been clearly demonstrated. In 1897, Osler indicated that heart disease "runs" in families. More recently, epidemiological studies have shown that this genetic tendency is due largely to the clustering in certain families of risk factors such as hyperlipemia, diabetes, and hypertension (Gertler and White, 1954; Simborg, 1970; Slack and Evans, 1966; Thomas and Cohen, 1955). Several recent reports suggest that the genetic defect common to all these risk factors may reside in the absence or structure of the functional receptor molecules on the surfaces of either secretory or target cells (Cerasi and Luft, 1974; Goldstein and Brown, 1975; Goldstein et al., 1975; Kones, 1974; Lacy, 1974, 1975; Robertson and Porte, 1973). If these suggestions are valid, it may then be possible to attribute the multifaceted carbohydrate metabolic disorders such as hyperlipemia and diabetes to an error in the genetic code responsible for membrane structure and function.

Carbohydrate consumed in excess of caloric need is converted and stored as glycogen and lipid. The synthesis of lipid from carbohydrate takes place primarily in the liver in humans (Patel et al., 1975; Shrago et al., 1971) and is under hormonal control. The hormones insulin, glucagon, growth hormone, ACTH, epinephrine, norepinephrine, and glucocorticoid all influence carbohydrate utilization and energy balance. In the absence of insulin action, lipogenesis from glucose is impaired and lipolysis is enhanced. Abnormal glucose utilization results from the continued absence of insulin action and the disease diabetes mellitus results (see section on Errors in Glucose Utilization). Other hormonal abnormalities or imbalances can also result in deranged carbohydrate and lipid metabolism, but these defects will not be considered within the scope of this chapter.

After the liver has converted the glucose into lipid (primarily triglycerides and cholesterol), the lipids are then transported as lipoproteins to the periphery where the carrier proteins are removed and the lipids are transferred into the cells for storage. Genetic errors in the synthesis, transport, and clearance of these lipids from the blood have been suggested as explanations for the lipemia associated with high dietary carbohydrate intakes. Interest in hypertriglyceridemia has been greatly stimulated by reports of an association of elevated serum triglycerides and/or cholesterol with coronary heart disease (Albrink and Marr, 1959).

The plasma lipids include cholesterol, triglycerides, monoglycerides, diglycerides, free fatty acids, phospholipids, and other lipid-soluble constituents such as vitamin A and cerebrosides. The plasma serves as the transport medium for the translocation of these lipids from one tissue to another. The level of lipid in the plasma varies from individual to individual, depending on the time of the last meal, its composition, the time of day, and the physiologic status of the individual.

Phospholipids comprise the largest lipid fraction in the plasma. There is an age-related increase in the levels of phospholipid; in young males and females, plasma phospholipid levels average 215 mg/100 ml; in males and females 50–59 years old, the levels average 305 mg/100 ml (Stewart and Hendry, 1935). No relationship has been shown to implicate the phospholipids in the genesis of abnormal carbohydrate metabolism.

The second largest lipid fraction in the plasma is the sterol (primarily cholesterol) fraction. Cholesterol levels are also age related; young subjects have an average cholesterol level of 180 mg/100 ml and older (50–59 yr of age) subjects an average level of 250 mg/100 ml (Carlson, 1960a; Swell et al., 1960; Sperry and Webb, 1950). Most of the cholesterol in the circulation is esterified to long-chain, unsaturated fatty acids. Elevated cholesterol levels have been described as significant risk factors in coronary heart disease (Carlson and Bottiger, 1972; Epstein and Ostrander, 1971; Goldstein et al., 1973a, b; Kannel et al., 1971).

The glycerides (mono-, di-, and triglycerides) comprise the third largest plasma lipid class. The glycerides range in normal sera from 25–150 mg/100 ml (Carlson 1960a). More than any other lipid component, the glyceride level is dependent on the composition of the diet. Glycerides having a fatty acid composition of the dietary lipids and arising from the gut, via the thoracic duct are said to be exogenous glycerides; glycerides arising from hepatic or extrahepatic synthesis are said to be endogenous glycerides. As with cholesterol, elevated glyceride levels have been associated with coronary heart disease (Ahrens et al., 1961; Albrink and Marr, 1959; Brown et al., 1965; Carlson, 1960b; Carlson and Bottinger, 1972).

The free fatty acid component of the plasma reflects largely the net transport of lipid between the various lipid synthesizing and utilizing tissues. The free fatty acids serve as fuel in the absence of glucose; thus, free fatty acid levels are reciprocals of glucose and insulin levels. "Normal" levels of free fatty acids fluctuate widely, depending on many factors including age, diet, and psychic state. Fasting (12–16 hr) levels range from 0.3 to 0.7 meq/liter. The relationship of the changes in free fatty acid levels to lipid disorders has not been established.

The plasma lipids are usually transported as lipid–protein complexes. At least three polypeptides (albumin, α- and β-peptides) have been identified as lipid carrier proteins (Levy and Fredrickson, 1965; Scannu and Hughes, 1962; Shore, 1957). The different lipoproteins can be separated and identified on the basis of their antigenicity (Fredrickson and Gordon, 1958), their electrophoretic mobility, and their density (Fredrickson et al., 1967, 1975). The low-density or β-lipoproteins contain the β-peptide, cholesterol, and some phospholipids (most phospholipids are carried as α-lipoproteins). With age the lipid content of the plasma tends to rise (Carlson, 1960a) and this rise is reflected almost entirely as an increase in the β-lipoproteins. As the density of the lipoproteins decreases, the molecular weight and complexity of the lipid it carries decreases. Whereas the β-lipoproteins contain sterols and some phospholipid, the pre-β-lipoproteins carry mainly triglycerides. The pre-β-lipoproteins have a smaller protein content and can have from 20 to 60% glycerides. These glycerides are mainly of endogenous origin.

The exogenous glycerides are usually carried as chylomicrons. These particles are the largest and least dense of the lipid–protein complexes (Dole and Hamlin, 1962). When the lipoproteins are separated by paper electrophoresis, the chylomicrons remain near the point of origin. The α-lipoproteins migrate furthest from the origin whereas the β- and pre-β-lipoproteins migrate to points between the chylomicrons and the α-lipoproteins. Each band represents molecules under independent control, and the presence, absence, or change in concentration forms the basis for the segregation and identification of the various hyperlipoproteinemic states (Beaumont et al., 1970; Fredrickson et al., 1967). These states or types (I-V) are further characterized by blood lipid levels and by other distinguishing body characteristics.

A. Type I Hyperlipoproteinemia

Type I hyperlipoproteinemia (type I) is defined by the presence of large amounts of chylomicrons in the plasma of fasting (16 hr without food) patients on a normal diet. The normal diet is defined as containing 35–45% of calories from fat, 45–55% from carbohydrate, and 10–15% from proteins. The chylomicron levels in type I patients can be reduced significantly by a fat-restricted diet. In type I patients the α-, and β- and pre-β-lipoproteins are low; when dietary fat is restricted, the pre-β-lipoprotein levels tend to rise, indicating an increase in endogenous lipid synthesis. This disease is the least common of the lipemias and manifests itself early in life as a severe hyperlipemia. The lipemia is accompanied by eruptive xanthomas, abdominal discomfort, and perhaps hepatomegaly and splenomegaly. Despite elevated serum lipid levels, atherosclerosis is not a complication of this disorder. The chylomicronemia and eruptive xanthomas disappear with dietary fat restriction.

The disease is thought to be due to a defect in the removal of the chylomicrons and other lipid-rich complexes from the plasma (Havel and Goldfien, 1961; Havel and Gordon, 1960; Nestel, 1964). Usually the chylomicrons are rapidly removed by both hepatic and extrahepatic tissues (Nestel, 1964). In type I, it appears that the uptake of glycerides from the sera by the peripheral tissues is defective. This defect is due to the absence of the specific enzyme lipoprotein lipase (Fredrickson et al., 1967; Havel and Gordon, 1960; Kuo et al., 1965), an enzyme located in the capillary wall (Havel, 1965) and perhaps the membrane of the adipocyte (Rodbell, 1964). Since lipoprotein lipase is responsible for the hydrolysis of circulating glycerides at the site of removal (Robinson, 1963), a decrease in the activity of this enzyme imposes a severe limitation on the rate of chylomicron clearance. Type I patients have almost no fat tolerance as a result of having almost no threshold for fat removal. This presents somewhat of a problem in the management of these patients. While a fat-restricted diet will initially relieve the symptoms, the low-fat diet is necessarily high in carbohydrate. This carbohydrate is converted by the liver into glycerides that, in turn, are transported as pre-β-lipoproteins to the periphery for storage. These lipoproteins also cannot be adequately cleared from the blood, and the lipemia initially reduced by fat restriction returns. Since the lipemia is now due to an increase in the pre-β-lipoproteins, the patient could be classified as a type V hyperlipoproteinemic patient. The distinction must then be made as to the primary disease in question. Usually, this is resolved when consideration of the diet and age of onset is given. In type I patients, the lipemia is reduced on low-fat diets and increases gradually with time as the patient adapts his endogenous lipogenic systems to handle the increased dietary carbohydrate load; the lipemia is observed very early in life, perhaps within weeks of birth. Type V patients are not detected until much later in life.

Type I hyperlipemia is inherited via an autosomal recessive mode (Fredrickson et al., 1967). It is relatively rare but may occur in sibs of heterozygote asymptomatic parents. Heterozygotes may have subnormal lipoprotein lipase activity (Fredrickson et al., 1967; Nestel and Havel, 1962).

B. Type II Hyperlipoproteinemia

Familial hypercholesterolemia or type II hyperlipoproteinemia (type II) is characterized by elevated serum cholesterol levels and an elevation in β-lipoprotein levels. Several subclasses of this fairly common disorder have been described as well as hypercholesterolemia resulting from untreated hypothyroidism, nephrosis, or intermittent porphyria or myeloma (Cohen et al., 1966; Lees et al., 1970; Scott et al., 1970; Walton et al., 1965). Type II is frequently associated with lipid depositions in the skin, eyes, tendons, and vascular system (Fredrickson et al., 1967). The severity of the disease ranges from a moderate increase in β-lipoproteins to widespread atheromatous invasion of the vascular tissue, particularly the vessels of the heart.

It appears that type II occurs in several genetically and clinically identifiable forms (Brown and Goldstein, 1975; Fredrickson, 1971; Goldstein et al., 1975; Khachadurian, 1964). Type IIa or simple hypercholesterolemia appears to be related to the functionality of the β-lipoprotein receptor site. Two defects in receptor site function have been described (Goldstein et al., 1975). One of these defects results in the absence of a functional receptor site for the binding of the cholesterol carrying β-lipoprotein. In these receptor-negative homozygotes, none of the cholesterol-carrying lipoprotein is bound to the cell providing cholesterol for transferral into the cell. Since cholesterol is an inhibitor of hydroxymethyl-glutaryl CoA (HMGCoA) reductase, this means that this enzyme is not suppressed and cholesterol synthesis continues unabated. In addition, cholesterol esterification is not stimulated. The cell continuously synthesizes cholesterol, contributing to the already overloaded intracellular and extracellular cholesterol pool. The receptor-negative phenotype is characterized by marked (600–1,000 mg/100 ml) hypercholesterolemia, cutaneous planar xanthomas observed in the latter part of the first decade of life, and premature coronary vascular disease (Brown and Goldstein, 1975; Fredrickson et al., 1967; Khachadurian, 1964).

According to Khachadurian (1964, 1971) the receptor-negative phenotype results when each parent contributes a mutant allele that may or may not be identical but affects the structure of the receptor site. Heterozygotes who inherit only one mutant allele are less severely affected than homozygotes. Whereas the homozygotes have no functional lipoprotein receptor sites, heterozygotes have less than half the number of receptor sites (Goldstein and Brown, 1975). It has been estimated that about 1 in 500 persons carries the trait for hypercholesterolemia (Brown and Goldstein, 1975; Goldstein et al., 1973a).

A second defect, also characterized by hypercholesterolemia and early death, involves the functionality of the lipoprotein receptor site. In these receptor-defective individuals, cholesterol ester formation and partial suppression of HMGCoA reductase can be shown indicating a reduced affinity of the receptor site for the lipoprotein (Goldstein et al., 1975). It is estimated that the defective receptors possess only 10% of the normal binding capacity for the cholesterol-carrying lipoprotein. The receptor-defective individual appears to possess at least one type of mutant allele that specifies the production of a receptor capable of a low level of function. Since this appears to be a dominant trait, it may be that the receptor-defective individual is the heterozygote for the receptor-negative homozygote since both phenotypic expressions involve the functionality of the receptor site.

Another type of hypercholesterolemia, designated as type IIb, is characterized by a moderate increase in serum triglycerides as well as an increased cholesterol level. Cholesterol balance studies have shown that patients with this defect synthesize almost three times as much cholesterol as hypercholesterolemic-normo-glyceridemic patients (Sodhi and Kudchodkar, 1973). The increase in sterol synthesis appears to take place primarily in the liver. Whereas type IIa has a pronounced β-lipoprotein band and elevated serum cholesterol levels, type IIb may have in addition a pre-β-band that is more intense than normal and elevated serum triglycerides. The cholesterol/triglyceride ratio is usually greater than two (Beaumont et al., 1970). It is altogether possible that this type also may have a defective receptor mechanism that allows for the accumulation of both lipid classes in the serum while enhancing the intracellular synthesis of these lipids. As yet, this type of error has not been reported.

C. Type III Hyperlipoproteinemia

Patients with type III hyperlipoproteinemia (type III) on a normal diet have elevated levels of cholesterol, phospholipids, and triglycerides. Upon electrophoresis, fasting sera have pronounced β- and pre-β-lipoprotein bands. The hyperglyceridemia is induced by feeding a carbohydrate-rich diet. Tuberous, planar, and tendon xanthomas, atheromas, ischemic heart disease, and glucose intolerance also are observed (Fredrickson et al., 1967, 1975). Types III and IIb may be related disorders, distinguished at present only by the lack of abnormal glucose tolerance in type IIb. It is possible that an additional allele is present next to the mutant allele for type IIb, thus accounting for the phenotype III.

The lipemia in type III can usually be reduced through caloric restriction at the expense of the carbohydrate and fat portions of the diet. With a lowering of serum lipids the xanthomas may disappear. While abnormal glucose tolerance is reported in type III patients, frank diabetes requiring insulin treatment is not common.

The biochemical defect in type III lipoproteinemia has not been well defined. However, as early as 1950, Watkin et al. reported that hypertensive patients placed on a rice and fruit diet became hyperlipemic. Later, Ahrens and co-workers (1961) conclusively showed that some hyperlipemics were very sensitive to dietary carbohydrate, exhibiting serum glyceride levels roughly proportional to their carbohydrate intakes. In normal man, high-carbohydrate feeding can induce increases in serum glycerides and the very-low-density (pre-β) lipoproteins (Antonis and Bersohn, 1961; Beveridge et al., 1964; Schonfeld, 1970). These increases are of importance, however, only when they occur in individuals consuming a normal, moderate carbohydrate diet.

Carbohydrate induction may be due to an increased diversion of the dietary glucose to lipid synthesis rather than to glycogen synthesis. Equally possible, however, may be the inability of the peripheral tissues to metabolize glucose (peripheral insulin insensitivity), forcing the burden of glucose metabolism on the liver. The liver in response would synthesize more lipid from the glucose sending this endogenously produced lipid to the periphery via the pre-β-lipoproteins. Coupled with decreased insulin sensitivity would be an increased lipolysis at the adipocyte, which would increase the free fatty acid flux from the adipocyte to the hepatocyte.

An inability to clear the plasma of the pre-β-lipoproteins is clearly implicated, and postheparin lipoprotein lipase activity is normal (Fredrickson et al., 1967). Adipose tissue lipoprotein lipase may be at fault as suggested by the inactivity of this enzyme in diabetic rats (Kessler, 1963). To date the cellular defect accounting for type III hyperlipoproteinemia has not been elucidated.

While type III has been considered a variant of type II (broad B), the evidence that both are different phenotypic expressions of the same mutant allele is incomplete. It has been suggested that the type III is inherited as an autosomal dominant trait with a gene frequency of 1 in 5,000 (Bierman, 1973; Morganroth et al., 1975).

D. Type IV Hyperlipoproteinemia

Several population surveys have revealed that type IV hyperlipoproteinemia (type IV) is the most common of the five types (Carlson and Lindstedt, 1968; Kuo et al., 1965; Miettinen, 1973; Schaefer, 1964). The abnormality is characterized by an increased pre-β-lipoprotein band with no increase in either the β-lipoproteins or the chylomicrons. The increase in plasma triglycerides in patients on a normal diet is thought to be due to an increased endogenous synthesis of lipid from carbohydrate rather than due to an impaired triglyceride removal (Kuo et al., 1967; Hagenfeldt et al., 1975). Patients with type IV hyperlipoproteinemia frequently have premature atherosclerosis, ischemic heart disease, obesity, impaired glucose tolerance, or mild diabetes (Fredrickson et al.,

1967). An increased insulin response after oral glucose is often observed in these patients before the appearance of overt diabetes (Eaton and Nye, 1973; Farquhar et al., 1966; Kuo and Feng, 1970; Tengo et al., 1967). No distinguishing xanthomas are present to differentiate type III from type IV patients, except those who have very high serum lipid levels. Type IV is sometimes diagnosed in uncontrolled diabetics (Camitta and Gray, 1969). In these patients the hypertriglyceridemia is secondary to the diabetic condition and disappears when the diabetes is brought under control. It has been difficult to distinguish type IV from type V since both conditions are characterized by an increased endogenous triglyceride synthesis and an increased pre-β-lipoprotein band. Some clinicians group the two together for convenience sake. In part, the overlap of the two types is due to the great variability in serum lipid levels in type IV patients. Since the pre-β-lipoprotein contains about 20% cholesterol, changes in serum cholesterol levels would affect the serum pre-β-lipoprotein level. Type IV patients appear to be more responsive in terms of elevations in serum lipids to increases in dietary sucrose than to dietary starch (Kuo et al., 1967). However, the effect of kind of dietary carbohydrate on serum lipids may depend on the kind of fat included in the diet (Little et al., 1970).

Type IV hyperlipoproteinemia is thought to be genetically heterogenous since relatives of type IV patients may have either type III or type V patterns (Lees and Wilson, 1971). The literature, to date, has very few family studies of clear-cut type IV disease. Nonetheless, it is thought to be inherited as an autosomal dominant trait with an estimated gene frequency of 2/1,000 (Bierman, 1973; Lees and Wilson, 1971; Schreibman et al., 1969).

E. Type V Hyperlipoproteinemia

This syndrome (type V), defined as a condition where both chylomicrons and endogenously synthesized triglycerides (pre-β-lipoproteins) are elevated, is fairly common. It is usually associated with obesity, eruptive xanthomas, recurrent abdominal discomfort, and hepatosplenomegaly. Atherosclerosis is more common in these patients than in the general population (Slack, 1969). Modest elevations in serum cholesterol and greatly elevated serum triglyceride levels are observed. Impaired glucose tolerance, which further deteriorates with age, is also observed. The lipemia is frequently discovered in late adolescence or early adulthood as a consequence of a hospital admission for acute abdominal pain.

The biochemical defect in type V may be a combination of those already discussed for types I, III, and IV. Certainly, both enhanced synthesis of endogenous lipid and reduced clearance of circulating lipid can be demonstrated (Fredrickson et al., 1967). While these defects may reflect a genetic error in cell metabolism, this error has yet to be described. The inheritance of the defect or defects has not been worked out, primarily due to the lack of understanding of the basic or primary defect involved. The condition has been described as being inherited as either an autosomal dominant or recessive trait with a gene frequency estimated as rare or as 2/1,000 (Bierman, 1973).

X. ERRORS IN GLUCOSE UTILIZATION

Defective glucose utilization, or diabetes mellitus—characterized by hyperglycemia, glycosuria, polyuria, excessive thirst and weight loss followed by ketoacidosis, coma, and death—has been known since the days of early civilization. Current evidence indicates that diabetes is not a single syndrome but a collection of syndromes having in common defective glucose utilization and some, none, or all of the above symptoms. Common to all the syndromes is a relative deficiency of insulin action. Whether insulin insufficiency is the primary cause of the above symptoms or secondary to a more basic matabolic cellular error remains to be elucidated.

Glucose oxidation by different tissues is dependent in varying degrees on the presence of insulin. Both adipose tissue and resting muscle require the binding of insulin to the receptor site prior to or concomitant with the passage of glucose into the cell (Cuatrecasas, 1969; Kono, 1969; Renner, 1973). In contrast, the liver and exercising muscle do not require insulin for glucose passage (Cahill et al., 1958; Hetenyi et al., 1969; Issekutz et al., 1966; Wierzuchowski, 1966). All tissues, however, do require insulin (bound to the receptor site) for glucose metabolism (Bergman and Buccolo, 1974; Hall and Ball, 1970; Mondon et al., 1975). The activities of hexokinase (Anderson and King, 1975; Hansen et al., 1970), glycogen synthetase (Gold, 1969; Miller and Larner, 1973), glycogen transferase (Bishop et al., 1971), glucose-6-phosphate dehydrogenase (Berdanier et al., 1971; Novello et al., 1969; Rudack et al., 1971), 6-phosphogluconate dehydrogenase (Berdanier et al., 1971; Novello et al., 1967), pyruvate dehydrogenase (Coore et al., 1971; Sica and Cuatrecasas, 1973; Taylor et al., 1973; Wieland et al., 1971), lipoprotein lipase (Borensztajn et al., 1972), lipogenic enzymes (Halperin, 1970, 1971; Murthy and Steiner, 1972; Saggerson and Greenbaum, 1970), and the enzymes of gluconeogenesis and glycogenolysis (Anderson and Zakim, 1970; Exton et al., 1966; Friedman et al., 1967; Glinsmann and Mortimore, 1968; Jefferson et al., 1968) are all regulated or affected by insulin. Thus, most reactions involving the degradation or resynthesis of energy-containing compounds require the presence of insulin (Greenbaum et al., 1971).

Since the presence of insulin bound to the receptor site is prerequisite for normal cellular function, all steps leading to and including this binding are logical sites for genetic errors that could result in diabetes. Dissecting this process permits the speculation as to the location of the primary defect or defects. Among these defects might be (1) an inability of the pancreas to synthesize, store, and release appropriate amounts of insulin in response to need; (2) errors in the transport of insulin to the target tissues; (3) incompetent insulin receptor sites that interfere with the normal binding of insulin; (4) a deficiency in glucose tolerance factor that facilitates insulin binding to the receptor site; (5) excess levels of other hormones that interfere or compete with insulin for the binding site; (6) an incompetent second messenger system that does not properly stimulate insulin release or the cellular metabolism of the target cell when insulin is bound to it. Errors in insulin synthesis (Elliott et al., 1965; Melani et al., 1970; Sherman et al., 1971), storage (Danowski et al., 1960; Wrenshall, 1958), and release (Cerasi and Luft, 1967; Fujita et al., 1975; Grodsky et al., 1974; Robertson and Porte, 1973) have been documented in diabetic patients and in experimental animals. Errors in synthesis and release are usually manifested early in life in terms of the health and well-being of the patient. Absolute deficits of insulin usually characterize the juvenile diabetic (Bornstein and Laurence, 1951; Murthy et al., 1968; Vallence-Owen et al., 1955; White, 1956; Wrenshall, 1958), a form of diabetes less common than the maturity-onset diabetes.

Defects in the form of insulin transported in the blood have been reported in diabetics (Antonaiades et al., 1962; Elliott et al., 1965), but whether these defects are primary defects leading to the diabetic state or whether they are secondary to a more fundamental problem is subject to question. The inability of some subjects to convert proinsulin (an insulin consisting of an A, B, and C peptide chains) to free or active insulin (the C chain removed) has been suggested as an explanation of diabetes that develops somewhat later than juvenile diabetes (Gorden and Roth, 1968). The presence of insulin antagonists and/or "synalbumin" has received attention as a factor in the development of diabetes (Baird and Bornstein, 1957; Davidson and Poffenbarger, 1970; Vargas et al., 1960; Vallence-Owen, 1960).

The elegant work of Cuatrecasas (1969, 1972) and Kono (1969) clearly indicates that incompetent binding or incompetent binding sites are related to the development of diabetes, particularly the diabetes or impaired glucose tolerance observed in the obese (Boshell et al., 1968; Butterfield et al., 1963; Rabinowitz and Zierler, 1961; Stunkard and Blumenthal, 1972). As the fat cell expands, the receptor sites are spread apart, and the cell becomes less responsive to insulin (Amatruda et al., 1975). When obese patients return to normal weight, their glucose tolerance also normalizes (Bagdade et al., 1974; Salans et al., 1968), thus implicating some change in cell structure affecting insulin reactivity as the fat cell shrinks to normal size.

Age-related impaired glucose tolerance has been shown to improve when glucose tolerance factor (an organic chromium compound) is supplied (Glinsmann and Mertz, 1966; Mertz, 1969, 1975). Apparently, these patients are unable to synthesize this factor or consume chromium-deficient diets. It has been suggested that many older mild diabetics do not have problems with insulin supply per se but are, in fact, glucose-tolerance-factor deficient (Mertz, 1975).

Diabetes that results from an excess of other hormones, such as glucocorticoid (Stadie et al., 1949), glucagon (Johansen et al., 1974; Muller et al., 1970; Unger and Orci, 1975), and growth hormone (Sabeh et al., 1969; Stadie et al., 1949), can be regarded as a secondary disease and perhaps should be omitted from the current discussion. However, inasmuch as diseases of one endocrine gland may be regarded as having a strong genetic component, one should also include diabetes that develops as a consequence of other endocrine malfunctions. Because the maintenance of blood glucose is a complex process involving hormones other than insulin, errors in hormone balance must be included in this list of possible genetic defects.

Lastly, errors in the second messenger system (see Chapter 4) involving cAMP, GMP, phosphodiesterase, adenyl cyclase, and other components may occur that may result in an inadequate release of insulin from the islet cells (Boquist et al., 1974; Grodsky et al., 1974) or a blunting of the effects of insulin on cellular metabolism. Reports of errors in this area, in diabetic man, are scarce. As our technology improves, however, it may be possible to classify some diabetics as having this kind of defect. Reports of changes in this system with experimental diabetes have been made in animals (Chang et al., 1974; Desai and Hollenberg, 1975; Kaplan et al., 1973).

The question of whether diabetes in its many forms can be classed as an inborn error in metabolism has yet to be resolved. Its inclusion in this chapter is justified by the fact that genetics plays an important role in its development. Genetic transmission of diabetes has been shown in a number of species of experimental animals (see Chapter 9) (Berdanier, 1974; Chick et al., 1970; Coleman and Hummel, 1967; Dulin and Wyse, 1970; Gerritsen and Dulin, 1967; Gonet et al., 1963, 1965; Hummel et al., 1966; Iwatsuka et al., 1970a, b; Shafrir et al., 1972). In the various species studied, diabetes has been shown to be transmitted as an autosomal dominant (yellow mice), autosomal recessive (obese mice, adipose mice, fatty rat diabetes mice), and/or polygenic (New Zealand and KK mice, Chinese hamster) (Renold and Burn, 1970) trait. Whether the genetic trait for diabetes results from a spontaneous mutation or a viral infection is not known. Viral infections have been shown to result in diabetes (Craighead, 1975; Maugh, 1975), and while the animal may recover from the virus with little or no aftereffects, glucose tolerance under physiologic stress may be impaired. This trait may then affect the glucose tolerance of succeeding generations even though these generations are not exposed to the inducing agent. Proof of the suggestion that environmental factors can give rise *de novo* to the disease that could then be transmitted genetically to succeeding generations was shown by Spergel et al. (1971).

From the studies of the genetic transmission of the diabetic trait in animals, it is clear that different genotypic errors may produce relatively similar phenotypic diseases. West (1975) has recently lamented the fact that the criteria for defining diabetes in population groups throughout the world are not uniform. Perhaps, unwittingly, different investigators have segregated different genotypes by their differing definition of diabetes. Differences in environment may either enhance or tend to obscure the presence of a genotypic lesion that might result in frank diabetes in another environment. The importance of both genetic and environmental (dietary) factors in the development of diabetes mellitus has been shown by Cohen et al. (1972; chapter 10) and by Medalie et al. (1975).

The overall incidence of diabetes is difficult to determine simply because (as West points out) our definition of the disease varies so broadly and also because the disease may not declare itself until late in life. In the United States it has been estimated that one person in 20 is or may be a diabetic (Remein, 1959; Sharkey, 1971). According to Sharkey (1971) the figures from the National Center for Health Statistics reveal that diabetes occurred in three successive generations in only 1% of the diabetic population. One in six diabetics had a diabetic mother; one in 12 had a diabetic father. In humans, different genotypes have been identified on the basis of age of onset (Tattersall and Fajans, 1975) and on the results of different glucose-tolerance tests (Beaven et al., 1974). Population studies indicate further differences in the modes of inheritance of these different forms of diabetes (Goodman and Chung, 1975). Whereas early juvenile diabetes appears to be inherited via a two-allele, single-locus mode, late-onset diabetes appears to be inherited via a multifactorial mode.

XI. SUMMARY

It is apparent that genetics plays an important role in the determination of how much and what kind of carbohydrate an individual can consume. The occurrence of so many inborn errors (see Fig. 1 for a summary of these errors) in carbohydrate metabolism is not remarkable considering the number of reactions

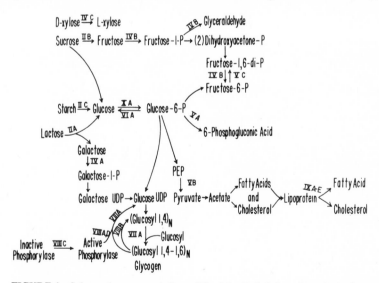

FIGURE 1 Schematic representation of the inherited defects in carbohydrate metabolism. Roman numerals and letter subscripts refer to the section of the text that describes the defect.

needed for the assimilation and utilization of this common class of dietary ingredients. As yet, nutritionists have not set any recommended daily allowance for carbohydrates. Yet it is clear from Chapter 6 that some dietary carbohydrate is required for optimal health and growth. Equally clear from Chapter 10 and this chapter is the concept that under certain conditions there is an upper limit or tolerance for carbohydrate, more specifically an upper limit for different carbohydrates that differs from person to person, depending on his or her genetic background. Sex and age (Chapter 9), as well as previous dietary states (Chapters 7 and 8), may also determine the optimal carbohydrate allowance. Future research may further dictate other considerations (perhaps even more subtle genetic errors) that will affect the recommended daily allowance for carbohydrate.

REFERENCES

Adelman, R. C., Ballard, F. J. and Weinhouse, S. 1967. *J. Biol. Chem.* 242:3360.

Ahrens, E. H., Jr., Hirsch, J., Oette, K., Farquhar, J. W. and Stein, Y. 1961. *Trans. Assoc. Am. Phys.* 74:134.

Albrink, M. J. and Marr, E. B. 1959. *Arch. Int. Med.* 103:4.

Amatruda, J. M., Livingston, J. N. and Lockwood, D. H. 1975. *Science* 188:264.

Andersen, A. L., Lund-Johansen, P. and Clausen, G. 1969. *Scand. J. Clin. Lab. Invest.* 24:105.

Anderson, C. M., Kerry, K. R. and Townley, R. R. W. 1965. *Arch. Dis. Child.* 40:1.

Anderson, D. H. 1956. *Lab. Invest.* 5:11.

Anderson, J. W. and King, P. 1975. *Biochem. Med.* 12:1.

Anderson, J. W. and Zakim, D. 1970. *Biochem. Biophys. Acta* 201:236.

Antonaiades, H. N., Bougas, J. A. and Pyle, H. M. 1962. *New Engl. J. Med.* 267:218.

Antonis, A. and Bersohn, I. 1961. *Lancet* 1:3.

Auriccho, S., Dahlqvist, A., Murset, G. and Prader, A. 1963. *J. Pediatr.* 62:165.

Bagdade, J. D., Porte, D., Jr., Brunzell, J. D. and Bierman, E. L. 1974. *J. Lab. Clin. Med.* 83:563.

Baird, C. W. and Bornstein, J. 1957. *Lancet* 1:1111.

Baker, L. and Winegrad, A. I. 1970. *Lancet* 2:13.

Ballard, F. J. C. 1966. *Biochem. J.* 101:70.

Bayless, T. M., Paige, D. M. and Ferry, G. D. 1971. *Gastroenterology* 60:605.

Bayless, T. M. and Christopher, N. L. 1969. *Am. J. Clin. Nutr.* 22:181.

Beaumont, J. L., Carlson, L. A., Cooper, G. R., Fejfar, Z., Fredrickson, D. S. and Strasser, T. 1970. *Bull. WHO* 43:891.

Beaven, D. W., Arcus, A. C., Bell, J. P. and Smith, J. R. 1974. *N.Z. Med. J.* 80:291.

Berdanier, C. D. 1974. *Diabetologia* 10:691.

Berdanier, C. D., Szepesi, B., Diachenko, S. and Moser, P. 1971. *Proc. Soc. Exp. Biol. Med.* 131:861.

Bergman, R. N. and Buccolo, R. J. 1974. *Am. J. Physiol.* 227:1314.

Bergren, W. R., Ng, W. G. and Donnell, G. N. 1972. *Science* 176:683.

Beutler, E. 1965. In *Metabolic basis of inherited disease,* ed. J. B. Stanbury, J. B. Wyngaarden and D. S. Fredrickson, 2d ed., pp. 1060–1089. New York: McGraw-Hill.

Beutler, E., Baluda, M. C., Sturgeon, P. and Day, R. 1965. *Lancet* 1:353.

Beutler, E., Johnson, C., Powars, D. and West, C. 1974. *New Engl. J. Med.* 290:826.

Beveridge, J. M. R., Jagannathan, S. N. and Connell, W. F. 1964. *Can. J. Biochem.* 42:999.

Bierman, E. L. 1973. *Scope monograph,* p. 8. Kalamazoo, Mich.: The Upjohn Company.

Bishop, J. S., Goldberg, N. D. and Larner, J. 1971. *J. Biol. Chem.* 220:499.

Bollman, J. L. and Mann, F. C. 1931. *Am. J. Physiol.* 96:683.

Borensztajn, J., Samols, D. R. and Rubenstein, A. H. 1972. *Am. J. Physiol.* 223:1271.

Bornstein, J. and Laurence, R. D. 1951. *Br. Med. J.* 2:1541.

Boquist, L., Hellman, B., Lernmark, A. and Taljedal, I. 1974. *Biochem. Biophys. Res. Commun.* 60:1391.

Boshell, B. R., Chandalia, H. B., Kreisberg, R. A. and Roddam, R. F. 1968. *Am. J. Clin. Nutr.* 21:1419.

Bowie, M. D., Barbezat, G. O. and Hansen, J. D. L. 1967. *Am. J. Clin. Nutr.* 20:89.

Bretthauer, R. K., Hansen, R. G., Donnell, G. and Bergren, R. W. 1959. *Proc. Natl. Acad. Sci. U.S.A.* 45:328.

Brown, B. I. and Brown, D. H. 1966. *Proc. Natl. Acad. Sci. U.S.A.* 56:725.

Brown, D. H. and Illingworth, B. 1964. In *Control of glycogen metabolism,* ed. W. J. Whelan and M. P. Cameron, pp. 139–150. London: Churchill.

Brown, D. F., Kinch, A. S. and Doyle, J. T. 1965. *New Engl. J. Med.* 273:947.

Brown, M. S. and Goldstein, J. L. 1975. *Adv. Intern. Med.* 20:273.

Burgess, E. A., Levin, B., Mahalanabis, D. and Tonge, R. E. 1964. *Arch. Dis. Child.* 39:431.

Butterfield, W. J. H., Garratt, C. J. and Wichelow, M. J. 1963. *Clin. Sci.* 24:331.

Cady, A. B., Rhodes, J. B., Littman, A. and Crane, R. K. 1967. *J. Lab. Clin. Med.* 70:279.

Cahill, G. F., Ashmore, J., Earle, A. S. and Zotter, S. 1958. *Am. J. Physiol.* 192:491.

Cain, A. R. R. and Ryman, B. E. 1971. *Gut* 12:929.

Camitta, F. D. and Gray, T. K. 1969. *Diabetes* 18:44.

Carlson, L. A. 1960a. *Acta Med. Scand.* 167:377.

Carlson, L. A. 1960b. *Acta Med. Scand.* 167:399.

Carlson, L. A. and Bottiger, L. E. 1972. *Lancet* 1:865.

Carlson, L. A. and Lindstedt, S. 1968. *Acta Med. Scand. Suppl.* 493.

Cerasi, E. and Luft, R. 1967. *Acta Endocrinol.* 55:330.

Cerasi, E. and Luft, R. 1974. In *Advances in metabolic disorders,* ed. R. Levine and R. Luft, pp. 193–212. New York: Academic Press.

Chang, K., Marcus, N. A. and Cuatrecasas, P. 1974. *J. Biol. Chem.* 249:6854.

Chick, W. L., Lavine, R. L. and Like, A. A. 1970. *Diabetologia* 6:257.

Cohen, A. M., Teitelbaum, A. and Saliternik, R. 1972. *Metabolism* 21:235.

Cohen, L., Blaisdell, R. K., Djordjevech, J., Ormiste, V. and Dobrilovic, L. 1966. *Am. J. Med.* 40:399.

Coleman, D. L. and Hummel, K. P. 1967. *Diabetologia* 3:238.

Coore, H. G., Denton, R. M., Martin, B. R. and Randle, P. J. 1971. *Biochem. J.* 125:115.

Corbeel, L. M., Eggermont, E., Bettens, W., Castedo-Van Daele, M. and Timmermaus, J. 1970. *Helv. Paediatr. Acta* 42:626.

Cori, C. F. and Illingworth, B. 1957. *Proc. Natl. Acad. Sci. U.S.A.* 43:547.

Cori, G. T. and Cori, C. F. 1952. *J. Biol. Chem.* 199:661.

Cori, G. T., Ochoa, S., Slein, M. W. and Cori, C. F. 1951. *Biochim. Biophys. Acta* 7:304.

Court, J. M. and Dunlop, M. 1975. *Adolescent Med.* 86:453.

Courtecuisse, V., Royer, P., Habib, R., Monnier, C. and Demos, J. 1965. *Pediatrics* 22:1153.

Craighead, J. E. 1975. *Am. J. Pathol.* 78:537.

Cuatrecasas, P. 1969. *Proc. Natl. Acad. Sci. U.S.A.* 63:450.

Cuatrecasas, P. 1972. *J. Biol. Chem.* 247:1980.

Dahlqvist, A. 1962. *J. Clin. Invest.* 41:463.

Dahlqvist, A. 1966. *J. Am. Med. Assoc.* 165:38.

Dahlqvist, A. 1974. In *Sugars in nutrition,* ed. H. L. Sipple and K. W. McNutt, pp. 187–214. New York: Academic Press.

Dahlqvist, A., Auricchio, S., Semenza, G. and Prader, A. 1963. *J. Clin. Invest.* 42:556.

Danowski, T. S., Lombardo, Y. B., Mendelsohn, L. V., Corredor, D. G., Morgan, C. R. and Sabeh, G. 1969. *Metabolism* 18:731.

Davis, A. E. and Bolin, T. 1967. *Nature* 216:1244.

Davidson, M. B. and Poffenbarger, P. L. 1970. *Metabolism* 19:688.

Dawson, D. M., Spong, L. L., and Harrington, J. F. 1968. *Ann. Int. Med.* 69:229.

Desai, K. and Hollenberg, G. 1975. *Is. J. Med. Sci.* 11:540.

Dill, J., Levy, M. and Wells, R. 1972. *Am. J. Clin. Nutr.* 25:869.

Dole, V. P. and Hamlin, J. T. 1962. *Physiol. Rev.* 42:674.

Dubois, R., Loeb, H., Eggermont, E. and Mainguet, M. 1966. *Helv. Paediatr. Acta* 21:577.

Dulin, W. E. and Wyse, B. M. 1970. *Diabetologia* 6:371.

Duncan, L. W. and Scott, E. M. 1972. *Am. J. Clin. Nutr.* 25:867.

Eaton, R. P. and Nye, W. H. R. 1973. *J. Lab. Clin. Med.* 81:682.

Elliott, R. B., O'Brien, D. and Roy, C. C. 1965. *Diabetes* 14:780.

Engel, A. G. 1970. *Brain* 93:599.

Epstein, F. H. and Ostrander, L. D., Jr. 1971. *Progr. Cardiovasc. Dis.* 13:324.

Esmann, V., Hobolth, N. and Jorgensen, J. 1969. *J. Pediatr.* 74:90.

Euser, M., Shapiro, S. and Horecker, B. L. 1969. *Arch. Biochem. Biophys.* 129:377.

Exton, J. H., Jefferson, L. S., Jr., Butcher, R. W. and Park, C. R. 1966. *Am. J. Med.* 40:709.

Farquhar, J. W., Frank, A., Gross, R. C. and Reaven, G. M. 1966. *J. Clin. Invest.* 45:1648.

Fernandes, J. and Huijing, F. 1968. *Arch. Dis. Child.* 43:347.

Fernandes, J. and Pikaar, N. A. 1969. *Am. J. Clin. Nutr.* 22:617.

Fernandes, J., Huijing, F. and Vande-Kamer, J. H. 1969. *Arch. Dis. Child.* 44:311.

Fine, R. N., Frasier, S. N. and Donnell, G. N. 1969. *Am. J. Dis. Child.* 117:169.

Fischer, E. H. and Stein, E. A. 1960. In *The enzymes,* ed. P. D. Boyer, H. Lardy, and K. Myrback, vol. IV, pp. 313–330. New York: Academic Press.

Flatz, G., Saegudom, C. and Sanguanbhokhai, T. 1969. *Nature (London)* 221:758.

Forget, P. P., Fernandes, J. and Haverkamp-Begemann, P. 1974. *Pediatr. Res.* 8:114.

Fredrickson, D. S. 1971. *Br. Med. J.* 2:187.

Fredrickson, D. S. and Gordon, R. S., Jr. 1958. *Physiol. Rev.* 38:585.

Fredrickson, D. S., Levy, R. I. and Lees, R. S. 1967. *New Engl. J. Med.* 276:32, 148, 215, 273.

Fredrickson, D. S., Morganroth, J. and Levy, R. I. 1975. *Ann. Int. Med.* 82:150.

Freedberg, I. M., Feingold, D. S. and Hiatt, H. H. 1959. *Biochem. Biophys. Res. Commun.* 1:328.

Friedman, B., Goodman, E. H. and Weinhouse, S. 1967. *J. Biol. Chem.* 242:3620.

Froesch, E. R. 1966. In *Metabolic basis of inherited disease*, ed. J. B. Stanbury, J. B. Wyngaarden and D. S. Fredrickson, p. 124. New York: McGraw-Hill.

Fujita, Y., Herron, A. L. and Seltzer, H. S. 1975. *Diabetes* 24:17.

Gabbay, K. H. and Snider, J. J. 1972. *Diabetes* 21:295.

Gaetani, G. D., Parker, J. C. and Kirkman, H. N. 1974. *Proc. Natl. Acad. Sci. U.S.A.* 71:3584.

Garancis, J. C. 1968. *Am. J. Med.* 44:289.

Garrod, A. C. 1908. *Lancet* 2:214.

Gaviser, D. 1948. *Surgery* 24:873.

Gerritsen, G. C. and Dulin, W. E. 1967. *Diabetologia* 3:74.

Gertler, M. M. and White, P. D. 1954. *Coronary heart disease in young adults: A multidisciplinary study.* Cambridge, Mass.: Harvard University Press.

Gitzelmann, R. 1967. *Pediatr. Res.* 1:14.

Gitzelmann, R. 1972. *Helv. Paediatr. Acta* 27:125.

Gitzelmann, R., Curtius, H. C. and Schneller, I. 1967. *Exp. Eye Res.* 6:1.

Glinsmann, W. H. and Mertz, W. 1966. *Metabolism* 15:510.

Glinsmann, W. H. and Mortimore, G. E. 1968. *Am. J. Physiol.* 215:553.

Gold, A. H. 1969. *J. Biol. Chem.* 245:903.

Goldstein, J. L. and Brown, M. S. 1975. *J. Lab. Clin. Med.* 85:15.

Goldstein, J. L., Hazzard, W. R., Schrott, H. G., Bierman, E. L. and Motulsky, A. G. 1973a. *J. Clin. Invest.* 52:1533.

Goldstein, J. L., Schrott, H. G. and Hazzard, W. R. 1973b. *J. Clin. Invest.* 52:1544.

Goldstein, J. L., Dana, S. E., Brunschede, G. Y. and Brown, M. S. 1975. *Proc. Natl. Acad. Sci. U.S.A.* 72:1092.

Gonet, A. E., Mougin, J. and Renold, A. E. 1963. *Acta Endocrinol.* 100:135.

Gonet, A. E., Stauffacher, W., Pictet, R. and Renold, A. E. 1965. *Diabetologia* 1:165.

Goodman, M. J. and Chung, C. S. 1975. *Clin. Genet.* 8:66.

Gorden, P. and Roth, J. 1968. *Diabetes* 17:310.

Greenbaum, A. L., Gumaa, K. A. and McLean, P. 1971. *Arch. Biochem. Biophys.* 143:617.

Grodsky, G. M., Sando, H., Levin, S., Gerich, J. and Karam, J. 1974. In *Advances in metabolic disorders*, ed. R. Levine and R. Luft, p. 155. New York: Academic Press.

Grunfeld, J. P., Ganeval, D., Chanard, J., Fardeau, M. and Dreyfus, J. C. 1972. *New Engl. J. Med.* 286:1236.

Gudmand-Høyer, E., Dahlqvist, A. and Jarnum, S. 1970. *Am. J. Gastroenterol.* 53:460.

Hagenfeldt, L., Hellstrom, K. and Wahren, J. 1975. *Clin. Sci. Mol. Med.* 48:247.

Hall, C. L. and Ball, E. G. 1970. *Biochim. Biophys. Acta* 210:209.
Hallgren, P., Hanson, G., Henriksson, K. G., Hager, A., Lundblad, A. and Svensson, S. 1974. *Eur. J. Clin. Invest.* 4:429.
Halperin, M. L. 1970. *Can. J. Biochem.* 48:1228.
Halperin, M. L. 1971. *Biochem. J.* 124:615.
Hansen, R. J., Pilkis, S. J. and Krahl, M. E. 1970. *Endocrinology* 86:57.
Havel, R. J. 1965. In *Handbook of physiology, section 5, Adipose tissue*, ed. A. E. Renold and C. F. Cahill, Jr., p. 499. Washington, D.C.: Am. Physiol. Soc.
Havel, R. J. and Goldfien, A. 1961. *J. Lipid Res.* 2:389.
Havel, R. J. and Gordon, R. S. 1960. *J. Clin. Invest.* 39:1777.
Hedrick, J. L., Shaltiel, S. and Fischer, E. H. 1966. *Biochemistry* 5:2117.
Hers, H. G. 1952a. *Biochim. Biophys. Acta* 8:416.
Hers, H. G. 1952b. *Biochim. Biophys. Acta* 8:424
Hers, H. G. 1959. *Rev. Int. Hepat.* 9:35.
Hers, H. G. 1963. *Biochem. J.* 86:11.
Hers, H. G. 1964. In *Control of glycogen metabolism*, ed. W. J. Whelan and M. P. Cameron, pp. 354–374. Boston, Mass.: Little, Brown Co.
Hers, H. G. 1974. In *Sugars in nutrition*, ed. H. L. Sipple and K. W. McNutt, pp. 337–356. New York: Academic Press.
Hers, H. G. and Joassin, G. 1961. *Enzymol. Biol. Clin.* 1:4.
Hers, H. G. and Kusaka, T. 1953. *Biochim. Biophys. Acta* 11:427.
Hers, H. G., DeBarsy, T., Lederer, B., Hue, L. and Van Hoof, F. 1974. *Biochem. Trans.* 2:1051.
Hetenyi, G., Jr., Norwich, K. H., Studney, D. R. and Hall, J. D. 1969. *Can. J. Physiol. Pharmacol.* 47:361.
Hiatt, H. A. 1965. In *Metabolic basis of inherited disease*, ed. J. B. Stanbury, J. B. Wyngaarden and D. S. Fredrickson, pp. 109–115. New York: McGraw-Hill.
Holzel, A. 1968. *Proc. R. Soc. Med.* 61:1095.
Holzel, A., Schwarz, V. and Sutcliffe, K. W. 1959. *Lancet* 1:1126.
Holzel, A., Mereci, T. and Thomson, M. L. 1962. *Lancet* 2:1346.
Howell, R. R., Kaback, M. M. and Brown, B. I. 1971. *J. Pediatr.* 78:638.
Huang, S. S. and Bayless, J. M. 1968. *Science* 160:83.
Hug, G. 1962. *Pediatrics* 60:545.
Hug, G. and Schubert, W. K. 1970. *Biochem. Biophys. Res. Commun.* 41:1187.
Hug, G., Schubert, W. K. and Chuck, G. 1966. *Science* 153:1534.
Hug, G., Schubert, W. K. and Chuck, G. 1969. *J. Clin. Invest.* 48:704.
Hug, G., Schubert, W. K. and Chuck, G. 1970. *Biochem. Biophys. Res. Commun.* 40:982.
Hug, G., Chuck, G., Walling, L. and Schubert, W. K. 1974. *J. Lab. Clin. Med.* 84:26.
Hugh-Jones, K., Newcomb, A. L. and Hsia, D. Y. Y. 1960. *Arch. Dis. Child.* 35:521.
Huijing, F. 1967. *Biochim. Biophys. Acta* 148:601.
Huijing, F. 1968. In *Control of glycogen metabolism*, ed. W. J. Whelan, pp. 115–128. London: Academic Press.
Huijing, F. 1970. *Biochem. Gen.* 4:187.
Huijing, F. and Fernandes, J. 1969. *Am. J. Hum. Genet.* 21:275.
Hulsmann, W. C., Oei, T. L. and Van Creveld, S. 1961. *Lancet* 2:581.
Hulsmann, W. C., Eijkenboom, W. H. M., Koster, J. F. and Fernandes, J. 1970. *Clinica. Chem. Acta* 30:775.

Hummel, K. P., Dickie, M. M. and Coleman, D. L. 1966. *Science* 153:1127.

Illingworth, B. and Cori, C. F. 1965. *Biochem. Biophys. Res. Commun.* 19:10.

Illingworth-Brown, B. and Zellweger, H. 1966. *Biochem. J.* 101:16.

Issekutz, B., Miller, H. I. and Rodahl, K. 1966. *Fed. Proc.* 25:1415.

Iwatsuka, H., Matsuro, T., Shino, A. and Suzuoki, Z. 1970a. *J. Takeda Res. Lab.* 29:685.

Iwatsuka, H., Shino, A. and Suzuoki, A. 1970b. *Endocrinol. Jap.* 17:23.

Jacovic, S., Khachadurian, A. K. and Hsia, D. Y. Y. 1966. *J. Lab. Clin. Med.* 68:769.

Jefferson, L. S., Exton, J. H., Butcher, R. W., Sutherland, E. W. and Park, C. R. 1968. *J. Biol. Chem.* 243:1031.

Johanson, K., Soeldner, J. S. and Gleason, R. E. 1974. *Metabolism* 23:1185.

Johnstone, R. W. 1906. *Edinburg Med. J.* 20:138.

Jolly, J. G., Sarup, B. M. Bhatnagar, D. P. and Maini, S. C. 1972. *J. Indian Med. Assoc.* 58:196.

Kalckar, H. M. 1965. *Science,* 150:305.

Kanaghinis, T., Hatzioannori, J., Deliarggris, N., Danos, N., Zografos, N., Katsas, K. and Gardikas, C. 1974. *Dig. Dis.* 19:1021.

Kannel, W. B., Castelli, W. P., Gordon, T., and McNamara, P. M. 1971. *Ann. Intern. Med.* 74:1.

Kaplan, J. C., Pichard, A. L., Laudat, M. H. and Laudat, P. 1973. *Biochem. Biophys. Res. Commun.* 51:1008.

Kellermeyer, R. W., Carson, P. E., Schier, S. L., Tarlov, A. R. and Alving, A. S. 1961. *J. Lab. Clin. Med.* 58:715.

Kern, F., Struthers, J. E. and Attwood, W. L. 1963. *Gastroenterology* 45: 477.

Kerry, K. R. and Townley, R. R. W. 1965. *Aust. Paediatr.* 1:223.

Kessler, J. J. 1963. *J. Clin. Invest.* 42:362.

Khachadurian, A. K. 1964. *Am. J. Med.* 37:402.

Khachadurian, A. K. 1971. *Protides Biol. Fluids Proc. Colloq.* 19:315.

Kirkman, H. N. and Henderson, E. M. 1963. *Am. J. Hum. Genet.* 15:241.

Knox, W. E. 1958. *Am. J. Hum. Genet.* 10:385.

Koluiska, J. and Semenza, G. 1967. *Biochim. Biophys. Acta* 146:181.

Komrower, G. M., Schwarz, V., Holzel, A. and Goldberg, L. 1956. *Arch. Dis. Child.* 31:254.

Kones, R. J. 1974. *Ann. N.Y. Acad. Sci.* 36:738.

Kono, T. 1969. *J. Biol. Chem.* 244:1772.

Koster, J. F., Slee, R. G. and Fernandes, J. 1975. *Biochem. Biophys. Res. Commun.* 64:289.

Kranhold, J. F., Loh, D. and Morris, R. C. 1969. *Science* 165:402.

Krebs, E. G., Kent, A. B. and Fischer, E. H. 1958. *J. Biol. Chem.* 231:73.

Kretchmer, N., Ransonie-Kuti, O., Hurwitz, R., Dungy, C. and Alakya, W. 1971. *Lancet* 2:392.

Krivit, W., Sharp, H. L., Lee, J. C., Larner, J. and Edstrom, R. 1973. *Am. J. Med.* 84:88.

Kuo, P. Bassett, D., DiGeorge, A. and Carpenter, G. 1965. *Circ. Res.* 16:221.

Kuo, P. T. and Feng, L. Y. 1970. *Metabolism* 19:372.

Kuo, P. T., Feng, L. Y., Cohen, N. N., Fitts, W. T. and Miller, L. D. 1967. *Am. J. Clin. Nutr.* 20:116.

Lacy, P. E. 1974. In *Advances in metabolic disorders,* ed. R. Levine and R. Luft, pp. 171–182. New York: Academic Press.

Lacy, P. E. 1975. *Am. J. Pathol.* 79:170.

Landau, B. R., Marshall, J. S., Craig, J. W., Hosletter, K. Y. and Genuth, S. M. 1971. *J. Lab. Clin. Med.* 78:606.

Laplane, R., Polovsky, C., Etienne, M., Debray, P., Lods, J. C. and Pessarro, B. 1962. *Arch. Fr. Pediatr.* 19:895.

Larner, J. 1953. *J. Biol. Chem.* 202:491.

Larson, H. W., Blatherwick, N. R., Bradshaw, P. J., Ewing, M. E. and Sawyer, S. D. 1941. *J. Biol. Chem.* 138:353.

Layzer, R. B., Rowland, L. P. and Ranney, H. M. 1967. *Arch. Neurol.* 17:512.

Lebenthal, E., Antonowicz, I. and Shwachman, H. 1975. *Am. J. Clin. Nutr.* 28:595.

Lees, R. S. and Wilson, D. S. 1971. *New Engl. J. Med.* 284:189.

Lees, R. S., Song, C. S., Levere, R. D. and Kappas, A. 1970. *New Engl. J. Med.* 282:432.

Legum, C. P. and Nitowsky, H. M. 1969. *J. Pediatr.* 74:84.

Lejeune, N., Thines-Sempoux, D. and Hers, H. G. 1963. *Biochem. J.* 86:16.

Leloir, L. F. 1951. *Arch. Biochem. Biophys.* 33:186.

Leloir, L. F. and Cardini, C. E. 1957. *J. Am. Chem. Soc.* 79:6340.

Leichter, J. 1971. *Dig. Dis.* 16:1123.

Leuthardt, F., Testa, E. and Wolf, H. P. 1953. *Helv. Chim. Acta* 36:227.

Levine, R. and Huddleston, B. 1947. *Fed. Proc.* 6:151.

Levy, R. I. and Fredrickson, D. S. 1965. *J. Clin. Invest.* 44:426.

Lindquist, B. 1967. Symposium on Intestinal Absorption. Zurich.

Lindquist, B. and Meeuwisse, G. W. 1962. *Acta Paediatr. Scand.* 51:674.

Lindquist, B. and Meeuwisse, G. W. 1963. *Acta Paediatr. Scand. Suppl.* 146:110.

Lindquist, B., Meeuwisse, G. W., and Melin, K. 1963. *Acta Paediatr. Scand.* 52:217.

Linneweh, F., Schaumloffel, E., Graul, E. H. and Bode, H. H. 1966. *Schweiz. Med. Wochenschr.* 96:424.

Lisker, R., Topez-Habib, G., Daltabruit, M., Rostenberg, I. and Arroys, P. 1974. *Am. J. Clin. Nutr.* 27:756.

Little, J. A., Birchwood, B. L., Simmons, D. A., Antar, M. A., Kallos, A., Buckley, G. C. and Cisma, A. 1970. *Atherosclerosis* 11:173.

Littman, A. and Hammond, J. B. 1965. *Gastroenterology* 48:237.

Lockwood, D. H., Merimee, T. J., Edgar, P. J., Greene, M. L., Fujimoto, W. J., Seegmiller, J. E. and Howell, R. R. 1969. *Diabetes* 18:755.

Mackler, B. and Guest, G. M. 1953. *Proc. Soc. Exp. Biol. Med.* 83:327.

Marks, P. A. 1966. *Proc. XI Congr. Int. Soc. Haemat.* p. 271.

Mason, H. H. and Anderson, D. H. 1955. *Pediat.* 16:785.

Matsuura, N., Cheng, J. S. and Kalant, N. 1975. *Can. J. Biochem.* 53:28.

Maugh, T. H., Jr. 1975. *Science* 188:347.

McArdle, B. 1951. *Clin. Sci.* 10:13.

McMichael, H. H., Webb, J. and Dawson, A. M. 1965. *Lancet* 1:717.

Medalie, J. H., Papier, C. M., Goldbourt, U. and Herman, J. B. 1975. *Arch. Intern. Med.* 135:811.

Melani, F., Rubenstein, A. H. and Steiner, D. F. 1970. *J. Clin. Invest.* 49:497.

Mellick, R. S., Mahler, R. F. and Hughes, B. P. 1961. *Lancet* 2:1045.

Melin, K. and Meeuwisse, G. W. 1969. *Acta Paediatr. Scand. Suppl.* 188:19.

Mendeloff, A. D. and Weichselbaum, T. E. 1953. *Metab. Clin. Exp.* 2:450.

Mertz, W. 1969. *Physiol. Rev.* 49:163.

Mertz, W. 1975. *Nutr. Rev.* 33:129.

Miettinen, T. A. 1973. *Adv. Cardiol.* 8:85.

Miller, D. and Crane, R. K. 1961. *Biochim. Biophys. Acta* 52:293.

Miller, T. B. and Larner, J. 1973. *J. Biol. Chem.* 248:3483.

Mondon, C. E., Dolkas, C. B., Olefsky, J. M. and Reaven, G. M. 1975. *Diabetes* 24:225.

Morganroth, J., Levy, R. and Fredrickson, D. S. 1975. *Ann. Int. Med.* 82:158.

Morris, R. C., Jr., Ueki, I., Loh, D., Eanes, R. Z. and McLin, P. 1967. *Nature* 214:920.

Moses, S. W., Chayoth, R., Levin, S., Lazarowitz, E. and Rubinstein, D. 1968. *J. Clin. Invest.* 47:1343.

Motulsky, A. G. and Stamatoyannopoulos, G. 1966. *Ann. Intern. Med.* 65:1329.

Motulsky, A. G., Yosida, A. and Stamatoyannopoulos, G. 1971. *Ann. N.Y. Acad. Sci.* 179:636.

Muller, W. A., Faloona, G. R., Aguilar-Parada, E. and Unger, R. H. 1970. *New Engl. J. Med.* 283:109.

Murphy, J. R. 1960. *J. Lab. Clin. Med.* 55:286.

Murthy, D. Y. N., Guthrie, R. A. and Womack, W. N. 1968. *J. Pediatr.* 72:567.

Murthy, V. K. and Steiner, G. 1972. *Am. J. Physiol.* 222:983.

Nakada, H. J. 1956. *J. Biol. Chem.* 219:319.

Nandi, M. A. and Parham, E. S. 1972. *J. Am. Diet. Assoc.* 61:258.

Nelson, T. E., Kolb, E. and Larner, J. 1969. *Biochem.* 8:1419.

Nestel, P. J. 1964. *J. Clin. Invest.* 43:943.

Nestel, P. J. and Havel, R. J. 1962. *Proc. Soc. Exp. Biol. Med.* 109:985.

Newcomer, A. D. and McGill, D. B. 1967. *Gastroenterology* 53:890.

Nisell, J. and Linden, L. 1968. *Scand. J. Gastroenterol.* 3:80.

Nishikawa, M., Tsukiyama, K., Enomoto, T., Tarui, S., Okuno, G., Uede, K., Ikura, T., Tsujii, T., Sugase, T., Suda, M. and Tanaka, T. 1965. *Proc. Jap. Acad.* 41:350.

Novello, F., Gumaa, J. A. and McLean, P. 1969. *Biochem. J.* 111:713.

Ockerman, P. A. 1972. *Acta Paediat. Scand.* 61:533.

Olambiwonnee, N. O., McVie, R., Ng, W. G., Frasier, S. D. and Donnell, G. N. 1974. *Pediatrics* 53:314.

Oski, F. A. and Diamond, L. K. 1963. *New Engl. J. Med.* 269:763.

Oski, F. A., Nathan, D. G., Sidel, V. W. and Diamond, L. K. 1964. *New Engl. J. Med.* 270:1023.

Osler, W. 1897. *Lectures on angina pectoris and allied states.* New York: Appleton-Century-Crofts.

Paes, I. C., Searl, P., Rubert, M. W. and Taloon, W. W. 1967. *Gastroenterology* 53:49.

Pagliara, A. S., Karl, I. E., Keating, J. P., Brown, B. I. and Kipnis, D. M. 1972. *J. Clin. Invest.* 51:2115.

Paige, D. M., Bayless, T. M., Ferry, G. D. and Graham, G. C. 1971. *Hopkins Med. J.* 129:163.

Paige, D. M. and Graham, G. C. 1971. *Gastroenterology* 61:798.

Patel, M. S., Owen, O. E., Goldman, L. I. and Hanson, R. W. 1975. *Metabolism* 24:161.

Pearson, C. M., Rimer, D. G. and Mommaerts, W. 1961. *Am. J. Med.* 30:502.

Pickering, W. R. and Howell, R. R. 1972. *J. Pediatr.* 81:50.

Piomelli, S. and Siniscalco, S. 1969. *Br. J. Haemat.* 16:537.

Plotkin, G. R. and Isselbacher, K. J. 1964. *N. Engl. J. Med.* 271:1033.

Pompe, J. C. 1932. *Nederl. T. Geneesk.* 76:304.

Porte, D., Grawford, D. W., Jennings, D. B., Aber, C. and McIlroy, M. B. 1966. *New Engl. J. Med.* 275:406.

Prader, A., and Auricchio, S. 1965. *Annu. Rev. Med.* 16:345.

Prader, A., Auricchio, S. and Murset, G. 1961. *Schweiz. Med. Wochenschr.* 91:465.

Putschar, W. 1932. *Beitr. Pathol. Anat.* 90:222.

Rabinowitz, D. and Zierler, K. L. 1961. *Lancet* 2:690.

Reddy, V. and Pershad, J. 1972. *Am. J. Clin. Nutr.* 25:114.

Reinecke, R. M. 1944. *J. Physiol.* 14:669.

Remein, Q. R. 1959. *Ann. N.Y. Acad. Sci.* 82:229.

Renner, R. 1973. *FEBS Lett.* 32:87.

Renold, A. E. and Burn, I. 1970. *Calif. Med.* 112:23.

Robertson, R. P. and Porte, D., Jr. 1973. *J. Clin. Invest.* 52:870.

Robinson, D. S. 1963. *Adv. Lipid Res.* 1:183.

Robinson, M. A., Loder, P. B. and de Gruchy, G. C. 1961. *Br. J. Haematol.* 7:327.

Rodbell, M. 1964. *J. Biol. Chem.* 239:753.

Rosensweig, N. S. and Herman, R. H. 1967. *Clin. Res.* 15:419.

Rowland, L. P., Fahn, S. and Schotland, D. L. 1963. *Arch. Neurol.* 9:325.

Roth, J. C. and Williams, H. E. 1967. *J. Pediatr.* 71:567.

Rudack, D., Chisholm, E. M. and Holten, D. 1971. *J. Biol. Chem.* 246:1249.

Sabeh, G., Mendelsohn, L. V., Corredor, D. G., Sunder, J. H., Friedman, L. M., Morgan, C. R. and Danowski, T. S. 1969. *Metabolism* 18:748.

Sadeghi-Nejad, A., Loridan, L. and Senior, B. 1970. *J. Pediatr.* 76:561.

Saggerson, E. D. and Greenbaum, A. L. 1970. *Biochem. J.* 119:221.

Sahi, T., Isokoski, M., Jussila, J., Launiala, K. and Pyrala, K. 1973. *Lancet* 2:823.

Salans, L. B., Knittle, J. L. and Hirsch, J. 1968. *J. Clin. Invest.* 47:153.

Sanchez, J. J. Gorzalez, N. S. and Pontis, H. G. 1971. *Biochim. Biophys. Acta* 227:67.

Sarcione, E. J., Sokal, J. E. and Lowe, C. U. 1970. *Biochem. Med.* 3:337.

Scannu, A. and Hughes, W. L. 1962. *J. Clin. Invest.* 41:1681.

Schaefer, L. E. 1964. *Am. J. Med.* 36:262.

Schapira, F., Schapira, G. and Dreyfus, J. C. 1961. *Enzymol. Biol. Clin.* 1:170.

Schmid, R. and Mahler, R. 1959. *J. Clin. Invest.* 38:2044.

Schonfeld, G. 1970. *J. Lab. Clin. Med.* 75:206.

Schreibman, P. H., Wilson, D. E. and Arky, R. A. 1969. *New Engl. J. Med.* 281:981.

Schwartz, D., Savin, M., Drash, A. and Field, J. B. 1970. *Metabolism* 19:238.

Schwartz, R., Ashmore, J. and Renold, A. 1957. *Pediatrics* 19:585.

Scott, P. J., White, B. M., Winterbourn, C. C. and Hurley, P. J. 1970. *Aust. Ann. Med.* 1:1.

Scriver, C. R. 1967. In *Symposium on intestinal absorption and malabsorption*, ed. H. Shmerling, H. Berger and A. Prader. University of Zurich.

Selwyn, J. G. and Dacie, J. V. 1954. *Blood* 9:414.

Semenza, G., Auricchio, S. and Rubino A. 1965. *Biochim. Biophys. Acta* 96:487.

Senior, B. and Loridan, L. 1968. *New Engl. J. Med.* 279:958.

Shafrir, E., Teitelbaum, A. and Cohen, A. M. 1972. *Is. J. Med. Sci.* 8:990.

Sharkey, T. P. 1971. *J. Am. Diet. Assoc.* 58:201.

Shen, L. C., Edstrom, R. D. and Larner, J. 1972. *Physiol. Chem. Phys.* 4:56.

Sherman, B. M., Gordon, P. and Roth, J. 1971. *J. Clin. Invest.* 50:849.

Shore, B. 1957. *Arch. Biochem.* 71:1.

Shrago, E., Glennon, J. A., and Gorden, E. S. 1971. *Metabolism* 20:54.

Sica, V. and Cuatrecasas, P. 1973. *Biochemistry* 12:2282.

Sidbury, J. B., Jr. 1957. *J. Clin. Invest.* 36:929.

Sidbury, J. B., Jr., Mason, J., Burns, W. B., Jr. and Ruebner, B. H. 1962. *Bull. Johns Hopkins Hosp.* 3:157.

Simborg, D. W. 1970. *J. Chron. Dis.* 22:515.

Slack, J. 1969. *Lancet* 2:1380.

Slack, J. and Evans, K. A. 1966. *J. Med. Genet.* 3:239.

Smith, E. E., Taylor, P. M. and Whelan, W. J. 1968. In *Carbohydrate metabolism and its disorders,* ed. F. Dickens, P. J. Randle and W. J. Whelan, vol. I, pp. 89–138. New York: Academic Press.

Sodhi, H. S. and Kudchodkar, B. J. 1973. *Metabolism* 22:895.

Sokal, J. E., Lowe, C. U. and Sarcione, E. J. 1962. *Arch. Int. Med.* 109:612.

Sols, A. and Crane, R. K. 1954. *J. Biol. Chem.* 210:581.

Sowers, M. F. and Winterfeld, E. 1975. *Am. J. Clin. Nutr.* 28:704.

Spach, M. S., Martin, A. M., Sidbury, J. B., Jr., Hackel, D. B. and Canent, R. V., Jr. 1966. *Am. Heart J.* 72:265.

Spergel, G., Levy, L. J. and Goldner, M. G. 1971. *Metabolism* 20:401.

Sperry, W. M. and Webb, M. 1950. *J. Biol. Chem.* 187:97.

Stadie, W. C., Haugaard, N., Hills, A. G. and Marsh, J. B. 1949. *Am. J. Med. Sci.* 218:275.

Steinitz, K. 1962. *J. Med. Assoc. Is.* 62:272.

Stewart, C. P. and Hendry, 1935. *Biochem. J.* 29:1683.

Stunkard, A. J. and Blumenthal, S. A. 1972. *Metabolism* 21:599.

Swaiman, K. F., Kennedy, W. R. and Sauls, H. S. 1968. *Arch. Neurol.* 18:642.

Swell, L., Field, H., Jr., and Treadwell, C. R. 1960. *Proc. Exp. Biol. Med.* 105:129.

Tanaka, K. R., Valentine, W. N. and Mirva, S. 1962. *Blood* 19:267.

Tarui, S., Okuno, G., Ikura, Y., Tanaka, T., Suda, M. and Nishikawa, M. 1965. *Biochem. Biophys. Res. Commun.* 19:517.

Tarui, S., Kono, N., Nasu, T. and Nishikawa, M. 1969. *Biochem. Biophys. Res. Commun.* 34:77.

Tattersall, R. B. and Fajans, S. S. 1975. *Diabetes* 24:44.

Taylor, P. M. and Whelan, W. J. 1968. *Control of glycogen metabolism.* New York: Academic Press.

Taylor, S. I., Mukherjee, C. and Jungas, R. L. 1973. *J. Biol. Chem.* 248:73.

Tengo, A., Crepaldi, G., Muggeo, M., Avogaro, P., Engi, G., Trisotto, A. and Federspil, G. 1967. *Acta Diabetol. Lat.* 4:591.

Tobin, R. B. and Coleman, W. A. 1965. *Ann. Int. Med.* 62:313.

Touster, O. 1959. *Am. J. Med.* 26:724.

Unger, R. H. and Orci, L. 1975. *Lancet* 1:14.

Vallance-Owen, J. 1960. *Br. Med. Bull.* 16:214.

Vallance-Owen, J., Hurlock, B. and Pease, M. W. 1955. *Lancet* 2:68.

Vallee, B. L., Stein, E. A., Sumerwell, W. N. and Fisher, E. H. 1959. *J. Biol. Chem.* 234:2901.

Van Creveld, S. and Huijing, F. 1964. *Metabolism* 13:191.

Van Hoof, F. and Hers, H. G. 1968. *Eur. J. Biochem.* 7:34.

Vargas, L., Taylor, K. W. and Randle, P. J. 1960. *Biochem. J.* 77:43.

Von Gierke, E. 1929. *Beitr. Pathol. Anat.* 82:497.

Wahren, J., Felig, P., Havel, R. J., Jorfeldt, L., Pernow, B. and Saltin, B. 1973. *New Engl. J. Med.* 288:774.

Walker, G. J. and Whelan, W. J. 1960. *Biochem. J.* 76:257.

Walton, K. W., Scott, P. J., Dyres, P. W. and Davies, S. W. L. 1965. *Clin. Sci.* 29:217.

Wang, Y. M. and van Eys, J. 1970. *New Engl. J. Med.* 282:892.

Watkin, D. M., Froeb, H. F., Hatch, F. T. and Gutman, A. B. 1950. *Am. J. Med.* 9:441.

Weijers, H. A., van de Kanier, J. H., Dicke, W. K. and Ijsseling, J. 1961. *Acta Paediatr.* 50:55.

Weijers, H. A., van de Kanier, J. H., Mossel, D. A. A. and Dicke, W. K. 1960. *Lancet* 2:296.

Wells, W. W., Pittman, T. A. and Egan, T. J. 1964. *J. Biol. Chem.* 239:3192.

Welsh, J. D. 1970. *Medicine* 49:257.

Welsh, J. D., Zschiesche, O. M., Willits, V. L. and Russel, L. 1968. *Arch. Intern. Med.* 122:315.

Welt, S. I., Jackson, E. H., Kirkman, H. N. and Parker, J. C. 1971. *Ann. N.Y. Acad. Sci.* 179:625.

West, K. 1975. *Diabetes* 24:641.

Whelan, W. J. 1960. *Die Starke* 12:358.

White, P. 1956. *Diabetes* 5:445.

Wieland, O., Siess, E., Schulze-Wethmar, F. H., Funcke, H. G. and Winton, B. 1971. *Arch. Biochem. Biophys.* 143:593.

Wierzuchowski, M. 1966. *Am. J. Physiol.* 211:19.

Williams, C. and Field, J. B. 1968. *J. Pediatr.* 72:214.

Williams, H. E. and Field, J. B. 1961. *J. Clin. Invest.* 40:1841.

Wolf, H., Zschokke, B., Wedemeyer, F. W. and Huelner, W. 1959. *Klin Wochenschr.* 37:693.

Wolfe, H. J. and Cohen, R. B. 1968. *Arch. Pathol.* 86:579.

Wrenshall, G. A. 1958. *Minn. Med.* 41:342.

Wright, W. T. 1961. *New Engl. J. Med.* 265:1154.

Yoshida, A. 1973. *Science* 179:732.

Yoshida, A., Beutler, E. and Motulsky, A. G. 1971. *Bull. WHO* 45:243.

AUTHOR INDEX

Numbers in italics refer to the pages on which the complete references are cited.

Long, J. M., 130, *147*
Longman, D., 226, *238*
Lopez-S., A., 8, *11*
Lorenzi, M., 98, 99, 100, *102*
Loridan, L., 255, 258, *200*
Loriette, C., 189, *203*
Lossow, W. J., 84, *102*
Loud, A. V., 169, *199*
Love, A. H. G., *75*
Lovinger, R., 98, *102*
Low, R. B., 163, *210*
Lowe, C. V., 254, 255, 280, *281*
Lowenstein, J. M., 157, *203*
Lubbe, A. M., 69, *75*
Lucas, P., 218, *220*
Luft, R., 95, 99, *101*, 132, *145*, 261, 273
Lundbaek, K., 99, 100, *100*, 234, *238*
Lundblad, A., 257, *276*
Lund-Johansen, P., 247, *259*
Lusk, G., 110, 119, *126*
Lutz, W., 197, *201*
Luyckx, A., 80, 84, 95, *102*, 167, *204*
Luyken, R., 69, *73*
Lynch, A., 88, *102*
Lynen, F., 157, 183, *199, 205*
Lyon, J. B., Jr., 182, *202*

Mabuchi, H., 98, 100, *103*
Macdonald, I., 9, *11*, 57, 61, 63, *72, 75*, 212, 213, 215, 217, 218, 219, 220, *221, 222*, 224, 225, *238*
MacDonald, W. C., 63, *75*
Macfadyen, B. V., 139, 140, 141, *146, 147*
Mach, D., 184, 192, *203*
Mackler, B., 249, *278*
MacKrell, D. J., 80, 84, 93, 95, 97, *102*
MacLean, W. C., Jr., 174, *201*
Macrae, A. R., 50, 57, *75*
Madappally, M. M., 107, *126*
Madison, L. L., 95, 99, *102, 104*, 153, 167, *209*
Mahalanabis, D., 246, *273*
Mahler, R., 153, *204, 259, 278, 280*
Mahy, M., 95, *103*
Mainguet, M., 246, *274*
Majerus, P. W., 182, 184, *204*
Makman, M. H., 85, *103*
Malaisse, W., 95, *103*, 132, *147*, 153, 154, *204*
Malaisse-Lagae, F., 95, *103, 153, 204*

Malathi, P., 50, 59, *75, 76*
Mallette, L. E., 87, *103, 132, 146*
Manchester, K. L., 182, *210*
Mancini, R. E., 234, *237*
Mann, F. C., 249, *273*
Mann, G. V., 234, *237*
Mann, J. I., 217, *222*
Manome, S. H., *75*
Mansford, K. R. L., 59, 65, *72, 75*
Manzoli, F. A., 194, *204*
Marco, J., 132, *147*
Marcus, N. A., 155, *199*, 270, *273*
Mardell, R. J., 152, *198*
Margen, S., 154, 170, *203, 209*
Margolis, S., 179, *200*
Marks, L. J., 131, *147*
Marks, V., 67, *77, 78*, 87, 94, 95, *100, 103*
Markscheid-Kaspi, L., 65, *73*
Marr, E. B., 262, *272*
Marsh, J. B., 269, *281*
Mart, M., 216, *221*
Marliss, E., 119, *126*, 132, 144, *147*, 170, 172, *201, 204*
Marshall, J. S., 250, *278*
Marshall, M. W., 93, *100*, 224, 225, *238*
Marston, R., 4, *11*, 46, *73*
Martin, B. R., 268, *273*
Martin, D. B., 91, 92, 95, *104*, 154, *201*
Martin, D. M., 154, *205*
Martin, D. W., Jr., 186, 187, *209*
Martin, R. S., 226, *237*
Maruhama, Y., 9, *11*
Mason, H. H., 254, *278*
Masoro, E. J., 178, *203*
Mateu, L., 56, *71*
Mathur, K. S., 69, *75*
Matoba, T., 35, *44*
Matoush, L. D., 153, 197, *200*
Matschinsky, F., 154, 169, *204, 205*
Matsubara, S., 29, *43*
Matsuda, T., 184, *204*
Matsui, H., 56, *73*
Matthew, F. S., 234, *236*
Matthews, J., 53, *71*
Matthew, W. T., 196, *203*
Matthews, D. M., 61, 64, *75*
Matzelt, D., 122, 124, *127*
Maugh, T. H., Jr., 270, *278*
Maumenee, A. E., 234, *238*
Mavrias, D. A., 56, 57, 63, *75*
Mayer, J., 8, *11*
Mayer, R. J., 56, 57, 63, 64, *75*, 163, *203*

SUBJECT INDEX

Sweetness, 23, 25, 27
  ethylene glycol and, 24
  intensity of, 29
  of the amino acids, 30
  of amino acid enantiomers, 33
  of sugar enantiomers, 33
Sweet taste, 31
  of aldohexoses, 32
  of β-D-fructopyranose, 32
  receptor site, 25, 26, 29, 32
  stereochemistry of, 28

Taste receptors, stereospecificity of, 34
Tendon xanthomas, 265
Thermal mutarotation, 26
Tolbutamide, 153
Trace element balances, 139
Transcription, 185
Transfer RNA, 194
Trauma
  basal energy requirements and, 137
  catabolic response to, 137
  decreased food intake and, 136
  fat tolerance and, 135
  glycosuria and, 135
  hormonal responses to, 131
  hyperglycemia and, 135
  lipolysis and, 131
  metabolic responses to, 133
  metabolism, effect on, 130
  protein
    catabolism and, 131
    requirement and, 137
  secretion
    of epinephrine, 131
    of norepinephrine, 131
Triacinolone, 124
Tricarboxylic acid (TCA) cycle, 110, 167
Triglycerides, 106, 212, 261
  diminished clearance, 254

growth and nitrogen retention with the
    use of, 107–108
lipase, 258
net protein utilization with the use of,
    108
as a source of glycerol, 108
Tryptophan pyrrolase, 159
Type I glycogenosis (*see* Von Gierke's
    disease)
Type II glycogenosis (*see* Pompe's
    disease)
Type III glycogenosis (*see* Forbe's disease)
Type IV glycogenesis (*see* Amylopectinosis)
Type V glycogenosis (*see* McArdle's disease)
Type VI glycogenosis, 259
Type IX glycogenosis, 259

UDP (uridine diphospho)-galactose
    pyrophosphatase, 247–248
UDPG pyrophosphorylase, 255
Uridine diphosphate glucose, 255
Urokinase, 159

Vascular complications, 232, 233
Vitamin A, requirements for, 138
Vitamin C, requirements for, 138
Von Gierke's disease, 254, 258

Water intake, 152

Xylose, 250
Xylulose, 250

Zinc
  deficiency, 142
  requirements for, 138